Controversies in Neurological Surgery: Neurovascular Diseases

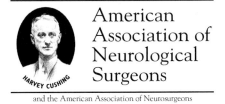

American Association of Neurological Surgeons

and the American Association of Neurosurgeons

American Association of Neurosurgeons • Rolling Meadows, Illinois

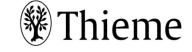

Controversies in Neurological Surgery: Neurovascular Diseases

Michael T. Lawton, M.D.
Associate Professor
Chief of Cerebrovascular Surgery, Tong-Po Kan Endowed Chair
Department of Neurological Surgery
University of California, San Francisco School of Medicine
San Francisco, California

Daryl R. Gress, M.D.
Associate Professor
Lynchburg General Hospital
Lynchburg, Virginia

Randall T. Higashida, M.D.
Clinical Professor
Department of Radiology, Neurological Surgery, Neurology, and Anesthesiology
University of California, San Francisco School of Medicine
San Francisco, California

Thieme
New York • Stuttgart

American Association of Neurosurgeons
Rolling Meadows, Illinois

Thieme Medical Publishers, Inc.
333 Seventh Ave.
New York, NY 10001

American Association of Neurosurgeons (AANS)*
5550 Meadowbrook Drive
Rolling Meadows, Illinois 60008-3852

Associate Editor: Birgitta Brandenburg
Executive Editor: Timothy Hiscock
Vice-President, Production and Electronic Publishing: Anne T. Vinnicombe
Production Editor: Shannon Kerner
Associate Marketing Manager: Verena Diem
Sales Director: Ross Lumpkin
Chief Financial Officer: Peter van Woerden
President: Brian D. Scanlan
Compositor: Alden Pre-Press Services
Printer: Maple-Vail Book Manufacturing Group
Cover illustration: © 2006 Chris Gralapp, M.A., C.M.I.
* The acronym AANS refers to both the American Association of Neurological Surgeons
and the American Association of Neurosurgeons

Library of Congress Cataloging-in-Publication Data

Controversies in neurological surgery : neurovascular diseases/[edited by] Michael T.
Lawton, Daryl R. Gress, Randall T. Higashida.
   p.   ; cm.
   Includes bibliographical references and index.
   ISBN 1-58890-400-8 (TMP ISBN : hardcover : alk. paper) — ISBN 3-13-141881-8 (GTV ISBN :
hardcover : alk. paper)   1. Nervous system–Surgery.
   [DNLM: 1. Cerebrovascular Disorders–surgery.   2. Vascular Surgical Procedures. WL 355
C764 2006]   I. Lawton, Michael T.   II. Gress, Daryl R.   III. Higashida, Randall T.
   RD593.C66   2006
   617.4′ 8—dc22   2006002264

Important note: Medical knowledge is ever-changing. As new research and clinical experience broaden our knowledge, changes in treatment and drug therapy may be required. The authors and editors of the material herein have consulted sources believed to be reliable in their efforts to provide information that is complete and in accord with the standards accepted at the time of publication. However, in view of the possibility of human error by the authors, editors, or publisher of the work herein or changes in medical knowledge, neither the authors, editors, nor publisher, nor any other party who has been involved in the preparation of this work, warrants that the information contained herein is in every respect accurate or complete, and they are not responsible for any errors or omissions or for the results obtained from use of such information. Readers are encouraged to confirm the information contained herein with other sources. For example, readers are advised to check the product information sheet included in the package of each drug they plan to administer to be certain that the information contained in this publication is accurate and that changes have not been made in the recommended dose or in the contraindications for administration. This recommendation is of particular importance in connection with new or infrequently used drugs.

Some of the product names, patents, and registered designs referred to in this book are in fact registered trademarks or proprietary names even though specific reference to this fact is not always made in the text. Therefore, the appearance of a name without designation as proprietary is not to be construed as a representation by the publisher that it is in the public domain.

Printed in the United States of America

5 4 3 2 1

TMP ISBN 1-58890-344-3
TMP ISBN 978-1-58890-344-0
GTV ISBN 3 13 141881-8
GTV ISBN 978-3-13-141881-4

Dedication

To Suzanne, for your steady love and support

To Alexandra, Simone, and Blake, for reminding me always about balance

Michael T. Lawton, M.D.

CME Credit Information

The AANS is accredited by the Accreditation Council for Continuing Medical Education to sponsor continuing medical education for physicians.

The American Association of Neurosurgeons designates this continuing medical education activity for a maximum of 15 credits in Category I of the Physician's Recognition Award of the American Medical Association.

The Home Study Examination is online on the AANS Web site at http://www.aans.org/education/books/controversy.asp

Participants have until February 28, 2009 to complete and pass the examination. No CME will be available after this date. For more information on CME credits, visit the AANS Web site http://www.aans.org/education/cme.asp or contact the Member Services Department of the AANS at

Phone: (888) 566-AANS (2267) or (847) 378-0500
E-mail: memberservices@aans.org

Contents

Foreword

One of the most gratifying aspects of a long career in medicine is enjoying the clinical and academic successes of one's students, especially those actively involved in charting the future of the discipline. Such successes have been abundant in the case of Michael Lawton. Even as a resident, it was clear that he would assume a place among the leaders pushing the boundaries of neurosurgery. During his training, more than one colleague remarked that Michael had the "best pair of hands" in the operating room. And his expertise was not confined to the clinical arena. I believe that Michael still holds the record for the number of research articles published by a neurosurgical resident at Barrow Neurological Institute—more than 60 as I recall and a phenomenal level of productivity by anyone's standards. His research was both solid and innovative—he had a decided knack for bringing a fresh perspective to data whose analysis others might have already considered completed—pushing the envelope just a bit further in the process to uncover novel and heuristic interpretations. Not surprisingly then, within a few years of assuming his position at the University of California, San Francisco, Michael has doubled the number of his publications and obtained tenure while continuing to advance his clinical level of excellence.

Now Michael, along with his talented co-editors Daryl Gress and Randall Higashida, has compiled and edited this textbook devoted to some of the thorniest issues that cerebrovascular surgeons currently confront and will confront in the future. The impressive list of contributors to *Controversies in Neurological Surgery: Neurovascular Disease*, includes experts both old and new—those who have defined neurosurgery as we know it today and those who will do so in the future. Readers will benefit from the frank discussions of treatment strategies for the most challenging cerebrovascular diseases by some of our foremost practitioners. Equally important they will find thoughtful analyses on the economics and patterns of neurosurgical practice. Few neurosurgeons receive adequate formal training on these issues. Nonetheless, they are issues that can affect a clinical practice as much as, if not more, than clinical or technological advances. Indeed, we do well to remember that we do not operate in a vacuum; larger social concerns can literally determine how we practice medicine, if at all. Both established practitioners and trainees pursuing their goal of becoming neurosurgeons will benefit from this discussion.

I note with particular satisfaction the contribution from my own neurosurgical mentor, Charles Wilson, to this text, his chapter, "The Medical Marketplace." On a personal level, joining Dr. Wilson and Dr. Lawton in this volume feels rather like a portrait of my extended family—a satisfying one at that.

Robert F. Spetzler, M.D.
Phoenix, Arizona

Preface

The practice of neurological surgery is becoming increasingly complex. Sophisticated molecular techniques increase our understanding of neurological diseases and evolving technology expands our therapeutic armamentarium. This increasing complexity demands neurosurgical subspecialization to augment clinical volume and foster expertise. However, narrow clinical focus can also breed bias, competition, and controversy. These responses can be positive when they spur innovation, improve patient outcomes, and heighten standards of excellence, but can also be negative when they ignite discord, engender suspicion, and impede progress. Nowhere are these elements more pervasive than in the field of neurovascular surgery, where endovascular techniques have become a legitimate alternative to open neurosurgical techniques.

In this textbook we explore some of the controversies in neurovascular surgery. Leaders in neurosurgery, endovascular surgery, and interventional neuroradiology were invited to express openly their perspectives and practices, with an emphasis on decision-making and the "art" of medicine, rather than on the techniques and results, which are elaborated abundantly in so many other textbooks. Some of the most challenging moments occur in the office, after explaining the various treatment options and published reports, when an anxious and overwhelmed patient begs for a recommendation or guidance, and the clinician must leap beyond evidence and steer a patient safely, ethically, and without bias. This book is intended to help in those moments, because the exploration of controversy often defines critical issues and clarifies hard choices that we ask our patients to make today, choices that we once made for them or that did not exist before.

The book has three sections. The first section examines future trends in open cerebrovascular surgery, endovascular techniques, molecular and genetic therapies, and finally economic factors. The second section focuses on specific clinical controversies associated with aneurysms, arteriovenous malformations, dural arteriovenous fistulas, cavernous malformations, and atherosclerotic diseases, presenting the differing perspectives of cerebrovascular surgeons and endovascular surgeons. The third section examines organizational issues, like structuring a practice to integrate different subspecialists, and training specialists for the future. Hopefully, this textbook will paint a picture of the future of this rapidly evolving, interdisciplinary, and highly controversial specialty. The specialty's future will be bright if we share experiences, remain flexible in our approaches, and work together closely despite our differences. Controversy should not threaten collaboration, but should spark creativity, thoughtful analysis of current practices, and innovative therapies for patients with cerebrovascular diseases.

Michael T. Lawton, M.D.
San Francisco, California

Contributors

Arun P. Amar, M.D.
Assistant Professor
Department of Neurosurgery
Yale University School of Medicine
New Haven, Connecticut

Stanley L. Barnwell, M.D., Ph.D.
Chief, NeuroInterventional Radiology
Oregon Health and Science University
Portland, Oregon

Daniel Louis Barrow, M.D.
MBNA, Bowman Professor and Chairman
Department of Neurosurgery
Emory University School of Medicine
Atlanta, Georgia

Mustafa K. Baṣkaya, M.D.
Assistant Professor
Department of Neurological Surgery
University of Wisconsin-Madison
Madison, Wisconsin

H. Hunt Batjer, M.D.
Michael J. Marchese Professor and Chair
Department of Neurological Surgery
Northwestern University, Feinberg
    School of Medicine
Chicago, Illinois

Joshua B. Bederson, M.D.
Professor
Department of Neurosurgery
Mount Sinai Medical Center
New York, New York

Bernard R. Bendok, M.D.
Assistant Professor
Department of Neurological Surgery and Radiology
Northwestern University, Feinberg School of Medicine
Chicago, Illinois

Alejandro Berenstein, M.D.
Director
Hyman-Newman Institute for Neurology
    and Neurosurgery
Roosevelt Hospital Center for Endovascular Surgery
New York, New York

Mitchell F. Berman, M.D., M.P.H.
Associate Professor of Clinical Anesthesiology
Department of Anesthesiology
Columbia University
New York, New York

Alan S. Boulos, M.D.
Assistant Professor of Surgery and Radiology
Department of Surgery
Albany Medical College
Albany, New York

Bob S. Carter, M.D., Ph.D.
Assistant Professor of Surgery
Department of Neurosurgery
Massachusetts General Hospital
Boston, Massachusetts

Patricia Cassidy, B.A., M.B.A.
Senior Vice President
Loyola University Health System
Maywood, Illinois

C. Michael Cawley, M.D.
Assistant Professor of Neurosurgery and Radiology
Department of Neurosurgery
Emory University School of Medicine
Atlanta, Georgia

E. Sander Connolly Jr, M.D.
Associate Professor
Department of Neurological Surgery
Columbia University
New York, New York

Edwin J. Cunningham, M.D.
Endovascular Fellow
Department of Neurosurgery
Cleveland Clinic Foundation
Cleveland, Ohio

Arthur L. Day, M.D., F.A.C.S.
Professor, Program Director and
   Associate Chairman
Department of Neurological Surgery
Brigham and Women's Hospital
Boston, Massachusetts

Michael Louis DiLuna, M.D.
Department of Neurosurgery
Yale University School of Medicine
New Haven, Connecticut

Jacques E. Dion, M.D., F.R.C.P. (C)
Professor
Department of Radiology and Neurosurgery
Emory University Hospital
Atlanta, Georgia

Gary Duckwiler, M.D.
Professor of Interventional Neuroradiology
Department of Radiology
University of California, Los Angeles
Los Angeles, California

Joseph M. Fitzgerald, M.B.A.
Vice President of Electrophysiology
Boston Scientific
Fremont, California

Mary T. Fitzgerald, B.A., R.N.
Vice President of Service Lines
Department of Hospital Administration
Loyola University Health System
Maywood, Illinois

John C. Flickinger, M.D., F.A.C.R.
Professor of Radiation Oncology
Department of Radiation Oncology
University of Pittsburgh School of Medicine
Pittsburgh, Pennsylvania

Chirag D. Gandhi, M.D.
Chief Resident
Department of Neurosurgery
Mount Sinai Medical Center
New York, New York

Christopher C. Getch, M.D.
Assistant Professor
Department of Neurological Surgery
Northwestern University,
Feinberg School of Medicine
Chicago, Illinois

Steven L. Giannotta, M.D.
Professor
Department of Neurological Surgery
Keck School of Medicine of University of Southern
   California
Los Angeles, California

Cole B. Graham III, M.D.
Assistant Professor
Section of Neurointerventional Radiology
Department of Radiology
Miami School of Medicine
Miami, Florida

Daryl R. Gress, M.D.
Associate Professor
Lynchburg Neurology Associates
Lynchburg, Virginia

Murat Gunel, M.D.
Associate Professor
Chief, Section of Neurovascular Surgery and
   Neurovascular/Neuroscience Intensive Care Unit
Department of Neurosurgery
Yale Neurovascular Surgery Program
Yale University School of Medicine
New Haven, Connecticut

Lee R. Guterman, Ph.D., M.D.
Associate Professor of Neurosurgery
   and Radiology
Department of Neurosurgery and Toshiba Stroke
   Research Center
School of Medicine and Biomedical Sciences
University at Buffalo,
The State University of New York
Buffalo, New York

Roberto C. Heros, M.D.
Professor and Co-Chairman
Department of Neurosurgery
University of Miami School of Medicine
Jackson Memorial Medical Center
Miami, Florida

Randall T. Higashida, M.D.
Clinical Professor
Department of Radiology, Neurological Surgery,
    Neurology and Anesthesiology
University of California, San Francisco Medical Center
San Francisco, California

L. Nelson Hopkins, M.D.
Professor of Neurosurgery, Radiology
Chairman of Neurosurgery
Department of Neurosurgery and Toshiba Stroke
    Research Center
School of Medicine and Biomedical Sciences
University at Buffalo, The State University of New York
Buffalo, New York

Reza Jahan, M.D.
Assistant Professor of Interventional Neuroradiology
Department of Radiology
University of California, Los Angeles
Los Angeles, California

Andrew Jea, M.D.
Chief Resident of Neurosurgery
Department of Neurological Surgery
University of Miami
Miami, Florida

S. Claiborne Johnston, M.D., Ph.D.
Assistant Professor
Department of Neurology and Epidemiology
University of California, San Francisco
San Francisco, California

Stanley H. Kim, M.D.
Director of Neuroendovascular Surgery
Department of Neurosurgery
St. David's Medical Center
Austin, Texas

Nerissa U. Ko, M.D.
Assistant Professor
Department of Neurology
University of California, San Francisco
San Francisco, California

Douglas Kondziolka, M.D., M.Sc., F.R.C.S.C., F.A.C.S.
Professor
Department of Neurological Surgery
University of Pittsburgh Medical Center
Pittsburgh, Pennsylvania

Mark J. Kupersmith, M.D.
Chief
Division of Neuro-Ophthalmology
Hyman-Newman Institute for Neurology and
    Neurosurgery
Roosevelt Hospital Center for Endovascular Surgery
New York, New York

Sean D. Lavine, M.D.
Assistant Professor of Neurological Surgery and Radiology
Department of Neurosurgery
Columbia-Presbyterian Medical Center
New York, New York

Michael T. Lawton, M.D.
Associate Professor
Chief of Cerebrovascular Surgery
Tong-Po Kan Endowed Chair
Department of Neurological Surgery
University of California, San Francisco Medical Center
San Francisco, California

Italo Linfante, M.D.
Associate Professor of Radiology and Neurology
Department of Radiology
University of Massachusetts Memorial Medical Center
Worcester, Massachusetts

Charles Y. Liu, M.D., Ph.D
Assistant Professor of Neurological Surgery
Department of Neurological Surgery
Keck School of Medicine of University of Southern
    California
Los Angeles, California

Christopher M. Loftus, M.D., F.A.C.S.
Professor and Chairman
Department of Neurosurgery
Temple University Hospital
Philadelphia, Pennsylvania

Demetrius K. Lopes, M.D.
Assistant Professor
Department of Neurosurgery and Radiology
Rush University Medical Center
Chicago, Illinois

George Luh, M.D.
Assistant Professor
Director of Interventional Neuroradiology
Department of Radiology
Loma Linda University Medical Center
Loma Linda, California

L. Dade Lunsford, M.D., F.A.C.S.
Lars Leksell Professor and Chairman
Department of Neurological Surgery
University of Pittsburgh Medical Center
Pittsburgh, Pennsylvania

Marc R. Mayberg, M.D.
Executive Director
Seattle Neuroscience Institute
Seattle, Washington

Colin T. McDonald, M.D.
CEO and Chief Medical Officer
Brainsaving Technologies, Inc.
Wellesley Hills, Massachusetts

Cameron G. McDougall, M.D., F.R.C.S.C.
Director of Endovascular Neurosurgery
Department of Neurosurgery
Barrow Neurological Institute
Phoenix, Arizona

Philip M. Meyers, M.D.
Associate Professor
Department of Radiology and Neurosurgery
Columbia and Cornell University Medical Centers
New York, New York

Jacques J. Morcos, M.D., F.R.C.S.,
Associate Professor
Department of Neurological Surgery
University of Miami
Miami, Florida

Gary M. Nesbit, M.D.
Associate Professor
Department of Radiology, Neurosurgery,
    and Neurology
The Dotter Interventional Institute
Oregon Health and Science University
Portland, Oregon

Yasunari Niimi, M.D.
Attending Physician
Hyman-Newman Institute for Neurology and
    Neurosurgery
Roosevelt Hospital Center for Endovascular Surgery
New York, New York

Christopher S. Ogilvy, M.D.
Professor
Department of Neurosurgery
Massachusetts General Hospital
Harvard Medical School
Boston, Massachusetts

T. C. Origitano, M.D., Ph.D.
Professor and Chair
Department of Neurological Surgery
Loyola University Medical Center
Maywood, Illinois

Brian A. O'Shaughnessy, M.D.
Resident
Department of Neurological Surgery
Northwestern University, Feinberg School of Medicine
Chicago, Illinois

Richard J. Parkinson, M.D.
Fellow
Department of Neurological Surgery
Northwestern University, Feinberg School of Medicine
Chicago, Illinois

Aman B. Patel, M.D.
Assistant Professor
Department of Neurosurgery and Radiology
Director of Endovascular Neurosurgery
Mount Sinai School of Medicine
New York, New York

Katie Lynn Pricol
Department of Neurosurgery
Yale University School of Medicine
New Haven, Connecticut

Christopher M. Putman, M.D.
Director, Interventional Neuroradiology
Fairfax Radiology Associates
Inova Fairfax Hospital
Falls Church, Virginia

Howard A. Riina, M.D., F.A.C.S.
Assistant Professor Neurological Surgery, Neurology
    and Radiology
Department of Neurological Surgery
Weill Medical College of Cornell University
New York Presbyterian Hospital
New York, New York

Andrew J. Ringer, M.D.
Associate Professor
Department of Neurosurgery
The Neuroscience Institute, Mayfield Clinic
University of Cincinnati
Cincinnati, Ohio

Avi Setton, M.D.
Director
Department of Neurointerventional Radiology
Northshore University Hospital
Manhasset, New York

Ganesh Shankar, B.S.
Department of Neurological Surgery
Harvard Medical School
Boston, Massachusetts

Harish N. Shownkeen, M.D.
Assistant Professor
Department of Neurological Surgery and Radiology
Loyola University Medical Center
Maywood, Illinois

Vineeta Singh, M.D.
Assistant Clinical Professor
Division of Stroke and Neurocritical Care
Department of Neurology
University of California, San Francisco School of Medicine
San Francisco, California

Brian E. Snell, M.D.
Department of Neurosurgery
University of Oklahoma College of Medicine
Oklahoma City, Oklahoma

Robert A. Solomon, M.D.
Byron Stookey Professor and Chairman
Department of Neurological Surgery
College of Physicians and Surgeons
Neurological Institute of New York Columbia University
New York, New York

Robert F. Spetzler, M.D., F.A.C.S.
Director
Barrow Neurological Institute
J. N. Harber Chairman of Neurological Surgery
Phoenix, Arizona
Professor
Section of Neurosurgery
University of Arizona
Tucson, Arizona

Raymond Tien, M.D., Ph.D.
The Center, Orthopedic and Neurosurgical
    Care and Research
Bend, Oregon

Daniel Tuden, Ph.D.
Boston Scientific Neurovascular
Fremont, California

G. Edward Vates, M.D., Ph.D.
Assistant Professor
Department of Neurological Surgery
University of Rochester Medical Center
Rochester, New York

Hunaldo Villalobos, M.D.
Clinical Assistant Instructor of Neurosurgery
Department of Neurosurgery and
    Toshiba Stroke Research Center

School of Medicine and Biomedical Sciences
University at Buffalo,
    The State University of New York
Buffalo, New York

Fernando Vinuela, M.D.
Professor of Interventional Neuroradiology
Department of Radiology
University of California, Los Angeles
Los Angeles, California

Ajay K. Wakhloo, M.D., Ph.D.
Professor of Radiology and Neurosurgery
Director, Division of Neuroimaging and
    Interventional Neuroradiology
Department of Radiology
University of Massachusetts
    Memorial Medical Center
Worchester, Massachusetts

Michael Y. Wang, M.D.
Assistant Professor
Department of Neurological Surgery
Keck School of Medicine of the
    University of Southern California
Los Angeles, California

Robert J. Wienecke, M.D.
Neuroscience Specialists
Oklahoma City, Oklahoma

Charles B. Wilson, M.D., M.S.H.A., Sc.D.
Professor Emeritus
Department of Neurosurgery
Senior Advisor, Health Technology Center
Senior Advisor and Surgery Program Coordinator,
    Global Health Sciences
University of California San Francisco
San Francisco, California

Y. Jonathan Zhang, M.D.
Instructor
Department of Neurological Surgery
Emory University School of Medicine
Atlanta, Georgia

Trends in Neurovascular Medicine

1

Trends in Neurovascular Surgery

BRIAN A. O'SHAUGHNESSY, RICHARD J. PARKINSON, BERNARD R. BENDOK,
CHRISTOPHER C. GETCH, AND H. HUNT BATJER

Objectives: Upon completion of this chapter, the reader should be able to identify advances in the microsurgical management of aneurysms, arteriovenous malformations, dural arteriovenous fistulas, cavernous malformations, and ischemic diseases of the brain.

Accreditation: The AANS* is accredited by the Accreditation Council for Continuing Medical Education (ACCME) to sponsor continuing medical education for physicians.

Credit: The AANS designates this educational activity for a maximum of 15 credits in Category 1 credit toward the AMA Physician's Recognition Award. Each physician should claim only those hours of credit that he/she spent in the educational activity.

The Home Study Examination is online on the AANS Web site at: http://www.aans.org/education/books/controversy.asp

* The acronym AANS refers to both the American Association of Neurological Surgeons and the American Association of Neurosurgeons.

The last decade has met with remarkable advances in the surgical treatment of neurovascular disease as well as an improved comprehension of the neurophysiology that underpins its basic science. Many of the advances in clinical neurovascular disease have resulted from the considerable refinements in neuroendovascular techniques, which have paved the way for a variety of new and exciting treatment options for complex diseases of the cerebral vasculature. Terms such as superselective angiography, microcatheter-based embolization, and stent-assisted coiling are now commonplace in both our literature and daily vernacular. While many of us have been quick to educate ourselves about new technologies in an attempt to provide the best possible therapies for our patients, we must adopt these treatments carefully and do so with a degree of cautious optimism. New strategies for the management of disease, while very intriguing and increasingly promising, must measure up to the existing techniques with regard to safety and efficacy to earn a firm place in modern treatment practices. We must strike the proper balance between technical innovation and patient safety.

The multitude of recent technological innovations developed for the management of neurovascular disease has created a paradigm shift with regard to our practice environment. A multidisciplinary group of physicians, each possessing a subspecialized training background, is now making the important therapeutic decisions, as opposed to a single individual. The modern neurovascular group is typically composed of neurovascular surgeons, neuroendovascular surgeons, neuroradiologists, neuroanesthesiologists, stroke neurologists, critical care physicians, and physiatrists. By discussing the challenging problems we face in our practices in a collaborative manner, we can consider a variety of different perspectives in a professional setting, thereby facilitating a more integrative approach to disease management. With the increased development of these combined neurovascular groups throughout the world, as well as the costly technology needed to support them, patients with complex neurovascular lesions disease routinely will be referred to large tertiary referral centers for the treatment of their disease. In concert with this recent paradigm shift in practice environment, there is a similar and analogous change in the training of today's neurovascular surgeon. Several programs, in fact, now provide single fellowships in which proficiency in both "open" surgery and neuroendovascular techniques is acquired. The various pros and cons of such programs are beyond the scope of this chapter, but they are debated actively within the medical community. In this chapter, we attempt to distill the significant recent achievements in each of the principal fields of neurovascular surgery described in this book. This is truly a formidable task and one that might be tackled differently by other authors, as it is subjective in nature. Nevertheless, several important events have occurred in nearly every aspect of neurovascular therapeutics, many of which have affected our current practice. Our goal is to briefly and accurately describe these achievements, illustrate certain points of controversy, and reflect on the historical context in which these recent advances are situated.

■ Aneurysms

The treatment of cerebral aneurysms has evolved over the last 10 years more than any other disease in neurovascular surgery. Not only have there been substantial technical advances, including innovative revascularization techniques, improved aneurysm clip design, and more sophisticated metabolic and hypothermic cerebral protection techniques, but also important changes with respect to treatment strategy. Several significant developments in neuroendovascular technology have fueled the refinement in therapeutics for cerebral aneurysms, and the quality of this treatment modality appears to be steadily improving. In fact, the success of endovascular therapy for cerebral aneurysms has resulted in considerable controversy as to the best available therapy for this disease. Microsurgical clipping as the primary treatment of choice recently has been challenged. Still, as we proceed into the 21st century, there remains an important role for open surgery in the treatment of intracranial aneurysms. Interestingly, because of advances in endovascular therapy, the clinical problems treated by open microsurgery at major referral centers for neurovascular disease have become even more challenging and complex in many respects. Sophisticated cranial base surgery techniques and cerebral revascularization procedures are now widely utilized for the treatment of complex aneurysms. This knowledge and skill set, still rigorously studied microanatomically in the laboratory, will continue to play an important role in neurovascular surgery in the future.

Currently, a multicenter prospective randomized trial is underway to compare clipping and coiling for ruptured intracranial aneurysms. Although the preliminary 1 year clinical outcome data for endovascular coiling of ruptured aneurysms from the International Subarachnoid Aneurysm Trial (ISAT)[1] appears promising, these results must be cautiously interpreted and properly situated in the context of a previously proven durable therapy that has "stood the test of time" with remarkably rare recurrences. Specifically, the ISAT investigators found that, after 1 year of follow-up, there was an absolute risk reduction for attaining a poor outcome of 6.9% in the endovascularly treated patients. However, the rate of rehemorrhage in the endovascular arm was 2.6 times that of the patients who underwent microsurgical clipping. In addition, endovascularly allocated patients were 3.7 times more likely to require an additional treatment procedure for their aneurysm compared with those treated initially with microsurgery.

Based on these current data, there are a number of key questions and concerns. Is the early gain in periprocedural morbidity and mortality made by undergoing an endovascular procedure acceptable given the future risk of rebleeding and the profound implications of such an event? What will be the relative morbidity and mortality rates 10 years from now? What are the medical costs incurred by each of the study groups given the need for repetitive follow-up procedures (angiography with or without additional coiling) in endovascularly treated patients? Poor surgical results, published in the interim ISAT report, have not been borne out in other large, multicenter trials.[2] Only approximately 22% of all patients admitted to participating hospitals were ever randomized to the ISAT, a factor clearly leading to inherent selection bias, and one that will ultimately impair the extrapolation of this outcome data to daily practice. Despite the known low incidence of complete aneurysm occlusion and the high risk of recurrence at 1 year with endovascular treatment, no follow-up angiography was required or reported at 1 year. How many of the "good outcome" endovascular patients harbor incompletely occluded or growing aneurysms that will manifest later? In addition, the ISAT trial is Europe based; what is the data applicability to North American centers with high levels of subspecialty staffing?

In a differently designed, yet valuable study, Murayama and colleagues[3] reported the results of the endovascular treatment of 818 patients with 916 aneurysms at the University of California–Los Angeles using Guglielmi detachable coils (GDCs). Their study was retrospective and nonrandomized; however, it is a candid and detailed account of the safety and efficacy of aneurysm coiling (in both ruptured and unruptured lesions) in a large number of patients by leaders in the field, with multiyear follow-up. Interestingly, these authors found that complete occlusion was achieved in only 55% of the aneurysms treated. In addition, the overall recanalization rate approached 21%. Even more compelling, however, was the discovery that for aneurysms considered ideal for microsurgical clipping (i.e., small aneurysms with small necks), the rate of complete obliteration with coiling was only 75%. These figures stand in stark contrast to a microsurgical series in which a remaining aneurysmal neck after surgery is estimated to be 3 to 6%.[4,5] These data have not only been revealing but have forced neurovascular specialists to consider the natural history and optimal management of a posttreatment aneurysmal remnant. For instance, what is the risk of bleeding from an incompletely obliterated aneurysm? Is the risk of future hemorrhage from an aneurysm remnant dependent on the type of previous treatment or the location and morphology of the aneurysm? Finally, how frequently should asymptomatic angiographic recurrences be followed, and by what imaging modality?

Enabled by the endovascular advances in the past decade, we now commonly see aneurysms treated with a combination of modalities in a so-called hybrid approach. It is not uncommon for a complex, ruptured aneurysm of the posterior circulation to be incompletely coiled purposefully to prevent early rebleeding, with the plan of treating the lesion with microsurgical clipping once the major risk period for developing edema or vasospasm has elapsed. Conversely, some lesions are clipped intentionally so that a small remnant remains, particularly in cases where complete access to the neck is obscured by vital perforating arteries or skull base structures. In such cases, the remnant is coiled postoperatively to complete the aneurysm occlusion. We have successfully implemented this strategy in the management of complex paraclinoidal aneurysms in which a portion of the lesion extends into the cavernous sinus, but the fundus is in the subarachnoid space.

In concert with the greater application of endovascular therapy, neurovascular surgeons will need to manage patients with previously coiled aneurysms. These lesions pose a unique set of challenges that have only recently been appreciated and described in the literature.[6,7] The treatment of these patients, while not uniform and clearly multifactorial, can be broadly dichotomized based on the time and nature of recurrence. In patients who acutely recanalize following coiling, temporary trapping followed by aneurysmorrhaphy and coil evacuation often enables straightforward clip reconstruction and exclusion of the aneurysm. Such a strategy, however, is significantly more difficult to carry out in patients who recur more than 6 months after coiling. By this time, the coils have become firmly adhered to the fundus of the aneurysm and may extrude from the aneurysm tissue itself. The coil mass frequently stents open the residual aneurysm wall, making gathering of the sac and parent artery reconstruction quite challenging even with prolonged periods of temporary occlusion. In these "chronic" coiling patients presenting with asymptomatic recurrence, we therefore prefer to wait for the remnant to expand enough so that a surgically clippable neck is present and the parent artery is more amenable to reconstruction. The risk of hemorrhage during this time is unknown.

In relation to aneurysm therapeutics, the management of lesions that cannot be clipped has substantially evolved recently (**Fig. 1–1A–C**). Parent cerebral artery sacrifice for the treatment of complex cerebral aneurysms was used and refined by Dr. Charles Drake[8–10] in the early 1990s; it is still used successfully today. This treatment is now being compared with attractive endoluminal strategies of parent artery reconstruction made possible by the development of flexible intracranial stents.[11,12] Aneurysms with no reconstructible neck are treated from the inside out, with an endoluminal stent serving to reconstruct the parent vessel as well as to prevent herniation of the coil mass out of the aneurysm sac. Despite the numerous theoretical advantages of this approach and a multitude of successes, reports of aneurysm recurrence, thromboembolic ischemia, parent vessel thrombosis, and subarachnoid hemorrhage following the application of stent-based therapies currently exist.[13–17] Moreover, some concerns exist with regard to the need for potent antithrombotic regimens in patients treated with a stent who have a ruptured aneurysm. In cases of incomplete aneurysm occlusion with a stent, does the patient on powerful antithrombotic agents have an increased risk of rebleeding? Is the outcome significantly worse if this patient does bleed again? These controversies notwithstanding, we are very much encouraged by this novel way to treat aneurysms untreatable by conventional clipping methods; we look forward to future developments in this methodology as well as additional studies assessing its utility.

Several additional areas of development, both surgical and conceptual, exist today in the management of cerebral aneurysms and deserve mention. In concert with the profound advances in neuroimaging, surgical treatment of cerebral aneurysms using computerized tomographic angiography (CTA) alone in preoperative planning has been recently described.[18] Despite its controversy, experienced neurovascular teams have documented the feasibility of this approach. In cases of the poor-grade or moribund aneurysmal subarachnoid hemorrhage patient possessing a concomitant life-threatening intracerebral hematoma, surgery based on only CTA prior to catheter angiography may prove life saving by avoiding the delay imposed by angiography. Indeed, we treat the majority of our patients with unruptured aneurysms and an increasing number of patients with ruptured lesions without cerebral angiography. It is our opinion that cerebral angiography will become the province of the endovascular surgeon and angiography will be performed only when endovascular intervention is considered or for follow-up after intervention.

Current trends include a recognition of the value of screening asymptomatic patients who demonstrate identifiable risk factors for harboring a cerebral aneurysm

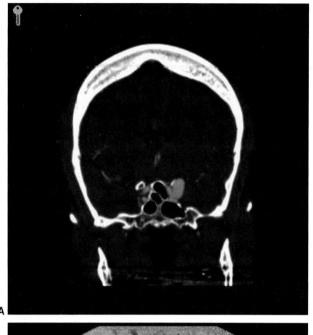

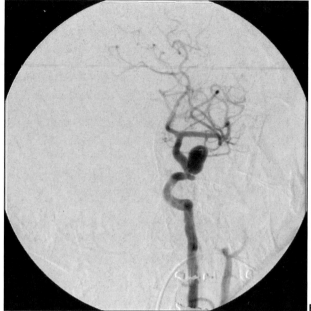

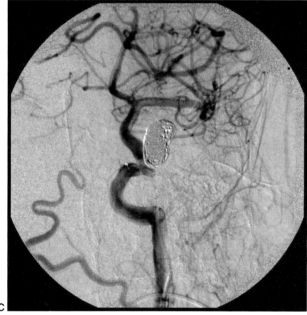

FIGURE 1–1 This is a 52-year-old right-handed female who presented with sudden-onset headache following exercise. (**A**) Coronal CT angiographic reconstruction reveals an aneurysm arising from the petrous carotid artery, which extends into the subarachnoid space. Because of the relative inaccessibility of the neck surgically an endovascular strategy was pursued. (**B**) Digital subtraction angiography shows the petrous aneurysm. (**C**) Postcoiling angiography demonstrates complete occlusion of the aneurysm with preservation of the afferent and efferent arterial circulation.

and who have a higher risk of rupture, such as family history, smoking, hyperlipidemia, coronary artery disease, or inherited conditions associated with severe vasculopathies such as autosomal dominant polycystic kidney disease or Marfan syndrome. We still must identify the overall benefits of screening patients at risk, the modality of choice, and the time of initial evaluation as well as follow-up. Also, if an aneurysm is detected in a patient in a high-risk category, should data from the International Study of Unruptured Intracranial Aneurysms (ISUIA)[2] be applied to treatment decisions, or is this data not applicable in the high-risk patient population? Several important questions in terms of aneurysm natural history and screening deserve critical analysis in the decade to come.

■ Arteriovenous Malformations

Cerebral arteriovenous malformations (AVMs), lesions composed of a dynamic array of arteries and veins linked by a central nidus, are among the most challenging entities in all of neurovascular surgery. A key review of the unique practice of Professor Troupp[19] helped to clarify the behavior of symptomatic AVMs of the brain in the absence of treatment, revealing a 4% annual risk of hemorrhage. Each hemorrhagic episode was shown to be associated with an approximately 10% risk of death and a 30% risk of major neurological morbidity.[20] With the potentially severe natural history associated with an untreated cerebral AVM in mind, several significant advances have been made in the neuroendovascular and neuroimaging arena as well as in radiosurgical methods. These have resulted in a greater breadth of available treatment options for simple as well as the most complex cerebral AVMs. The modern treatment of AVMs, particularly large lesions embedded within eloquent tissue, has truly evolved into a multidisciplinary effort in which several treatment strategies are integrated synergistically to render the best possible intervention. A broader range of AVMs is now curable with better safety than was possible a decade ago.

The most valuable current application of endovascular therapy in the treatment of AVMs is goal-directed embolization of arterial feeders prior to either operative resection or, much less commonly, radiosurgical obliteration (**Fig. 1–2A–F**). Initially pioneered by Luessenhop in the 1960s,[21,22] the application of selective endoluminal devascularization of arterial inflow to a large AVM can frequently allow a safer and less time-consuming microsurgical resection. Preoperative embolization of deep arterial feeders that are accessible only with significant parenchymal retraction now is possible using softer, smaller, and more trackable microcatheters, safer microwires, and better embolic agents. Super-selective intranidal embolization techniques when compared with earlier-generation flow-directed prenidal arterial occlusion, are a dramatic improvement in the treatment of complex AVMs. Many complex AVMs that would be otherwise too formidable for safe microsurgical resection alone are now treatable through this combined approach. Moreover, preembolization significantly reduces the incidence of postoperative hyperperfusion and intracranial hemorrhage. In fact, the potential benefits of preoperative embolization may have created an environment in which the technique is over-applied. In general, the use of embolization as a preoperative adjunct should be restricted to situations in which the risk of microsurgery and embolization combined is less than the risk of microsurgery alone. In stating this, preembolization is usually considered unnecessary for the majority of grade I and II AVMs, which can be treated with microsurgery alone, yielding excellent results.[23,24]

In addition to its role as an adjunct, embolization is used as a curative measure for certain small AVMs that are fed by a limited number of accessible arterial pedicles. In choosing embolization as either a preoperative adjunct or a stand-alone therapy, the neurovascular surgeon must be keenly aware of the wide spectrum of possible complications, which include but are not limited to stroke, hemorrhage, arterial dissection or perforation, and death. Taylor and colleagues[25] recently reported the complications they accrued over an 11-year period in the embolization of 201 patients with cerebral AVMs at the University of Texas Southwestern Medical Center in Dallas. These data revealed a 2% risk of death and 9%

risk of permanent neurological morbidity, comparable figures to those of other large, well-respected centers.

A current point of controversy is the role of embolization as a palliative measure for symptomatic AVMs that are not safely treated with complete excision and are too sizeable for radiosurgical obliteration. The reduction of flow may, in some cases, reduce the mass effect and arterial steal associated. with large, high-flow AVMs. Despite this possibility, we would argue against the common practice of palliative embolization as there is no literature available to suggest a better outcome. In fact, several reports suggest that staged embolization without complete AVM obliteration may alter the nidal hemodynamics in such a manner that an increased risk of hemorrhage is produced.[26,27] In the face of the significant risks associated with embolization therapy, a persistent and possibly increased risk of future hemorrhage is simply not acceptable in the overwhelming majority of cases.

In addition to the increasing role of endovascular techniques in the treatment of cerebral AVMs, stereotactic radiation has also proven very useful in properly selected patients. Radiosurgery, which may be delivered by gamma knife, a linear accelerator, or heavy charged particle, has been used successfully both alone and in concert with other therapeutic options for many years. With its initial introduction as a treatment modality for cerebral AVMs by Steiner in 1972,[28] the avoidance of potential morbidity and mortality associated with a craniotomy was appealing to both patients and physicians alike. When the AVM is deep within subcortical gray matter, radiosurgery may be the only rational therapeutic choice available. Several decades later, we now have a greater (but still incomplete) understanding of the various advantages as well as disadvantages of this treatment strategy, as well as its role in the treatment of AVMs.

In radiosurgical therapy for an AVM, there is a 2- to 3-year latency period during which time the patient is still at risk of hemorrhage. In addition, there have been numerous reports of angiographic recurrence of cerebral AVMs following previously documented radiosurgical obliteration[29,30]; this is an extremely uncommon event after angiographically verified microsurgical excision.[24] Further, the development of postradiosurgery neoplasms (particularly meningiomas) has also been demonstrated.[31,32] This certainly impacts treatment decisions in children and young adults with AVMs who have an otherwise normal life expectancy. Radiosurgery, while clearly efficacious for certain AVMs, requires further study with regard to the long-term effects of radiation to neighboring parenchyma, the incidence and clinical effects of potentially subtle neuropsychological sequelae of radiation, and the true risk of later recurrence with clinically significant hemorrhage or neurological decline.

The size of an AVM as well as the radiosurgical dosage utilized, are integral factors in predicting the overall success of radiosurgery. An angiographic cure can be expected in up to 85% of patients harboring lesions with a diameter smaller than 3 cm. Larger lesions, which have a poor rate of obliteration with a single radiosurgical treatment, have been approached with either preradiation embolization or staged radiosurgery. Both of these approaches lack long-term efficacy data. While we have used both approaches in our practice, we have applied them very selectively. Endovascular embolization followed by radiosurgery is limited by the potential for subsequent arterial recanalization in regions of an AVM previously considered to be obliterated.

Perhaps the most interesting and promising advance in cerebral AVM therapeutics has been the development

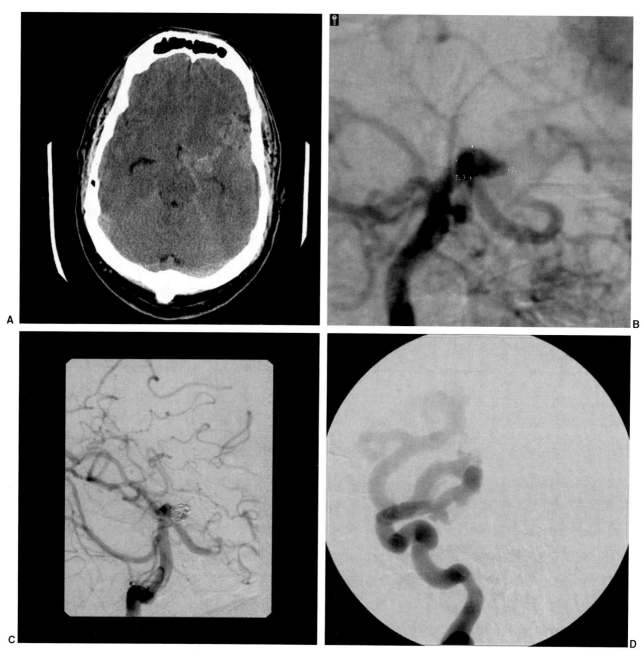

FIGURE 1–2 This is a 50-year-old right-handed male who presented with a Hunt and Hess Grade 1 subarachnoid hemorrhage (SAH). Angiography showed a large left frontotemporal arteriovenous malformations (AVM), which had feeding vessel aneurysms on the left supraclinoid carotid artery as well as the left P1 segment. The P1 aneurysm appeared to have been the source of hemorrhage and was therefore treated first by coiling. The aneurysms on the carotid artery were subsequently clipped. After treatment of the aneurysms, the AVM was sequentially embolized, then treated with stereotactic radiosurgery. (**A**) An initial CT scan shows SAH due to rupture of the left P1 aneurysm. These are precoiling (**B**) and postcoiling (**C**) working views of the P1 aneurysm. Preclipping (**D**) and postclipping angiograms.

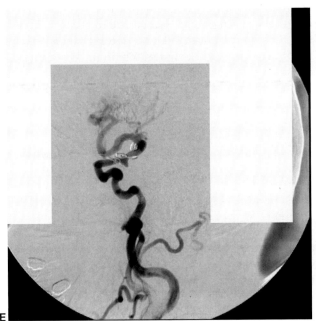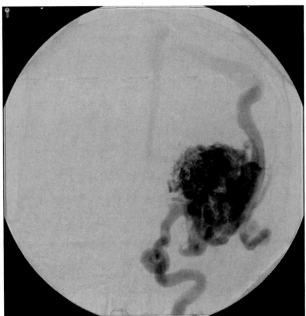

FIGURE 1–2 (continued) (**E**) of the left carotid artery (note also that there is a posterior communicating artery infundibulum present) are shown. (**F**) An early arterial-phase angiogram shows the AVM nidus.

of functional magnetic resonance imaging (fMRI). Much research is under way to determine how this modality can allow us to determine the relationship of the AVM to the patient's cortex. Traditional neuroanatomic landmarks may be completely unreliable in patients with these congenital lesions. Regarding motor function, we have seen patients with AVMs in the motor cortex demonstrate migration of function to the supplemental motor area or to the contralateral motor cortex. Such patients usually develop a deficit after resection, but it remarkably clears within a few days. The technique of fMRI has expanded the universe of potentially curable AVMs.

■ Dural Arteriovenous Fistulas

Dural arteriovenous fistulas (DAVFs), complex neurovascular lesions that display a great deal of clinical and angiographic heterogeneity, have become more completely understood over the last two decades.[33–37] The origin of cranial DAVFs is most commonly attributed to dural venous sinus injury and subsequent sinus thrombosis. Ignited by the sinus injury is an inflammatory cascade that presumably involves stimulation of angiogenesis, a sequence of events that ultimately results in sinus recanalization and the recruitment of dural arterioles. Because of the arteriovenous shunting, directly into a dural sinus, its wall, or neighboring cortical veins, the hallmark of a DAVF is the detection of early venous filling through these channels during the arterial phase on cerebral angiography.

Traditional treatment strategies for DAVFs were previously reserved for patients who were unfortunate enough to present with intracranial hemorrhage, progressive neurological deficit, or symptoms related to venous hypertension (such as severe headache, elevated intracranial pressure, or seizure). Surgical interruption of the draining vein at the level of the fistula was often quite successful. Several reports in the last 10 to 15 years, however, have greatly improved our understanding of the natural history of DAVFs,[33–39] and consequently their treatment.

In 1990, Awad and colleagues[33] reported a meta-analysis of 377 patients harboring DAVFs, including 17 cases of their own. This report, as well as several others that followed, demonstrated the integral role of cortical venous drainage with regard to the clinical presentation of DAVFs. Specifically, DAVFs that possessed retrograde leptomeningeal drainage exclusively or in addition to sinus drainage were demonstrated to have a dramatically more ominous natural history than those draining into a venous sinus alone. This distinction is so significant that DAVFs have recently been considered "aggressive" or "benign" based on the presence of cortical venous drainage.[38,39] In fact, some DAVFs have been associated with a mortality rate as high as 30% after rupture,[35] a figure rendering the prognosis in these cases more devastating than that following hemorrhage from a parenchymal AVM. Certain locations for a DAVF, a factor not distinct from the venous drainage pattern, also result in a worse natural history, as do disturbances of the venous angioarchitecture such as the presence of venous congestion or frank variceal dilatation.[33] Despite several studies that showed these features as they related to a hemorrhagic presentation as well as the development of two important classification systems by Borden et al[34] and Cognard et al,[37] little was previously known about the natural history of DAVFs *after* initial presentation.

In 2002, the Toronto neurovascular group made two very significant contributions to our understanding of DAVFs.[38,39] In one article,[39] they described their experience following 118 patients with DAVFs having cortical venous drainage for a mean of 4.3 years. They found an annual mortality rate of 10.4% and an annual event rate of 15.0%. The annual risk of hemorrhage or the development of a nonhemorrhagic neurological deficit was 8.1% and 6.9%, respectively. Their study confirmed the previously reported information regarding the severity of clinical course associated with a DAVF that has cortical venous drainage.

In a different, yet equally important, publication,[38] the same Toronto group looked at 117 patients with "benign" cranial DAVFs, namely those without cortical venous drainage at presentation or initial angiography. In a mean follow-up period of 27.9 months, these authors found that 98% of these patients followed a benign course while only 2% converted from benign to aggressive. A subject of some degree of controversy, therefore, is what imaging modality should be used to follow patients with benign disease. Because noninvasive modalities like CT angiography or magnetic resonance angiography (MRA) may miss the early development of cortical venous drainage,

are these modalities enough to assess potentially subtle yet crucial angiographic changes? Based on this information, it is the practice of our group and others simply to follow patients with benign DAVFs in an expectant manner with periodic MRA until a sudden or unexpected change in symptoms occurs. Should the patient experience a symptomatic event, he or she should undergo another six-vessel cerebral angiogram for complete analysis of the cerebral vasculature.

Treatment strategies for DAVFs, which often are reserved for patients harboring aggressive lesions or benign fistulas that result in truly disabling symptoms, have also evolved considerably over the last several years. Several reports have emerged in which stereotactic radiosurgery has been used to treat DAVFs successfully. Such an approach, as with parenchymal AVMs, is associated with a 2- to 3-year latency period prior to realizing any benefits. Because of the enormous annual risk of a lesion with cortical venous drainage, this delay of possible obliteration is far from optimal and generally is not advocated.

The most compelling advances in the therapy for DAVFs are in neuroendovascular surgery. A transvenous approach is commonly preferred to a transarterial route because of the unpredictable number of arterial feeders to the fistula and the likelihood of persistent shunting posttreatment. There are several reports of cases in which a combined transarterial and transvenous approach cured a complex DAVF. In cases involving a stenosed

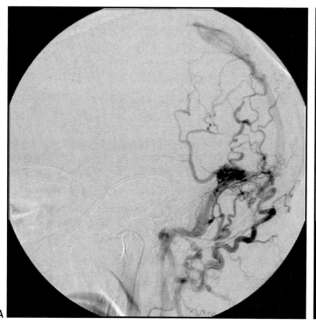
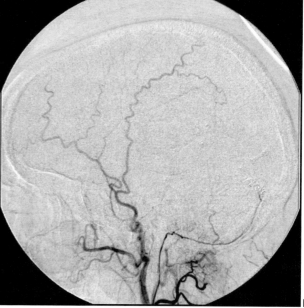

FIGURE 1–3 This is a 73-year-old male with a history of mild headache who was referred for treatment of this dural AV fistula. The diseased transverse sinus was initially embolized with coils; however, when the lesion recurred, the sinus was successfully surgically excised. (**A**) An occipital artery selective angiography shows the fistula fed at multiple regions by this vessel. Feeding vessels also include the middle meningeal artery, meningohypophyseal trunk, and ascending pharyngeal artery. Cortical venous drainage is present. (**B**) Postembolization angiogram of the fistula with GDC coils shows the initial satisfactory occlusion.

segment of involved dural sinus, the use of endoluminal intracranial stents have been used to augment an endovascular occlusive solution. The development of super-selective microcatheter angiography has also promoted a transvenous approach to aggressive DAVFs trapped within a region of sinus through a cortical draining vein, if a surgical solution is not feasible. Despite many achievements in treatment for these lesions, however, open neurosurgical techniques are still commonly employed today for challenging DAVFs in which endoluminal access to the fistula or nidus is either not feasible or carries an unacceptably high risk to the patient. In fact, the highest rates of DAVF cures in large series have

often involved a treatment regimen consisting of surgical interruption of the cortical venous drainage preceded by transarterial embolization to reduce intraoperative bleeding. Using this strategy, success rates of close to 90% are achieved, even in the treatment of the most formidable fistulas (**Figs. 1–3A,B and 1–4A–C**).

■ Extracranial Carotid Artery Surgery

Stroke prevention related to carotid artery atherosclerotic disease has traditionally relied on open surgery in cases of severe occlusive disease. The carotid endarterectomy

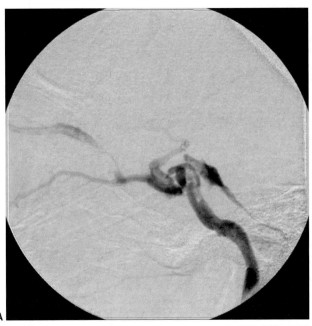

A

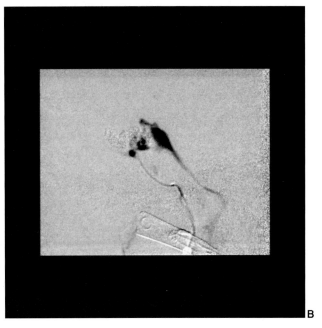

B

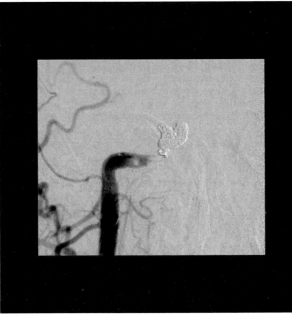

C

FIGURE 1–4 This is a 54-year-old left-handed male who experienced a dissection of his right internal carotid artery that was treated with an attempted stenting procedure. One month later, the patient presented with visual decline. (**A**) A lateral carotid angiogram shows a direct carotid-cavernous fistula with filling of the ophthalmic veins and inferior petrosal sinus. Poor flow through the dissected right internal carotid artery was noted. Treatment of the fistula was attempted, and only partial coiling was achieved. (**B**) Residual filling of the fistula was present following endovascular coiling. As such, the patient underwent a balloon test occlusion, which he passed clinically. The internal carotid artery, therefore, immediately proximal to the ophthalmic artery, was then occluded with multiple coils. (**C**) Complete occlusion of the fistula is shown.

(CEA), first performed successfully in 1953 by Dr. Michael DeBakey,[40] is one of the most widely performed surgical procedures in the United States. Its merits in the treatment of both symptomatic and asymptomatic high-grade extracranial carotid artery stenosis have been definitively established; however, the procedure should only be performed when only a limited degree of perioperative morbidity is expected.[41,42] The North American Symptomatic Carotid Endarterectomy Trial (NASCET; published in 1991)[41] included patients under the age of 79 years who had experienced a transient retinal or cerebral ischemic attack or a nondisabling stroke within the past 120 days. The study excluded patients with serious medical comorbidities, previous carotid artery surgery, or a cardioembolic origin for their ischemic events. At 2-year follow-up, the NASCET data revealed a cumulative risk of ipsilateral stroke in the medically treated group of 26%, a figure reduced to 9% in the patients who underwent CEA. In the Asymptomatic Carotid Atherosclerosis Study (ACAS),[42] the largest of five major trials designed to examine the value of CEA in the asymptomatic patient, the risk of ipsilateral stroke at the 5-year follow-up in patients with greater than 60% stenosis was 11% in the medically treated arm, compared with 5% in those who underwent CEA. Obviously, to compete with the natural history in symptomatic or asymptomatic patients, the surgical morbidity must be very low. The combined perioperative morbidity and mortality rate should not exceed 3% to derive statistical benefits from the revascularization procedure.

Because of the increasing spectrum of patients with both extracranial carotid artery stenosis as well as severe medical comorbidities that render the use of general anesthesia hazardous, alternative endoluminal strategies that have been developed. Preliminary series have, in fact, demonstrated the relative safety and efficacy of carotid artery angioplasty and stenting.[43,44] Recently, Wholey and associates[43] reported a detailed account of 3047 endovascular stenting procedures with a technical success rate of 98.8%. During or within 30 days of the procedure, the complications were 77 (2.53%) minor strokes, 41 (1.35%) major strokes, and 30 (0.98%) deaths. Restenosis rates after carotid artery stenting were 2.23% at 6 months and 2.48% at 1 year. These figures, while suggesting that carotid artery stenting is a potentially valuable procedure for high-risk patients, should not deter one from treating most patients with CEA. The Carotid and Vertebral Artery Transluminal Angioplasty Study (CAVATAS)[45] evaluated 504 patients randomized to CEA or stenting, and found no difference in 3-year stroke-related mortality. There was, however, a significantly higher 12-month restenosis rate in the patients who had received stents. Interestingly, several recent studies of merit have reported the success of CEA for high-grade carotid stenosis in high-risk patients with comorbidities that would have precluded their entry into NASCET.[46,47] Such information, which stands to further establish the value of CEA, poses even more challenges to the medical community to define the role of endovascular techniques for carotid revascularization.

Technical advances in angioplasty and stenting coupled with the improvement of devices specifically tailored for the extracranial carotid bifurcation have paved the way for the success of this burgeoning discipline. As a corollary to the development of tools for treating extracranial carotid artery stenosis by endovascular means, other pathological processes affecting this vessel such as spontaneous and traumatic dissection have also been successfully managed using these techniques. Future technical progress in this field, described more completely elsewhere in this book, has and will continue to rely upon the development of specific solutions to thromboembolic phenomena occurring in the perioperative period as well as a more thorough comprehension of restenosis and its pharmacological prevention. Currently, however, stenting is a valid alternative to CEA in carefully selected patients. Until further study of the two procedures in a prospective, randomized clinical trial, CEA continues to be the treatment of choice for the majority of patients with occlusive extracranial carotid artery disease.

■ Extracranial–Intracranial Bypass Surgery

Since its introduction in 1967 by Professors Yasargil and Donaghy,[48,49] the extracranial–intracranial (EC–IC) bypass procedure has been invaluable in the management of neurovascular disease. The procedure was initially used to treat medically refractory occlusive cerebrovascular disease; however, its use for this indication fell off rapidly with the highly controversial results reported by the EC–IC Bypass Study Group in 1985.[50] Currently, it is a powerful and indispensable adjunctive tool in the treatment of patients with complex aneurysms and tumors who are clearly at risk of ischemia because of prolonged temporary occlusion during aneurysm surgery, or when parent vessel sacrafice is needed for tumor excision (**Fig. 1–5A,B**).[35,40,41,51] While the EC–IC bypass is less commonly performed today than in years past, it is probably more appropriately used now than ever before because of the availability of sophisticated neuroimaging modalities and provocative cerebrovascular reserve testing such as trial balloon occlusion. In fact, these new tools for cerebral perfusion assessment have not only facilitated stratification for adjunctive bypass in aneurysm and tumor surgery but have also fostered a renewed interest in the use of EC–IC bypass surgery in the management of patients with occlusive intracranial cerebrovascular disease.

Currently, a large multiinstitutional trial is underway to reexamine the role of the EC–IC bypass in the treatment

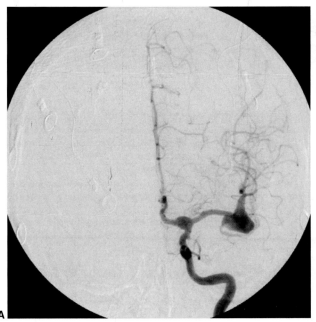

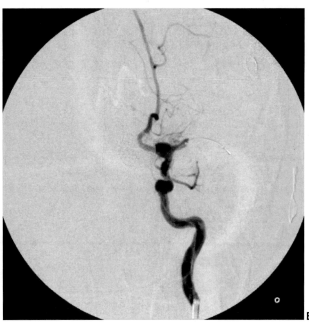

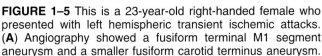

FIGURE 1–5 This is a 23-year-old right-handed female who presented with left hemispheric transient ischemic attacks. **(A)** Angiography showed a fusiform terminal M1 segment aneurysm and a smaller fusiform carotid terminus aneurysm.

(B) An intracranial balloon test occlusion was performed which failed. The aneurysm subsequently was trapped following a superficial temporal artery-middle cerebral artery bypass.

of occlusive cerebrovascular disease. The Carotid Occlusion Surgery Study (COSS)[52,53] seeks to impose stringent physiological criteria as well as clinical criteria to determine who might best benefit from EC–IC bypass. Inclusion criteria for COSS include catheter angiography demonstrating complete occlusion of the internal carotid artery and less than 50% stenosis of the contralateral internal carotid artery. For entry, patients must have had a transient ischemic attack or ischemic stroke within 120 days. Comorbidities that may affect the rate of stroke in the study populations such as diabetes mellitus and hypertension are factored in the data analysis. All patients in the trial will receive maximal medical therapy; the group that undergoes EC–IC bypass will therefore gauge the additional effect of this intervention in a select group of patients with regard to future risk of ischemic stroke. The primary endpoint of the trial is both an ipsilateral ischemic stroke within 2 years and any stroke within 40 days of entry into the study. The COSS is a much-anticipated investigation to elucidate the true value of stroke prevention with EC–IC bypass in a carefully selected group of patients based on the application of modern neuroimaging stratification.

■ Cerebral Cavernous Malformations

Advances over the last decade in both the understanding and surgical treatment of cerebral cavernous malformations have been profound. The advent and improvements in MR imaging have made this condition

recognized as a common clinical entity, affecting nearly 0.5% of the population.[54] Further, we have witnessed the successful integration of frameless stereotaxis into the microsurgical resection of these lesions. These navigational techniques have undoubtedly made approaches to cavernomas far more accurate and reproducible, while minimizing potential morbidity of resection. Beyond this, an improved appreciation for the natural history of cavernomas and their propensity to hemorrhage has occurred in recent years. As a true understanding of the natural history of cavernomas further develops, the management of deep lesions affecting the brainstem and deep gray matter could be enhanced with algorithms that are more specific. Currently, our indications for resection of a brainstem cavernoma include two clinically significant episodes of hemorrhage that result in progressive neurological deterioration as well as representation of the lesion at the pial surface, which is surgically accessible.

Even more remarkable than these surgical gains are the dramatic advances in the molecular genetics of cavernous malformations, particularly with regard to those of familial origin.[55] It is estimated that 10 to 20% of Caucasians with cavernous malformations have a first-degree relative with the condition, a figure that rises to 50% in Hispanic Americans.[56] Initial genetic linkage analysis performed in Hispanic Americans identified the the *CCM1* gene, which resides on chromosome 7q21.[57,58] Further experimentation utilizing positional cloning has enabled the recent discovery that one of the genes in this region, *KRIT1*, is in fact, the *CCM1* gene.[51,59,60] Additional studies have demonstrated a founder effect among both familial and sporadic cases in this population; all patients have an identical inherited mutation in this gene that is traceable to a common ancestor.[61,62] Currently, the function of the KRIT1 protein is unknown; studies to determine its biological role are being actively pursued.

Although the founder mutation in the *KRIT1* gene is responsible for apparently all cases of cavernous malformation seen in Hispanic Americans of Mexican descent, mutations in this gene are etiologically related to only approximately 30% of familial cases in the non-Hispanic population. Moreover, among non-Hispanic patients in whom there is no longer a family history of cavernomas, *KRIT1* mutations account for virtually none of the cases. In these patients, other chromosomal abnormalities not yet elucidated may play an important role in the disease pathogenesis. Recent linkage studies encompassing the entire genome have targeted two additional genes, *CCM2* on the short arm of chromosome 7 and *CCM3* on the long arm of chromosome 3.[55] Further study of the molecular genetics of these loci and the roles they play in the disease process appears promising. Such studies undoubtedly will occupy an important place in the copious amount of translational research in cerebrovascular disease.

■ Conclusion

Developments in neurovascular disease over the last decade have been as rich and poignant as the achievements of the neurosurgical legends that pioneered this field nearly a century ago. With the development of each new technology, traditional approaches to neurovascular problems are continually evolving. As we harness the numerous tangible and conceptual advances that will mark the coming years, we must do so with care and responsibility. The role of the neurovascular surgeon, while clearly changing, is not diminishing. In many respects, issues confronting neurovascular surgeons, now and in the near future, are more challenging than ever before. It is critical that the key points of controversy outlined in this chapter are studied in a scientific manner so that evidence-based principles are established for innovation in new technology. Possessing a new device or technique does not imply that it will be effective or safe. We must be diligent to ensure that our colleagues in industry do not influence the design of studies, the investigations involved, or the interpretation of data. These functions are the pure responsibility of our clinical neuroscience investigators.

■ References

1. Molyneux A, Kerr R, Stratton I, et al. International Subarachnoid Aneurysm Trial (ISAT) of neurosurgical clipping versus endovascular coiling in 2143 patients with ruptured intracranial aneurysms: a randomised trial. Lancet 2002;360:1267–1274

2. Wiebers DO, Whisnant JP, Huston J III, et al. Unruptured intracranial aneurysms: natural history, clinical outcome, and risks of surgical and endovascular treatment. Lancet 2003;362:103–110

3. Murayama Y, Nien YL, Duckwiler G, et al. Guglielmi detachable coil embolization of cerebral aneurysms: 11 years' experience. J Neurosurg 2003;98:959–966

4. Samson D, Batjer HH, Kopitnik TA Jr. Current results of the surgical management of aneurysms of the basilar apex. Neurosurgery 1999;44:697–702

5. Thornton J, Bashir Q, Aletich VA, et al. What percentage of surgically clipped intracranial aneurysms have residual necks? Neurosurgery 2000;46:1294–1298

6. Veznedaroglu E, Benitez RP, Rosenwasser RH. Surgically treated aneurysms previously coiled: lessons learned. Neurosurgery 2004;54:300–305

7. Zhang YJ, Barrow DL, Cawley CM, et al. Neurosurgical management of intracranial aneurysms previously treated with endovascular therapy. Neurosurgery 2003;52:283–293

8. Drake CG, Peerless SJ. Giant fusiform intracranial aneurysms: review of 120 patients treated surgically from 1965 to 1992. J Neurosurg 1997;87:141–162

9. Drake CG, Peerless SJ, Ferguson GG. Hunterian proximal arterial occlusion for giant aneurysms of the carotid circulation. J Neurosurg 1994;81:656–665

10. Steinberg GK, Drake CG, Peerless SJ. Deliberate basilar or vertebral artery occlusion in the treatment of intracranial aneurysms. Immediate results and long-term outcome in 201 patients. J Neurosurg 1993;79:161–173

11. Fiorella D, Albuquerque FC, Han P, et al. Preliminary experience using the Neuroform stent for the treatment of cerebral aneurysms. Neurosurgery 2004;54:6–17

12. Howington JU, Hanel RA, Harrigan MR, et al. The Neuroform stent, the first microcatheter-delivered stent for use in the intracranial circulation. Neurosurgery 2004;54:2–5

13. Kaku Y, Yoshimura S, Yamakawa H, et al. Failure of stent-assisted endovascular treatment for ruptured dissecting aneurysms of the basilar artery. Neuroradiology 2003;45:22–26

14. Levy EI, Boulos AS, Bendok BR, et al. Brainstem infarction after delayed thrombosis of a stented vertebral artery fusiform aneurysm: case report. Neurosurgery 2002;51:1280–1285

15. MacKay CI, Han PP, Albuquerque FC, et al. Recurrence of a vertebral artery dissecting pseudoaneurysm after successful stent-supported coil embolization: case report. Neurosurgery 2003;53:754–760

16. Sugiu K, Takahashi K, Muneta K, et al. Rebleeding of a vertebral artery dissecting aneurysm during stent-assisted coil embolization: a pitfall of the "stent and coil" technique. Surg Neurol 2004;61:365–370

17. Uhl E, Schmid-Elsaesser R, Steiger HJ. Ruptured intracranial dissecting aneurysms: management considerations with a focus on surgical and endovascular techniques to preserve arterial continuity. Acta Neurochir (Wien) 2003;145:1073–1083

18. Hoh BL, Cheung AC, Rabinov JD, et al. Results of a prospective protocol of computed tomographic angiography in place of catheter angiography as the only diagnostic and pretreatment planning study for cerebral aneurysms by a combined neurovascular team. Neurosurgery 2004;54:1329–1340

19. Ondra SL, Troupp H, George ED, et al. The natural history of symptomatic arteriovenous malformations of the brain: a 24-year follow-up assessment. J Neurosurg 1990;73:387–391

20. Samson D, Batjer HH. Preoperative evaluation of the risk/benefit ratio for arteriovenous malformations of the brain. In: Williams RH, Rengachary SS, eds. Neurosurgery Update II: Vascular, Spinal, Pediatric, and Functional Neurosurgery. New York, NY: McGraw-Hill; 1991: 129–133

21. Luessenhop AJ. Comments on experimental surgical techniques for cerebral aneurysms and A-V malformations. Med Ann Dist Columbia 1966;35:470–472

22. Luessenhop AJ, Velasquez AC. Observations on the tolerance of the intracranial arteries to catheterization. J Neurosurg 1964;21: 85–91

23. Hamilton MG, Spetzler RF. The prospective application of a grading system for arteriovenous malformations. Neurosurgery 1994;34:2–7

24. Heros RC, Korosue K, Diebold PM. Surgical excision of cerebral arteriovenous malformations: late results. Neurosurgery 1990;26: 570–578

25. Taylor CL, Dutton K, Rappard G, et al. Complications of preoperative embolization of cerebral arteriovenous malformations. J Neurosurg 2004;100:810–812

26. Han PP, Ponce FA, Spetzler RF. Intention-to-treat analysis of Spetzler-Martin grades IV and V arteriovenous malformations: natural history and treatment paradigm. J Neurosurg 2003;98:3–7

27. Kwon OK, Han DH, Han MH, et al. Palliatively treated cerebral arteriovenous malformations: follow-up results. J Clin Neurosci 2000;7(Suppl 1):69–72

28. Steiner L, Leksell L, Greitz T, et al. Stereotaxic radiosurgery for cerebral arteriovenous malformations. Report of a case. Acta Chir Scand 1972;138:459–464

29. Hladky JP, Lejeune JP, Blond S, et al. Cerebral arteriovenous malformations in children: report on 62 cases. Childs Nerv Syst 1994;10:328–333

30. Rodriguez-Arias C, Martinez R, Rey G, et al. Recurrence in a different location of a cerebral arteriovenous malformation in a child after radiosurgery. Childs Nerv Syst 2000;16:363–365

31. Ganz JC. Gamma knife radiosurgery and its possible relationship to malignancy: a review. J Neurosurg 2002;97:644–652

32. Shamisa A, Bance M, Nag S, et al. Glioblastoma multiforme occurring in a patient treated with gamma knife surgery. Case report and review of the literature. J Neurosurg 2001;94:816–821

33. Awad IA, Little JR, Akarawi WP, et al. Intracranial dural arteriovenous malformations: factors predisposing to an aggressive neurological course. J Neurosurg 1990;72:839–850

34. Borden JA, Wu JK, Shucart WA. A proposed classification for spinal and cranial dural arteriovenous fistulous malformations and implications for treatment. J Neurosurg 1995;82:166–179

35. Brown RD Jr, Wiebers DO, Nichols DA. Intracranial dural arteriovenous fistulae: angiographic predictors of intracranial hemorrhage and clinical outcome in nonsurgical patients. J Neurosurg 1994;81:531–538

36. Chaudhary MY, Sachdev VP, Cho SH, et al. Dural arteriovenous malformation of the major venous sinuses: an acquired lesion. AJNR Am J Neuroradiol 1982;3:13–19

37. Cognard C, Gobin YP, Pierot L, et al. Cerebral dural arteriovenous fistulas: clinical and angiographic correlation with a revised classification of venous drainage. Radiology 1995;194:671–680

38. Satomi J, van Dijk JM, Terbrugge KG, et al. Benign cranial dural arteriovenous fistulas: outcome of conservative management based on the natural history of the lesion. J Neurosurg 2002;97:767–770

39. van Dijk JM, terBrugge KG, Willinsky RA, et al. Clinical course of cranial dural arteriovenous fistulas with long-term persistent cortical venous reflux. Stroke 2002;33:1233–1236

40. DeBakey ME. Successful carotid endarterectomy for cerebrovascular insufficiency. Nineteen-year follow-up. JAMA 1975;233: 1083–1085

41. Beneficial effect of carotid endarterectomy in symptomatic patients with high-grade carotid stenosis. North American Symptomatic Carotid Endarterectomy Trial Collaborators. N Engl J Med 1991;325:445–453

42. Endarterectomy for asymptomatic carotid artery stenosis. Executive Committee for the Asymptomatic Carotid Atherosclerosis Study. JAMA 1995;273:1421–1428

43. Wholey MH, Eles G. Cervical carotid artery stent placement. Semin Interv Cardiol 1998;3:105–115

44. Yadav JS, Roubin GS, Iyer S, et al. Elective stenting of the extracranial carotid arteries. Circulation 1997;95:376–381

45. Endovascular versus surgical treatment in patients with carotid stenosis in the Carotid and Vertebral Artery Transluminal Angioplasty Study (CAVATAS): a randomised trial. Lancet 2001;357:1729–1737

46. Ballotta E, Da Giau G, Baracchini C, et al. Carotid endarterectomy in high-risk patients: a challenge for endovascular procedure protocols. Surgery 2004;135:74–80

47. Mozes G, Sullivan TM, Torres-Russotto DR, et al. Carotid endarterectomy in SAPPHIRE-eligible high-risk patients: implications for selecting patients for carotid angioplasty and stenting. J Vasc Surg 2004;39:958–965

48. Donaghy RMP, Yasargil MG. Extracranial blood flow diversion. In: Donaghy RMP, Yasargil MG, eds. Microvascular Surgery: Report of First Conference, October 6–7, 1966, Mary Fletcher Hospital, Burlington, Vermont. St. Louis: Mosby, 1967

49. Yasargil MG. Experimental small vessel surgery in the dog including patching and grafting of cerebral vessels and the formation of functional extra-intracranial shunts. In: Donaghy RMP, Yasargil MG, eds. Microvascular Surgery: Report of First Conference, October 6–7, 1966, Mary Fletcher Hospital, Burlington, Vermont. St. Louis: Mosby, 1967

50. Failure of extracranial-intracranial arterial bypass to reduce the risk of ischemic stroke. Results of an international randomized trial. The EC/IC Bypass Study Group. N Engl J Med 1985;313: 1191–1200

51. Couteulx SL, Brezin AP, Fontaine B, et al. A novel KRIT1/CCM1 truncating mutation in a patient with cerebral and retinal cavernous angiomas. Arch Ophthalmol 2002;120:217–218

52. Adams HP Jr, Powers WJ, Grubb RL Jr, et al. Preview of a new trial of extracranial-to-intracranial arterial anastomosis: the carotid occlusion surgery study. Neurosurg Clin N Am 2001;12:613–624 ix–x

53. Grubb RL Jr, Powers WJ, Derdeyn CP, et al. The Carotid Occlusion Surgery Study. Neurosurg Focus 2003;14:1–7

54. Robinson JR, Awad IA, Little JR. Natural history of the cavernous angioma. J Neurosurg 1991;75:709–714

55. Laurans MS, DiLuna ML, Shin D, et al. Mutational analysis of 206 families with cavernous malformations. J Neurosurg 2003;99: 38–43

56. Hayman LA, Evans RA, Ferrell RE, et al. Familial cavernous angiomas: natural history and genetic study over a 5-year period. Am J Med Genet 1982;11:147–160

57. Dubovsky J, Zabramski JM, Kurth J, et al. A gene responsible for cavernous malformations of the brain maps to chromosome 7q. Hum Mol Genet 1995;4:453–458

58. Gunel M, Awad IA, Anson J, et al. Mapping a gene causing cerebral cavernous malformation to 7q11.2-q21. Proc Natl Acad Sci U S A 1995;92:6620–6624

59. Cave-Riant F, Denier C, Labauge P, et al. Spectrum and expression analysis of KRIT1 mutations in 121 consecutive and unrelated patients with cerebral cavernous malformations. Eur J Hum Genet 2002;10:733–740

60. Verlaan DJ, Davenport WJ, Stefan H, et al. Cerebral cavernous malformations: mutations in Krit1. Neurology 2002;58:853–857

61. Gunel M, Awad IA, Finberg K, et al. A founder mutation as a cause of cerebral cavernous malformation in Hispanic Americans. N Engl J Med 1996;334:946–951

62. Gunel M, Awad IA, Finberg K, et al. Genetic heterogeneity of inherited cerebral cavernous malformation. Neurosurgery 1996;38:1265–1271

2

Trends in Endovascular Surgery

DEMETRIUS K. LOPES, ANDREW J. RINGER, STANLEY H. KIM, LEE R. GUTERMAN, AND L. NELSON HOPKINS

Objectives: Upon completion of this chapter, the reader should be able to identify with advances in the endovascular management of cerebral ischemic diseases, arteriovenous malformations, and aneurysms.

Accreditation: The AANS* is accredited by the Accreditation Council for Continuing Medical Education (ACCME) to sponsor continuing medical education for physicians.

Credit: The AANS designates this educational activity for a maximum of 15 credits in Category 1 credit toward the AMA Physician's Recognition Award. Each physician should claim only those hours of credit that he/she spent in the educational activity.

The Home Study Examination is online on the AANS Web site at: http://www.aans.org/education/books/controversy.asp

* The acronym AANS refers to both the American Association of Neurological Surgeons and the American Association of Neurosurgeons.

The development of endovascular surgery over the past two decades has dramatically affected methods for the management of cerebrovascular disease today. Endovascular surgery is in its infancy, and its potential for the future is great. In this chapter, we describe our perspective on the future of endovascular surgery in the management of cerebral ischemic disease, intracranial arteriovenous malformations (AVMs), and aneurysms.

■ Management of Cerebral Ischemic Disease

Patients who experience cerebrovascular ischemic symptoms today face a substantially lower risk of death, recurrent symptoms, and stroke than they did a decade ago. Progress in the management of cerebral ischemic disease is, in part, because of advances made in the treatment of coronary artery disease. Success observed in the management of coronary artery disease resulted from the rapid transfer of knowledge gained from laboratory investigations to the clinical setting; execution of well-designed, randomized, placebo-controlled trials; and technical innovation and refinement of percutaneous coronary intervention procedures. This systematic approach allowed the development of evidence-based management protocols. The three main strategies currently used in the management of cerebral ischemic disease reflect lessons learned from cardiology. The strategies are restoration and maintenance of blood flow at the site of occlusion, reduction of infarct size, and stabilization of the cerebrovascular vessel wall and vessel wall interaction with the bloodstream.

Restoration and Maintenance of Cerebrovascular Flow at the Lesion Site

This strategy aims to optimize the use of mechanical revascularization techniques and pharmacologic agents that affect coagulation, fibrinolysis, and platelet function to achieve timely, adequate, and durable cerebral reperfusion. In the past 10 years, significant progress has been made in the development and assessment of thrombolytic therapy for ischemic stroke. Recombinant tissue plasminogen activator (tPA) is currently the only drug approved by the FDA for acute thrombolysis in stroke. The National Institute of Neurological Disorders and Stroke trial demonstrated that patients treated with intravenously administered tPA within 3 hours of stroke symptom onset were 30% less likely than patients treated with placebo to have disabilities at 3 months.[1] Unfortunately, symptomatic intracranial hemorrhage occurred in 6.4% of patients, and the overall rate of mortality at 3 months was 17%.[1] The main limitations of systemic thrombolysis are the narrow therapeutic window of 3 hours, the need for high doses of thrombolytic agents leading to an increased risk of systemic or intracranial hemorrhage, and the inability to visualize the occlusion site by means of angiography or other imaging modality. In the cardiology literature, some evidence exists that a better strategy for acute myocardial revascularization may be prompt intra-arterial intervention.[2] Theoretically, intra-arterial delivery of thrombolytic agents is more likely to increase the reperfusion rates and decrease the morbidity and mortality rates associated with higher doses of thrombolytics administered for systemic treatment. These theoretical advantages have been evaluated in trials of intra-arterial thrombolysis with prourokinase, tPA, and urokinase for the management of acute ischemic stroke (**Table 2–1**). Although these agents did not receive FDA approval for clinical use, the results of these trials demonstrated therapeutic efficacy, even when the agent was administered late in the ischemic process. The average time from symptom onset to treatment was 5 hours.

The future of intra-arterial therapy for the management of acute stroke depends on improving recanalization rates and safety. At the University at Buffalo Department of Neurosurgery, we used reteplase, a third-generation recombinant tPA, for intra-arterial thrombolysis. Our preliminary results with the administration of heparin (activated coagulation time of 250 seconds) in combination with a maximum dose of 8 units of reteplase demonstrated neurological improvement (defined as a ≥ 4-point decrease in National Institutes of Health Stroke Scale score) in 7 (44%) of 16 patients at 24 hours.[8] Complete or near-complete recanalization (thrombolysis in myocardial infarction, TIMI; grade 3 or 4 flow) was achieved in 14 (88%) patients, and symptomatic intracerebral hemorrhage occurred in only one patient. Reteplase has a longer half-life and binds less to fibrin than alteplase (second-generation recombinant tPA). These improvements permit more penetration within the thrombus and prolonged thrombolytic activity. Despite the theoretical advantages of third-generation thrombolytic agents (reteplase), their efficacy in obtaining TIMI grade 3 or 4 flow is often limited. One limitation is that thrombolytic therapy stimulates the production of thrombin and the consequent reactivation of platelets. Platelet aggregation leads to the formation of a thrombolytic-resistant thrombus and the recurrence of thrombosis. In addition, platelets secrete plasminogen activator inhibitor (PAI)-1, which inhibits tPA penetration of thrombus.[9] We are evaluating the safety and effectiveness of mechanical thrombolysis using balloon angioplasty, snare, and stents in conjunction with intra-arterial reteplase for ischemic stroke.

In the cardiology experience, numerous advantages of administering adjunctive antiplatelet agents along with thrombolytic therapy were recognized. Among these advantages are accelerated reperfusion, decreased incidence of reocclusion, improved microvascular reperfusion, and enhanced safety and efficacy. Major trials have demonstrated the effects of the combination of a full

TABLE 2–1 Results of Major Intra-arterial Thrombolysis Trials for Stroke

Trial	Thrombolytic Agent	Angiographic Recanalization Rate (%)	Symptomatic Intracranial Hemorrhage (% of patients)
Prolyse in acute cerebral thromboembolism (PROACT) phase II[3]	ProUrokinase*	58	15
PROACT phase III[4]	ProUrokinase*	66	10
Emergency Management of Stroke (EMS) Bridging trial[5]	tPA† (intravenous + intra-arterial)	55	8.5
Universities Hospitals of Cleveland study[6]	Urokinase	72	9
Ehime University study[7]	Urokinase	76	5.3

*Prolyse (recombinant prourokinase), Abbott Laboratories, Abbott Park, IL.
†tPA – Activase (Alteplase), Genentech, San Francisco, CA.

dose of thrombolytic agents and IIb/IIIa inhibitors for the treatment of coronary artery disease (**Table 2–2**). Two trials have tested half-dose thrombolytic (alteplase or reteplase) therapy with full-dose abciximab for the management of acute myocardial infarction.[13,14] An added benefit of this approach might be a decreased risk of hemorrhagic complications. In the TIMI-14 trial,[14] the most effective regimen consisted of half-dose tPA (alteplase), full-dose abciximab, aspirin, and heparin. This regimen restored TIMI grade 3 flow in 77% of patients at 90 minutes, with a major hemorrhage rate of 1%. In the Strategies for Patency Enhancement in the Emergency Department (SPEED) trial,[13] the use of a half dose of reteplase (two 5-unit boluses 30 minutes apart) along with full-dose abciximab, aspirin, and heparin resulted in restoration of TIMI grade 3 flow in 62% of patients with myocardial infarction at 60 to 90 minutes after initiation of therapy. In Buffalo, we have started a prospective, nonrandomized, open-label trial to evaluate the safety of an escalating dose of intra-arterial reteplase in combination with intravenous abciximab for patients with acute ischemic stroke. According to the protocol, patients received intravenous heparin (30 units/kg bolus) to maintain an activated coagulation time between 180 and 250 seconds and then intravenous full-dose abciximab (0.25 mg/kg bolus followed by a 12-hour infusion at 0.125 mcg/kg/min to a maximum dose of 10 mg/min) and intra-arterial reteplase (maximum total dose of 2 U).[8] If the results from interventions for acute myocardial infarction are transferable to those for acute stroke, we can expect improvement in reperfusion rates with reduced rates of intracranial hemorrhage.

Another reperfusion strategy that has been explored for the treatment of coronary artery disease is the combination of fibrinolytic therapy with mechanical thrombolysis (stent and/or percutaneous transluminal coronary angioplasty).[15–17] TIMI grade 3 flow was achieved in 73% of patients who underwent percutaneous revascularization with primary angioplasty, and the average door-to-balloon time (interval from emergency room evaluation until treatment) was 114 minutes. In the Primary Angioplasty in Myocardial Infarction (PAMI) Stent trial (primary stenting),[18] TIMI grade 3 flow was achieved in 89% of patients, and the door-to-stent time was 135 minutes. In the Plasminogen-Activator Angioplasty Compatibility trial (PACT),[17] patients received half-dose tPA followed by immediate angiography and percutaneous revascularization if needed. At coronary angiography, 33% of patients had TIMI grade 3 flow in infarct-related arteries. This observation is of great importance because it suggests that patients can benefit from early intravenous thrombolysis while awaiting the initiation of percutaneous revascularization therapy. The combination of pharmacologic and mechanical intervention is a venue to be carefully explored in the management of acute stroke. The treatment of acute stroke is benefiting from future development of pharmacologic (heparinoid, antithrombin agents, and antiplatelet agents) and mechanical (using clot retrievers[18] and stents) thrombolysis strategies.

An interesting tendency observed in the cardiology literature is to perform early invasive revascularization therapy for non-ST segment elevation acute coronary syndromes. This syndrome involves nonocclusive coronary stenosis in patients with unstable angina. The lesions are more or less the equivalent of intracranial stenosis with "misery perfusion" or stage 2 hemodynamic failure (i.e., the presence of reduced blood flow and increased oxygen extraction fraction) documented by positron emission tomography (PET). New imaging technology (perfusion magnetic resonance imaging, PET) for the assessment of cerebral blood flow will improve our ability to identify those asymptomatic patients with intracranial stenosis who are at the greatest risk of stroke and who thus may derive the greatest benefit from revascularization therapies.

Reduction of Infarct Size

This strategy for the management of cerebral ischemic disease focuses on ways to attenuate the adverse functional consequences of ischemia and reperfusion. Ischemia induces the formation of a multitude of adaptive cellular responses. Some of these responses can

TABLE 2–2 Trials of IIb/IIIa Inhibitors with Full-dose Thrombolytic Therapy

Trial	Thrombolytic Agent	IIb/IIIa Inhibitor	TIMI Grade 3 Flow
Integrilin to Minimize Platelet Aggregation and Coronary Thrombosis in Acute Myocardial Infarction (IMPACT-AMI)[10]	TPA	Eptifibatide	66%
Ronner et al[11]	Streptokinase	Eptifibatide	53%
Platelet Aggregation Receptor Antagonist Dose Investigation and Reperfusion Gain in Myocardial Infarction (PARADIGM)[12]	tPA or streptokinase	Lamifiban	—

induce cell death. Among the more deleterious cell responses to ischemia are the formation of free radicals and the release of proteolytic enzymes and cytokines. There are many possible therapeutic targets for these pathways. Unfortunately, promising results obtained in the laboratory are not being replicated in the clinical arena, possibly because of differences in animal models and humans in anatomy and physiology that lead to differences in dose-response efficacy. At this point, it may be premature to draw conclusions about the influence of "brain protection" on the management of acute stroke.

Stabilization of the Cerebrovascular Vessel Wall and Vessel Wall Interaction with the Bloodstream

This strategy focuses on maintaining long-term vascular stability to prevent new strokes. The development and progression of atherosclerotic plaque seems to be an inflammatory process. The use of statin drugs to lower low-density lipoprotein levels to subnormal levels promotes stabilization of coronary plaque. Some evidence exists that a similar effect is seen in the carotid arteries.[19,20] Another important issue is the prevention of in-stent stenosis. The use of pharmacological coating for stents, β-radiation brachytherapy, and biodegradable stents to prevent in-stent stenosis is promising.

■ Management of Intracranial Arteriovenous Malformations

Endovascular embolization procedures have undergone dramatic evolution and improvement in recent years. The role of endovascular embolization in the treatment of AVMs is increasing as procedural safety and durability are demonstrated. The future of AVM embolization will involve a combination of advances in embolic materials, imaging technology, catheter designs, and embolization strategies.

Embolic Materials and Catheter Designs

A wide variety of embolic materials has been used for endovascular embolization of brain AVMs. The materials currently available include balloons, polyvinyl alcohol (PVA) particles, coils, and liquid embolic agents.

Balloons are effective for occlusion of the arteries that supply an AVM. Unfortunately, they have no effect on treating the AVM nidus. With the availability of embolic agents capable of penetrating the AVM nidus, the use of balloons became obsolete.

Polyvinyl alcohol particles are rarely used for AVM embolization in the United States since the approval of *n*-butyl cyanoacrylate (NBCA) for clinical use by the FDA in 2000. Currently, the use of PVA particles is reserved for presurgical embolization because the particles rarely provide permanent occlusion of the AVM.

Coils are used mainly as an adjunct to liquid embolic agents. They are placed in high-flow fistulas within the AVM. This strategy is very helpful to slow arterial flow to avoid premature penetration of liquid embolic agent in the venous portion of the AVM. Another application of coils is in the treatment of AVM flow-related aneurysms.

The use of liquid embolic agents is becoming the mainstay of endovascular strategies for the treatment of AVMs. Liquid agents currently used for AVM embolization include Trufill (NBCA; Cordis Neurovascular Inc., Miami Lakes, FL); Neuroacryl M[21]; Onyx, formerly called Embolyx E (Micro Therapeutics Inc., Irvine, CA), dissolved in dimethyl sulfoxide (DMSO), which is an organic solvent,[22] and ethyl alcohol.[23] These materials are substantially more effective than nonliquid embolic agents for long-term occlusion of an AVM. The focus for the next generation of embolic materials will be improved control of penetration of the material into the nidus to avoid premature occlusion of inflow or outflow areas of the AVM. Stereotaxis, Inc. (St. Louis, MO) is developing the concept of delivery of liquid embolics guided by a magnetic field. Compatibility with current magnetic resonance imaging technology is a limitation of this magnetic field technology. Nonadhesion to delivery catheters and long-term occlusion rates of liquid embolic materials must also be demonstrated.

The over-the-wire and flow-guided microcatheters used for AVM embolization can be positioned optimally (close to the nidus) in most instances. Technical advances in microcatheters will probably also involve the use of an external magnetic field to help guide the microcatheter to a wedge position whenever conventional techniques fail.

Embolization Strategies

Embolization has a significant role in the multimodality treatment of brain AVMs by either enabling or facilitating subsequent microsurgical or radiosurgical treatment. In selected cases, endovascular therapy alone may lead to a total and permanent cure. Appropriately targeted embolization in otherwise untreatable AVMs represents a reasonable form of palliative treatment by either ameliorating the patient's symptoms or reducing the potential risk of hemorrhage. The goal of the embolization should be determined before the procedure is begun. Embolization strategies such as distal coil protection, transvenous retrograde nidus sclerotherapy under controlled hypotensive anesthesia (TRENSH approach),[24] cardiac standstill,[25] and general anesthesia may increase the chances of reaching the predetermined goal.

A commonly used strategy for AVMs with high-flow fistulas is to embolize the fistula with "liquid coils" before injecting the glue. The liquid coils remain on the fistula side and prevent the migration of glue to the draining vein.

According to the proposed TRENSH treatment approach,[24] liquid embolic agent (sclerosant) is injected in a retrograde fashion through the venous side of the AVM after the induction of hypotensive anesthesia and with or without the aid of temporary balloon occlusion of the primary arterial feeder. Conceptually, the controlled hypotension leads to a reduction in arterial inflow such that the agent can permeate the nidus without filling arterial feeders and their branches to normal brain tissue. Hypothetically, the TRENCH approach may provide more complete permeation of the nidus while preventing ischemic complications associated with arterial delivery. Experimental studies directed at assessing the feasibility of this approach are justified before potential future clinical application.

Adenosine-induced cardiac pause may be a viable method of partial flow arrest in the treatment of brain AVMs.[25] The idea of flow arrest during injection of NBCA is to allow a more controlled, deep, and complete embolization.

Embolization of AVMs can be performed with or without general anesthesia. The use of general anesthesia is recommended for those cases in which the patient cannot cooperate with treatment, for instance, during pediatric cases.

Embolization of brain AVMs is a technical challenge that requires experience and skill on the part of the physician and further improvements in endovascular device technology. However, the endovascular surgeon can now choose from several strategies to achieve the goal of embolization, whether it is adjunctive, palliative, or curative.

■ Management of Intracranial Aneurysms

Endovascular techniques for the treatment of intracranial aneurysms have evolved in the past two decades. Serbinenko reported his experience with endovascular techniques in 1979,[26] when he described embolization with intravascular balloons. Balloon embolization became the endovascular procedure of choice in the 1980s[27–34] but was not ideally suited to selective occlusion of the aneurysm with preservation of the patency of the parent artery. Although it is sometimes possible to inflate a detachable balloon within the aneurysm while preserving flow through the parent artery, the disadvantage of this technique is that the size and shape of the balloon may not conform to that of the aneurysm, resulting in stretching of the aneurysm wall or incomplete filling of the aneurysm. The inability to customize a balloon to the configuration of an aneurysm led to the development of coil systems for aneurysm embolization.

Coil treatment permits conformation of the coil mass to the shape of the aneurysm, which represented a significant improvement over balloon embolization. Initially, pushable coils were used for treatment of cerebrovascular lesions.[35,36] The major disadvantage of this system was the inability to remove coils that did not assume a favorable position or configuration within the aneurysm. This problem was addressed by the introduction of mechanically detachable[37,38] and electrolytically detachable[39–42] coils. First described by Guglielmi et al[40,42] for the experimental treatment of cerebrovascular lesions, electrolytically detachable coils were favored by clinical interventionists because of concerns about the forces applied within the aneurysm for detachment of mechanically detachable coils. The design of the Guglielmi detachable coil (GDC; Boston Scientific/Target, Fremont, CA) combines the advantages of soft compliant platinum, retrievability (a coil can be withdrawn, repositioned, or replaced before detachment), and atraumatic detachment. Subsequent to the approval of the GDC system by the FDA in 1995, there has been a trend toward the preferential use of endovascular therapy for the treatment of intracranial aneurysms. Early series reported use of GDC embolization solely for high-risk surgical cases (i.e., for patients of poor clinical grade or those with aneurysms deemed inoperable).[43–48] Since that time, however, many centers have begun using endovascular treatment as first-line therapy for intracranial aneurysms.[49–51]

Evidence of the efficacy of endovascular treatment for patients with subarachnoid hemorrhage presenting in poor clinical condition[52] prompted some centers to adopt a policy of reserving clip ligation for aneurysms in patients felt to be at high risk for complications from coil embolization. At these centers, the anatomy of the aneurysm is evaluated with consideration for the ability to fill the aneurysm with coils without compromising the parent artery lumen. Favorable aneurysm anatomy includes a dome-to-neck ratio of greater than 2 and a small aneurysm neck diameter, usually less than 5 mm.[53] In addition, aneurysm location may be a factor involved in treatment decisions, with lower rates of technical success for coil embolization seen for middle cerebral artery aneurysms.[54] The size of the aneurysm dome and neck influences both the ability to occlude the aneurysm with coils and the rate of subsequent regrowth of the coil-treated aneurysm.[55] The presence of a large intraparenchymal hematoma with mass effect may favor a decision to perform open surgery to reduce intracranial pressure. Conversely, evidence of significant brain swelling without a mass lesion may increase the risk of surgical retraction, resulting in reduction in local blood flow and ischemic injury.[56] The overall trend has been to consider endovascular treatment first, reserving surgical therapy only for aneurysms with unfavorable geometry or other clear surgical indications, such as intraparenchymal hematoma.

One of the major shortcomings of endovascular therapy, despite the widespread enthusiasm for its indications, was the inability to treat wide-necked aneurysms adequately. The propensity for coil herniation and parent vessel compromise made complete filling of the aneurysm nearly impossible and coil compaction or aneurysm regrowth a significant concern. Currently, techniques available for treating wide-necked aneurysms include balloon-assisted coil embolization, direct stenting or stent-assisted coiling, liquid embolic agents, and modification of the standard coiling technique (such as three dimensional coils).

Researchers have described the treatment of wide-necked aneurysms with stent-assisted coiling in experimental models.[57,58] Hemodynamic evaluation in experimental aneurysm models demonstrated significant flow alterations within the aneurysm sac after stent placement across the ostium.[59–63] Flow models may be used to quantify flow velocity and bulk flow within the aneurysm or the parent vessel. Studies using these models demonstrated that the greatest shear stress occurs at the distal aneurysm neck, a common site for aneurysm regrowth after coiling. Also, bulk flow may be reduced after parent artery stenting to as little as 5% of the presenting baseline.[63] Clinical application of these findings followed soon afterward.[64–69] Successful deployment of a stent across the aneurysm ostium permits reconstruction of the parent vessel lumen and protects against coil prolapse. With this protection in place, coils may be packed more tightly within the aneurysm without fear of parent vessel compromise, thereby reducing the risk for residual aneurysm or aneurysm regrowth.

One concern about stent-assisted coiling is the fate of normal arterial branches after stents are placed across them. As most intracranial aneurysms occur at vessel bifurcations or branch points, a normal branch often arises near the aneurysm and may be difficult to avoid during stent positioning. In our experience, however, these branches do not become occluded after stenting. In a review of 10 patients with 10 branch arteries crossed by stents (to treat aneurysms in seven patients and intracranial stenosis in three patients) and angiographic follow-up ranging from 4 days to 35 months (average follow-up, 10 months), the branches remained angiographically patent, and no patient experienced an associated clinical ischemic episode.[70] Flow demand for angiographically demonstrable branch arteries is sufficient to maintain patency after stents are placed across them. Another concern about stent-assisted coiling is the ability to deliver a stent to the target site through the tortuous cerebral vessels. Stent delivery devices tend to be rigid—more rigid than balloon catheters without stents, and much more rigid than microcatheters. Accordingly,

it may be quite difficult to navigate a tortuous carotid siphon or cervical vertebral artery loop. In our series of intracranial stenting for all indications, we were able to successfully deploy a stent at the target site in 19 of 27 attempts.[71] Unsuccessful attempts were related to the inability to access the proximal vessel from a highly tortuous arch (one case), arterial injury (two cases), and inability to navigate the stent into position (five cases). In the difficult navigation cases, the loop of artery that was proximal to the target lesion tended to have a small radius of curvature in comparison with those cases in which stent deployment was successful. Therefore, when we are considering treatment by intracranial stenting, we give more consideration to proximal vascular anatomy than to the presence of normal branches that may be compromised during stent positioning.

Perhaps the most significant shortcoming of endovascular treatment for intracranial aneurysms is the potential for regrowth or recurrence of an aneurysm after coiling. Large series have reported angiographic recurrence or growth of a remnant after coiling in 10 to 15% of cases.[72–74] Although these same series report a low rate of recurrent hemorrhage for ruptured aneurysms treated with coiling and no cases of hemorrhage after coiling for unruptured aneurysms, hemorrhage remains the primary concern in cases of aneurysm regrowth. Current developments in the field of endovascular therapy for aneurysms are focusing on ways to reduce the incidence of aneurysm recurrence. Several design modifications primarily aimed at increasing the biological activity of GDCs have been proposed to stimulate the growth of endothelium over the aneurysm ostium at the coil surface. In a swine model, higher rates of aneurysm obliteration and re-endothelialization across the aneurysm ostium were achieved with collagen-coated platinum coils than with Dacron-fibered coils.[75] Additional coil modifications have included ion implantation, protein coating, and coating with growth-factor-secreting tissue grafts.[76,77] In vitro studies show increased endothelial cell-to-cell adhesion after exposure of coils to ion-implanted collagen coating than to nonimplanted collagen coating.[78] If the processes of cell adhesion and tissue growth at the aneurysm–coil interface are enhanced by coil modifications, improved tissue healing across the aneurysm ostium would, in theory, reduce the risk of aneurysm recurrence or regrowth.

Another technique under consideration for prevention of aneurysm growth is the use of liquid polymers to fill aneurysms. The concept stems from the fact that aneurysm recurrence is reduced with a greater density of coil packing.[79] In an in vitro study, Piotin et al[79] demonstrated that dense coil packing represented filling of only 30 to 40% of the volume of the aneurysm dome. The implication is that the less residual volume left unfilled after treatment (i.e., the greater the density of packing), the lower the risk of aneurysm recurrence. Because coil filling is incomplete even in the most densely packed aneurysms, increased filling may require the use of a different medium. Animal studies have demonstrated excellent filling of aneurysms using cellulose acetate polymer (CAP).[80,81] Subsequent clinical application was promising as well.[82–84] Histological evaluation suggests that reendothelialization is more rapid and complete with CAP than with GDC.[80] However, the same study suggests that complete filling of the aneurysm is more technically feasible with GDC than with CAP, underscoring the relative benefits of each. Another agent currently under clinical evaluation in the United States is the ethylene vinyl alcohol (EVAL) copolymer dissolved in dimethyl sulfoxide (DMSO). Clinical use of the ethylene vinyl alcohol mixture for aneurysm embolization was first reported by Nishi et al[85]; the parent vessel was occluded in two of three cases. Preservation of the parent artery requires temporary balloon occlusion during polymer delivery and precipitation, which may limit the use of polymers. The technology remains promising, however.

■ References

1. Tissue plasminogen activator for acute ischemic stroke. The National Institute of Neurological Disorders and Stroke rt-PA Stroke Study Group. N Engl J Med 1995;333:1581–1587

2. Weaver WD, Simes RJ, Betriu A, et al. Comparison of primary coronary angioplasty and intravenous thrombolytic therapy for acute myocardial infarction: a quantitative review. JAMA 1997;278: 2093–2098

3. del Zoppo GJ, Higashida RT, Furlan AJ, et al. PROACT: a phase II randomized trial of recombinant pro-urokinase by direct arterial delivery in acute middle cerebral artery stroke. PROACT Investigators. Prolyse in Acute Cerebral Thromboembolism. Stroke 1998;29:4–11

4. Furlan A, Higashida R, Wechsler L, et al. Intra-arterial prourokinase for acute ischemic stroke. The PROACT II study: a randomized controlled trial. Prolyse in Acute Cerebral Thromboembolism. JAMA 1999;282:2003–2011

5. Lewandowski CA, Frankel M, Tomsick TA, et al. Combined intravenous and intra-arterial r-TPA versus intra-arterial therapy of acute ischemic stroke: Emergency Management of Stroke (EMS) Bridging Trial. Stroke 1999;30:2598–2605

6. Suarez JI, Sunshine JL, Tarr R, et al. Predictors of clinical improvement, angiographic recanalization, and intracranial hemorrhage after intra-arterial thrombolysis for acute ischemic stroke. Stroke 1999;30:2094–2100

7. Ueda T, Sakaki S, Kumon Y, et al. Multivariable analysis of predictive factors related to outcome at 6 months after intra-arterial thrombolysis for acute ischemic stroke. Stroke 1999;30:2360–2365

8. Qureshi AI, Ali Z, Suri MF, et al. Intraarterial third-generation recombinant tissue plasminogen activator (reteplase) for acute ischemic stroke. Neurosurgery 2001;49:41–48:

9. White HD. Future of reperfusion therapy for acute myocardial infarction. Lancet 1999;354:695–697

10. Ohman EM, Kleiman NS, Gacioch G, et al. Combined accelerated tissue-plasminogen activator and platelet glycoprotein IIb/IIIa integrin receptor blockade with Integrilin in acute myocardial infarction. Results of a randomized, placebo- controlled, dose-ranging trial. IMPACT-AMI Investigators. Circulation 1997;95: 846–854

11. Ronner E, Dykun Y, van den Brand MJ, et al. Platelet glycoprotein IIB/IIIA receptor antagonists. An asset for treatment of unstable coronary syndromes and coronary intervention. Eur Heart J 1998,19.1608–1616

12. Combining thrombolysis with the platelet glycoprotein IIb/IIIa inhibitor lamifiban: results of the Platelet Aggregation Receptor Antagonist Dose Investigation and Reperfusion Gain in Myocardial Infarction (PARADIGM) trial. J Am Coll Cardiol 1998;32: 2003–2010

13. Trial of abciximab with and without low-dose reteplase for acute myocardial infarction. Strategies for Patency Enhancement in the Emergency Department (SPEED) Group. Circulation 2000;101: 2788–2794

14. Antman EM, Giugliano RP, Gibson CM, et al. Abciximab facilitates the rate and extent of thrombolysis: results of the thrombolysis in myocardial infarction (TIMI) 14 trial. The TIMI 14 Investigators. Circulation 1999;99:2720–2732

15. Grines CL, Cox DA, Stone GW, et al. Coronary angioplasty with or without stent implantation for acute myocardial infarction. Stent Primary Angioplasty in Myocardial Infarction Study Group. N Engl J Med 1999;341:1949–1956

16. McGuire DK, Hudson MP, East MA, et al. Highlights from the American Heart Association 72nd Scientific Sessions: November 6 to 10, 1999. Am Heart J 2000;139:359–370

17. Ross AM, Coyne KS, Reiner JS, et al. A randomized trial comparing primary angioplasty with a strategy of short-acting thrombolysis and immediate planned rescue angioplasty in acute myocardial infarction: the PACT trial. PACT investigators. Plasminogen-activator Angioplasty Compatibility Trial. J Am Coll Cardiol 1999;34: 1954–1962

18. Smith WS, Sung G, Starkman S, et al. Safety and efficacy of Mechanical embolectomy in acute ischemic stroke: results of the MERCI trial. Stroke 2005;36:1432–1438

19. Hebert PR, Gaziano JM, Chan KS, et al. Cholesterol lowering with statin drugs, risk of stroke, and total mortality. An overview of randomized trials. JAMA 1997;278:313–321

20. Rosenson RS. Biological basis for statin therapy in stroke prevention. Curr Opin Neurol 2000;13:57–62

21. Kerber CW, Wong W, Knox K, et al. Neuroacryl M: a new liquid embolic agent–Initial clinical results (abstr). J Neurosurg 2000;92: 196

22. Jahan R, Murayama Y, Gobin YP, et al. Embolization of arteriovenous malformations with Onyx: clinicopathological experience in 23 patients. Neurosurgery 2001;48:984–997

23. Yakes WF, Krauth L, Ecklund J, et al. Ethanol endovascular management of brain arteriovenous malformations: initial results. Neurosurgery 1997;40:1145–1154

24. Massoud TF, Hademenos GJ. Transvenous retrograde nidus sclerotherapy under controlled hypotension (TRENSH): a newly proposed treatment for brain arteriovenous malformations—concepts and rationale. Neurosurgery 1999;45:351–365

25. Pile-Spellman J, Young WL, Joshi S, et al. Adenosine-induced cardiac pause for endovascular embolization of cerebral arteriovenous malformations: technical case report. Neurosurgery 1999;44:881–887

26. Serbinenko FA. Six hundred endovascular neurosurgical procedures in vascular pathology. A ten-year experience. Acta Neurochir Suppl (Wien) 1979;28:310–311

27. Berenstein A, Choi IS. Surgical neuroangiography of intracranial lesions. Radiol Clin North Am 1988;26:1143–1151

28. Higashida RT, Halbach VV, Barnwell SL, et al. Treatment of intracranial aneurysms with preservation of the parent vessel: results of percutaneous balloon embolization in 84 patients. AJNR Am J Neuroradiol 1990;11:633–640

29. Higashida RT, Halbach VV, Cahan LD, et al. Detachable balloon embolization therapy of posterior circulation intracranial aneurysms. J Neurosurg 1989;71:512–519

30. Higashida RT, Halbach VV, Dowd C, et al. Endovascular detachable balloon embolization therapy of cavernous carotid artery aneurysms: results in 87 cases. J Neurosurg 1990;72:857–863
31. Higashida RT, Halbach VV, Dowd CF, et al. Intracranial aneurysms: interventional neurovascular treatment with detachable balloons–results in 215 cases. Radiology 1991;178:663–670
32. Higashida RT, Halback VV, Dormandy B, et al. Endovascular treatment of intracranial aneurysms with a new silicone microballoon device: technical considerations and indications for therapy. Radiology 1990;174:687–691
33. Pevsner PH, Doppman JL. Therapeutic embolization with a microballoon catheter system. AJR Am J Roentgenol 1980;134: 949–958
34. Zeumer H, Bruckmann H, Adelt D, et al. Balloon embolization in the treatment of basilar aneurysms. Acta Neurochir (Wien) 1985;78:136–141
35. Casasco AE, Aymard A, Gobin YP, et al. Selective endovascular treatment of 71 intracranial aneurysms with platinum coils. J Neurosurg 1993;79:3–10
36. Hanner JS, Quisling RG, Mickle JP, et al. Gianturco coil embolization of vein of Galen aneurysms: technical aspects. Radiographics 1988;8:935–946
37. Kinoshita A, Ito M, Skakaguchi T, et al. Mechanical detachable coil as a therapeutic alternative for cerebral aneurysm. Neurol Res 1994;16:475–476
38. Marks MP, Chee H, Liddell RP, et al. A mechanically detachable coil for the treatment of aneurysms and occlusion of blood vessels. AJNR Am J Neuroradiol 1994;15:821–827
39. Guglielmi G. Embolization of intracranial aneurysms with detachable coils and electrothrombosis. In: Vinuela F, Halbach V, Dion J eds. Interventional Neuroradiology: Endovascular Therapy of the Central Nervous System. New York: Raven Press; 1992: 63–75
40. Guglielmi G, Vinuela F, Dion J, et al. Electrothrombosis of saccular aneurysms via endovascular approach. Part 2: Preliminary clinical experience. J Neurosurg 1991;75:8–14
41. Guglielmi G, Vinuela F, Duckwiler G, et al. Endovascular treatment of posterior circulation aneurysms by electrothrombosis using electrically detachable coils. J Neurosurg 1992;77:515–524
42. Guglielmi G, Vinuela F, Sepetka I, et al. Electrothrombosis of saccular aneurysms via endovascular approach. Part 1: Electrochemical basis, technique, and experimental results. J Neurosurg 1991;75: 1–7
43. Byrne JV, Adams CB, Kerr RS, et al. Endosaccular treatment of inoperable intracranial aneurysms with platinum coils. Br J Neurosurg 1995;9:585–592
44. Byrne JV, Molyneux AJ, Brennan RP, et al. Embolisation of recently ruptured intracranial aneurysms. J Neurol Neurosurg Psychiatry 1995;59:616–620
45. Graves VB, Strother CM, Duff TA, et al. Early treatment of ruptured aneurysms with Guglielmi detachable coils: effect on subsequent bleeding. Neurosurgery 1995;37:640–648
46. Richling B, Gruber A, Bavinzski G, et al. GDC-system embolization for brain aneurysms—location and follow-up. Acta Neurochir (Wien) 1995;134:177–183
47. Standard SC, Guterman LR, Chavis TD, et al. Endovascular management of giant intracranial aneurysms. Clin Neurosurg 1995;42: 267–293
48. Vargas ME, Kupersmith MJ, Setton A, et al. Endovascular treatment of giant aneurysms which cause visual loss. Ophthalmology 1994;101:1091–1098
49. Gruber DP, Zimmerman GA, Tomsick TA, et al. A comparison between endovascular and surgical management of basilar artery apex aneurysms. J Neurosurg 1999;90:868–874
50. Leber KA, Klein GE, Trummer M, et al. Intracranial aneurysms: a review of endovascular and surgical treatment in 248 patients. Minim Invasive Neurosurg 1998;41:81–85
51. Steiger HJ, Medele R, Bruckmann H, et al. Interdisciplinary management results in 100 patients with ruptured and unruptured posterior circulation aneurysms. Acta Neurochir (Wien) 1999;141: 359–367
52. Martin N. Decision-making for intracranial aneurysm treatment: when to select surgery and when to select endovascular therapy. J Stroke Cerebrovasc Dis 1997;6:253–257
53. Debrun GM, Aletich VA, Kehrli P, et al. Aneurysm geometry: an important criterion in selecting patients for Guglielmi detachable coiling. Neurol Med Chir (Tokyo) 1998;38:1–20
54. Regli L, Uske A, de Tribolet N. Endovascular coil placement compared with surgical clipping for the treatment of unruptured middle cerebral artery aneurysms: a consecutive series. J Neurosurg 1999;90:1025–1030
55. Vinuela F, Duckwiler G, Mawad M. Guglielmi detachable coil embolization of acute intracranial aneurysm: perioperative anatomical and clinical outcome in 403 patients. J Neurosurg 1997;86:475–482
56. Yundt KD, Grubb RL Jr, Diringer MN, et al. Cerebral hemodynamic and metabolic changes caused by brain retraction after aneurysmal subarachnoid hemorrhage. Neurosurgery 1997;40:442–451
57. Geremia G, Haklin M, Brennecke L. Embolization of experimentally created aneurysms with intravascular stent devices. AJNR Am J Neuroradiol 1994;15:1223–1231
58. Szikora I, Guterman LR, Wells KM, et al. Combined use of stents and coils to treat experimental wide-necked carotid aneurysms: preliminary results. AJNR Am J Neuroradiol 1994;15:1091–1102
59. Aenis M, Stancampiano AP, Wakhloo AK, et al. Modeling of flow in a straight stented and nonstented side wall aneurysm model. J Biomech Eng 1997;119:206–212
60. Wakhloo AK, Lanzino G, Lieber BB, et al. Stents for intracranial aneurysms: the beginning of a new endovascular era? Neurosurgery 1998;43:377–379
61. Lieber BB, Stancampiano AP, Wakhloo AK. Alteration of hemodynamics in aneurysm models by stenting: influence of stent porosity. Ann Biomed Eng 1997;25:460–469
62. Sekhon LHS, Morgan MK, Sorby W, et al. Combined endovascular stent implantation and endovascular coil placement for the treatment of a wide-necked vertebral artery aneurysm: technical case report. Neurosurgery 1998;43:380–384
63. Yu SC, Zhao JB. A steady flow analysis on the stented and non-stented sidewall aneurysm models. Med Eng Physiol 21:133–141, 1999
64. Higashida RT, Halbach VV, Dowd CF, et al. Intracranial aneurysms. Evolution and future role of endovascular techniques. Neurosurg Clin N Am 1994;5:413–425
65. Higashida RT, Smith W, Gress D, et al. Intravascular stent and endovascular coil placement for a ruptured fusiform aneurysm of the basilar artery. Case report and review of the literature. J Neurosurg 1997;87:944–949
66. Lanzino G, Wakhloo AK, Fessler RD, et al. Efficacy and current limitations of intravascular stents for intracranial internal carotid, vertebral and basilar artery aneurysms. J Neurosurg 1999;91: 538–546
67. Lylyk P, Ceratto R, Hurvitz D, et al. Treatment of a vertebral dissecting aneurysm with stents and coils: technical case report. Neurosurgery 1998;43:385–388
68. Mericle RA, Lanzino G, Wakhloo AK, et al. Stenting and secondary coiling of intracranial internal carotid artery aneurysm: technical case report. Neurosurgery 1998;43:1229–1234
69. Wakhloo AK, Lanzino G, Lieber BB, et al. Stents for intracranial aneurysms: the beginning of a new era? Neurosurgery 1998;43: 377–379
70. Lopes D, Ringer A, Boulos A, et al. Fate of branch arteries after intracranial stenting. Neurosurgery 2003;52:1275–1279
71. Ringer A, Lopes D, Boulos A, et al. Current limitations to intracranial stent deployment (Abstract). J Neurosurg 2001;94:168A
72. Byrne JV, Sohn MJ, Molyneux AJ, et al. Five-year experience in using coil embolization for ruptured intracranial aneurysms: outcomes and incidence of late rebleeding. J Neurosurg 1999;90: 656–663

73. Cognard C, Weill A, Spelle L, et al. Long-term angiographic follow-up of 169 intracranial berry aneurysms occluded with detachable coils. Radiology 1999;212:348–356

74. Kuether TA, Nesbit GM, Barnwell SL. Clinical and angiographic outcomes, with treatment data, for patients with cerebral aneurysms treated with Guglielmi detachable coils: a single-center experience. Neurosurgery 1998;43:1016–1025

75. Dawson RC, Krisht AF, Barrow DL, et al. Treatment of experimental aneurysms using collagen-coated microcoils. Neurosurgery 1995;36:133–140

76. Murayama Y, Vinuela F, Suzuki Y, et al. Ion implantation and protein coating of detachable coils for endovascular treatment of cerebral aneurysms: concepts and preliminary results in swine models. Neurosurgery 1997;40:1233–1244

77. Nakagawa K, Touho H, Morisako T, et al. Long-term follow-up study of unruptured vertebral artery dissection: clinical outcomes and serial angiographic findings. J Neurosurg 2000;93:19–25

78. Murayama Y, Suzuki Y, Vinuela F, et al. Development of a biologically active Guglielmi detachable coil for the treatment of cerebral aneurysms. Part I: in vitro study. AJNR Am J Neuroradiol 1999;20:1986–1991

79. Piotin M, Mandai S, Murphy KJ, et al. Dense packing of cerebral aneurysms: an in vitro study with detachable platinum coils. AJNR Am J Neuroradiol 2000;21:757–760

80. Macdonald RL, Mojtahedi S, Johns L, et al. Randomized comparison of Guglielmi detachable coils and cellulose acetate polymer for treatment of aneurysms in dogs. Stroke 1998;29:478–486

81. Sugiu K, Kinugasa K, Mandai S, et al. Direct thrombosis of experimental aneurysms with cellulose acetate polymer (CAP): technical aspects, angiographic follow up, and histological study. J Neurosurg 1995;83:531–538

82. Kinugasa K, Mandai S, Terai Y, et al. Direct thrombosis of aneurysms with cellulose acetate polymer. Part II: Preliminary clinical experience. J Neurosurg 1992;77:501–507

83. Kinugasa K, Mandai S, Tsuchida S, et al. Direct thrombosis of a pseudoaneurysm after obliteration of a carotid-cavernous fistula with cellulose acetate polymer: technical case report. Neurosurgery 1994;35:755–760

84. Kinugasa K, Mandai S, Tsuchida S, et al. Cellulose acetate polymer thrombosis for the emergency treatment of aneurysms: angiographic findings, clinical experience, and histopathological study. Neurosurgery 1994;34:694–701

85. Nishi S, Taki W, Nakahara I, et al. Embolization of cerebral aneurysms with a liquid embolus, EVAL mixture: report of three cases. Acta Neurochir (Wien) 1996;138:294–300

3

Novel Approaches to Neurovascular Diseases

MICHAEL LOUIS DILUNA, KATIE PRICOLA, AND MURAT GUNEL

Objectives: Upon completion of this chapter, the reader should be able to report some of the molecular and genetic causes of neurovascular diseases, including cavernous malformations, hereditary hemorrhagic telangiectasia, aneurysms, hemorrhagic stroke, and ischemic stroke. The reader will be familiar with research to develop novel gene therapies and stem cell transplantation techniques.

Accreditation: The AANS* is accredited by the Accreditation Council for Continuing Medical Education (ACCME) to sponsor continuing medical education for physicians.

Credit: The AANS designates this educational activity for a maximum of 15 credits in Category 1 credit toward the AMA Physician's Recognition Award. Each physician should claim only those hours of credit that he/she spent in the educational activity.

The Home Study Examination is online on the AANS Web site at: http://www.aans.org/education/books/controversy.asp

* The acronym AANS refers to both the American Association of Neurological Surgeons and the American Association of Neurosurgeons.

The capacity to find and understand the underlying molecular and genetic causes of neurovascular disorders has led to advancements in our ability to devise means of halting and altering the natural history of these diseases. Molecular therapies are currently being developed that will enable a physician–scientist to identify, modify, and potentially stop disease progression. Since the discovery of the structure of DNA in 1953, never has there been such an abundance of technology and data available. Over the past 10 years, the amount of sequence accessible in the public access databases has grown exponentially. Through initiatives in the field of bioinformatics, namely all aspects of and resulting from The Human Genome Project, powerful technologies have evolved that have led to numerous novel disease therapy targets. Nascent approaches like gene expression studies (including differential display technologies), advanced cytogenetics, proteomics, and stem cell therapies are changing the form and focus of neurovascular surgery rapidly.

From the molecular genetics of Mendelian diseases such as cerebral cavernous malformations (CCM) and hereditary hemorrhagic telangiectasias (HHT) or Osler–Weber–Rendu syndrome to more complicated multifactorial disorders like cerebral aneurysms and even ischemic stroke, scientists are using neoteric technological means to identify and understand the underlying molecular pathways and pathology. In the next few decades, strategies using gene modification or replacement protocols, resulting from our understanding of disease processes at a molecular level and subsequent carefully controlled clinical studies, involving the existing architecture or stem cell transplantation, will greatly change the management and morbidity associated with many neurovascular disorders.

For most neurovascular diseases, we are now in the process of identifying novel molecular targets. The subsequent steps in this process involve defining approaches to manipulate these targets. In this chapter, the mechanisms of disease discovery will be briefly outlined.

Subsequently, seminal examples of molecular advances in Mendelian and non-Mendelian diseases will be presented followed by discussion of novel approaches to neurovascular diseases.

■ Means of Gene Discovery

In the mid-1980s, a consortium including the National Library of Medicine, the National Institutes of Health, and other public and private research facilities in this country and worldwide devised a protocol to create a detailed structural and genetic map of numerous animal genomes. Their discoveries include not only many bacteria and viruses but also complicated eukaryotes like yeast, *Candida elegans, Drosophila melanogaster,* mice, and humans. Through our understanding of the information available, powerful techniques to manipulate and examine the data, in vivo and in vitro, have evolved. Genetic linkage studies making use of distinct polymorphic nucleotide repeats throughout the genome, involving simple and complex Mendelian traits, have led to the identification of susceptibility loci enabling us to understand the underlying molecular genetic pathology of many diseases including neurovascular disorders like HHT and CCM. Through mutational screening involving single-strand conformation polymorphism (SSCP) (**Fig. 3–1A,B**), restriction fragment length polymorphism

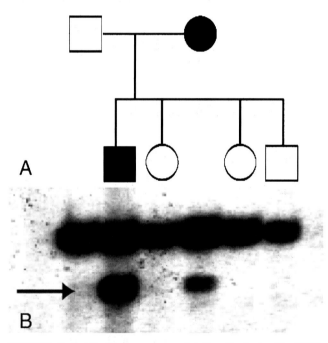

A

B

FIGURE 3–1 **(A)** Pedigree of a family affected with CCM. Open symbols denote unaffected individuals and filled symbols affected. **(B)** Photograph of a typical SSCP gel. Arrow notes the variant band corresponding to the genomic mutation. Note the one-to-one correlation between the affected individuals and the mutant band.

(RFLP), and sequencing, the molecular genetic mechanisms of disease grow even clearer. An emerging field of research is looking at the specific polymorphisms within genes that make us individuals but that also might lead to a disease phenotype. Single-nucleotide polymorphisms, or SNPs, are the most common genetic variations; they occur once every 100 to 300 bases. Currently, databases are being formed to determine which of these inheritable polymorphisms might lead to certain disease predilections. It is expected that the databases of SNPs will accelerate the disease gene discovery by enabling researchers to examine statistical associations between a disease and specific differences within populations. This differs from the more typical approach of pedigree genotyping.

Microarray or differential display technologies that look at the expression of all mRNAs in a tissue, normal compared with abnormal or diseased, have identified literally thousands of genes that are upregulated or downregulated, for instance, after ischemic stroke or hemorrhage and subsequent vasospasm, during gliosis or hypoxia, and during neoplastic change. Many of these isolated genes have become targets for therapy approach design, and some will be discussed later in this chapter. Studies in oncology showed the power of such an inquiry by looking at the gene expression profiles of breast cancer tumors. *BRCA1, BRCA2,* and sporadic tumors' RNAs were compared with a microarray of 6512 gene profiles revealing 176 specific genes differentially expressed by the *BRCA1* and *BRCA2* tumors.[1] One can clearly see the power of genetic discovery possible by differential display and microarray technologies. These techniques now are being applied to neurovascular disease.

The herald of a genetic contretemps is usually within the protein–protein interactions of a pathway. Faulty receptors, enzymes, oncogenes, or tumor suppressor genes fail to complete the cascade of events needed for the survival, replication, and turnover of healthy tissue. Despite the positional cloning of numerous genes causing a disease phenotype, the field of proteomics has proven to be a difficult one; where DNA studies are almost mathematical, protein function and folding involves an element of serendipity where many have struggled to achieve predictability. Recent in vivo and in vitro systems and methodologies for studying protein properties have opened some doors to discovery.

One such technology, yeast-2-hybrid studies (**Fig. 3–2**), have enabled scientists to clone a gene of interest into yeast and look for protein–protein interactions by yeast phenotype rescue through cotransformation with a cDNA library from a tissue of interest. For example, one could take the gene causing *CCM1,* the *Krit1* gene, clone it into a yeast expression vector, and cotransform the plasmid with a fetal brain cDNA library. The subsequent protein–protein interaction between Krit1 and the cDNA of interest will drive a promoter for the adenine

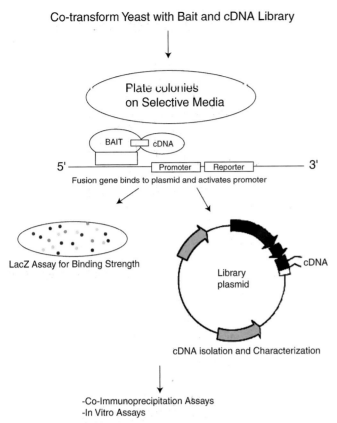

Co-transform Yeast with Bait and cDNA Library

Plate colonies
on Selective Media

BAIT   cDNA

5' ——————————[Promoter][Reporter]—————— 3'
Fusion gene binds to plasmid and activates promoter

LacZ Assay for Binding Strength

Library
plasmid

cDNA

cDNA isolation and Characterization

-Co-Immunoprecipitation Assays
-In Vitro Assays

FIGURE 3–2 Schematic of yeast-two-hybrid experiments. The gene of interest is cloned into a "bait" vector, which is subsequently transformed into competent yeast cells. A cDNA library is subsequently either cotransformed into the same yeast strain or transformed into another one to be mated with the "bait" strain. Once the yeast is plated on selective media (selective for "rescue" genes that will rescue the phenotype of yeast to enable growth on minimal media), colonies can be grown, and the plasmid encoding the interacting cDNA can be isolated, transformed into *Escherichia coli,* and sequenced. The interacting cDNA can be further analyzed for association with the bait gene through coimmunoprecipitation or in vitro expression assays.

synthetase gene on the yeast plasmid, rescuing the phenotype of the yeast on selective media. Subsequently, the strength of the interaction will be revealed by the binding of the protein–protein heterodimer to a *lacZ* promoter, causing the reporter enzyme β-galactosidase to be produced and allowing for a colorimetric assay of interaction strength (**Fig. 3–2**). The subsequent identification of the interacting cDNA could perspicaciously reveal novel pathways, as well as targets of gene therapies to be discussed later in this chapter.

■ Blood Vessel Formation

Central to the understanding of the underlying molecular and genetic pathology of neurovascular syndromes is the discernment of the processes that define and guide

vasculogenesis and angiogenesis. In the embryo, multipotential stem cells within the mesenchyme differentiate during vasculogenesis, the first of two stages, into a primitive vascular network: the vitelline capillary plexus of the yolk sac and the central vascular tree. This is followed by angiogenesis, the second stage, which enables preexisting immature vessels, including the central vascular tree and vitelline capillary plexus of the embryo, to sprout new vessels and capillary beds. It is during this stage, angiogenesis, that the primary plexus undergoes remodeling and organization. Thus, vasculogenesis refers to development of new microvessels from differentiating endothelial cells during embryogenesis, whereas subsequent sprouting from existing vessels to form new vascular channels is called angiogenesis. The process of vasculogenesis is an element exclusive to embryogenesis, but angiogenesis is a crucial process that continues to occur throughout the life of an organism.

During embryogenesis, the formation of the brain microvasculature dovetails with neural tube maturation. The first phase of this process is the growth of the primitive carotid arteries from the aortic arch, and subsequently the migration of these vessels to the ventral neural tube to form a primitive vascular plexus. Vessels originating from this plexus sprout and enter the brain parenchyma to form the microvasculature. Throughout this process, vascular endothelial growth factor (VEGF) appears to be a key figure as an angiogenic modulator. Its expression in the subependymal layer is accompanied by high levels of expression of VEGF receptors (*Flk-1* and *Flt-1*) on the surface of invading and proliferating endothelial cells.[2]

In general, angiogenesis can be divided into three stages, each of which is defined by activation of different sets of factors: initiation (induction of the differentiation of stem cells into angiogenic cells), invasion (cell proliferation, migration, and matrix degradation), and maturation (remodeling, lumen formation, and differentiation of endothelial cells) (**Fig. 3–3**). Four growth factor systems (VEGF, angiopoietins, ephrins, and transforming growth factor β [TGF-β]) are distinct players within all three stages of angiogenesis. The vascular phenotypes of various knockout and gain-of-function experiments showed that each signaling system, VEGF, angiopoietins, ephrins, or TGF-β signaling, appears to have an essential role during at least one particular phase of angiogenic growth of intersomitic veins and the embryonic vitelline capillary plexus. The complete list of molecules responsible for the angiogenesis pathways is complex and includes growth factors, membrane receptors, adhesive molecules, integrins, proteases, protease inhibitors, cytokines, tumor suppressor genes, and cytoskeleton elements.

Molecular Mechanisms of Angiogenesis

The construction and modeling of blood vessels begins with the initiation stage primarily through paracrine signaling through a group of transmembrane receptors that have either receptor tyrosine kinase (RTK) activity or homology. There are four essential RTKs in the angiogenesis pathways: VEGF-R1 and VEGF-R2 (receptors for VEGF, also known as Flt1 and Flk1, respectively), Tie1, and Tie2 (receptor for the proteins angiopoietin 1 and 2).[3] The balance between signals from the VEGF receptors and the angiopoietin receptors is a complex but necessary means of regulation throughout angiogenesis. A multipotential stem cell is differentiated into vascular cell types through signaling by VEGF and Flk1. Subsequently, primitive blood vessels are formed that are Tie1, Tie2, and Flt1 positive. The activation of these receptors allows for tube formation and branching, leading to the second phase of angiogenesis, invasion of blood vessels and endothelial recruitment (**Fig. 3–3**).

During the invasive phase of angiogenesis, the activated, recruited endothelial cells must cross through the basal lamina to migrate to their final destination. Proteases and extracellular matrix proteins accomplish this task through enzymes like urokinase (u-PA) and tissue-type (t-PA) plasminogen activators, along with several metalloproteinases. Through specific receptor activation, matrix proteins are broken down and subsequently remodeled for the passage of the migrating endothelium to the nascent site. During migration, plasminogen activator inhibitors and tissue inhibitors of metalloproteinases modulate endothelial cell behavior. This

process is crucial to our understanding of how blood vessels change with age, cellular insult, and cell death.

Acting in a complementary fashion, the TGF-β signaling complex, upon contact between endothelial and mesenchymal cells in the developing vessel, activates TGF-β receptor signaling pathways. This process is also essential to the continued invasive phase and the third, maturation phase. The TGF-β superfamily (includes TGF-βs, activins, bone morphogenic proteins, and a Mullerian-inhibiting substance) are multifunctional cytokines that regulate many aspects of cellular function like proliferation, differentiation, adhesion, migration, and extracellular matrix formation.[4] TGF-β signaling in angiogenesis induces differentiation of mesenchymal cells into pericytes and smooth muscle cells that surround the nascent tubes and stabilize them within the extracellular matrix.[5,6] Furthermore, during the invasive phase and maturation phases, the lumen becomes differentiated and the boundary between venous and arterial sides of circulation becomes distinct through TGF-β signal-induced processes. Later within the maturation phase, Tie1 and TGF-β receptors act in concert to maintain vessel integrity, structure, and strength in response to the increasing circulatory pressure.

In the mammalian CNS, angiogenesis occurs typically as a response to injurious or neoplastic insult. When ischemia or tumorigenesis occurs, endothelial cells, which are normally among the most quiescent cells in the

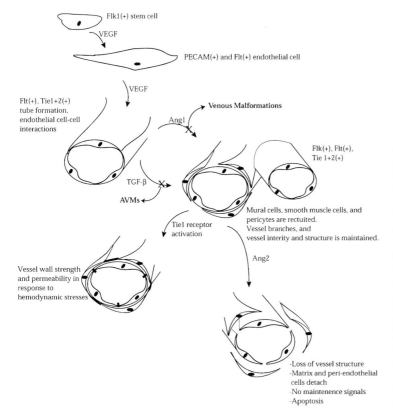

FIGURE 3–3 Angiogenesis begins with a totipotent stem cell. Extracellular signals convert this cell to a pluripotent Flk1+ vascular stem cell. Upon stimulation with VEGF, these cells differentiate into PECAM(+) and Flt+ endothelial cells. Further VEGF action on Flt, Tie1, and Tie2 organizes these endothelial cells into primitive vascular structures within which endothelial cell–endothelial cell interactions are strengthened. During the recruitment phase of angiogenesis, it appears as though TGF-β and Ang1 act in concert to have multiple effects on the nascent vascular structures. First, endothelial and vascular support cells are recruited to aid in blood vessel formation. Second, the strength of these vessels is maintained as they begin to branch and divide between the arterial and venous ends of circulation, with Tie1 receptor activation subsequently strengthening these interactions further. Ang2 can then play a role in vessel remodeling by detaching support cells, breaking down vessel structure, and in some cases, inducing endothelial cell apoptosis.

body, begin to proliferate rapidly in response to recruitment signals. The central cytokines and protein signals in this process are acidic and basic fibroblast growth factor (aFGF and bFGF), transforming growth factor superfamily members α and β (TGF-β and TGF-β), vascular endothelial growth factor (VEGF), and platelet-derived growth factor (PDGF).[7] Some of these angiogenic mediators and their receptors are also known to play an important role in central nervous system (CNS) vasculogenesis.

■ Molecular Genetics of Hemorrhagic Diseases

To understand why in certain patients the cerebral vasculature is prone to vascular malformations (VMs), stroke, aneurysm, or hemorrhage, one must first understand how normal blood vessels are built in the setting of the CNS. How vessels develop, differentiate the arterial side from the venous side of circulation, grow, remodel themselves in response to age and shear stresses, and maintain the blood–brain barrier (BBB) are seminal questions driving our pursuit of understanding neurovascular disease pathology. Through discoveries made in Mendelian models of stroke and aneurysm, much progress has been made toward our perception of the underlying genetic pathways involved in the development of the neurovasculature. **Table 3–1** lists some Mendelian forms of stroke and their underlying molecular pathologies.

Genetic examples of disease, although often less prevalent and more severe in phenotype than sporadic disease, provide a wealth of information to the understanding of disease provenance. From the results of genetic research, the physician–scientist has closed the gap between the clinic and the bench-top. This library of information has and will continue to lead to novel strategies and targets of therapy. Furthermore, we will be better able to screen those in the population believed to be at risk, whose stratification subsequently will have an impact as we plan a treatment protocol with newly gained foresight. The following are some examples of genetic diseases that led to the understanding of basic biological processes that have application to the more common forms of neurovascular disorders.

Venous Malformations

One example of a human disease phenotype caused by mutations in a gene involved in angiogenesis was found in the autosomal dominant disease, venous malformations, multiple cutaneous and mucosal (*VMCM1*). Although VMCM1 is a genetic syndrome that does not have a direct CNS phenotype, it is an excellent example of human vascular disease caused by defects in an element of the angiogenesis pathway. VMs are the most common errors of vascular morphogenesis in humans and are histologically composed of dilated, serpiginous channels containing variable amounts of smooth muscle.[8] The majority of the lesions in this disease are found on the mucosal surfaces and extremities with multiple lesions on visceral structures, including vascular tumors on the spleen, stomach, pancreas, and liver.[9] One large family enabled linkage mapping to locate a locus for *VMCM1* within a *24cM* interval on *9p*, specifically *9p21*, defined by the markers *D9S157* and *D9S163*, a different locus than *HHT1* or *HHT2* (a hotly pursued mapping target at that time, to be discussed later).[10] Missense, activating mutations in the *Tie2* gene (receptor for the proteins angiopoietin1 and 2, **Fig. 3–3**) were found in family members affected.[8] The mutation in *Tie2* disrupts the normal ability of endothelial cells to communicate with the extracellular matrix and smooth muscle cells, leading to these vascular dysmorphisms.

Sporadic cerebral arteriovenous malformations (AVMs) have a similar histologic structure to the lesions seen in VMCM1; they show abnormal expression of these vasculogenesis factors. Specifically, the expression of Tie2 and the VEGF receptors 1 and 2 (Flt1 and Flk1) is significantly lower in the lesions when compared with normal brain.[11] The generation of an AVM and its growth are likely influenced by an imbalance between the relative levels of VEGF and Tie2 signaling.

TABLE 3–1 Mendelian Forms of Neurovascular Diseases

Gene	Locus	Protein	Function
HHT1	*9q34.1*	Endoglin	TGF-β signaling,
HHT2	*12q11-q14*	Acvrl1	vessel maturation,
HHT3	Unknown	Unknown	and remodeling
CCM1	*7q11.2-q21*	Krit1	Integrin signaling
CCM2	*7p15-p13*	MGC4607	Unknown
CCM3	*3q25.2-q27*	PDCD10	Unknown
CADASIL	*19p13.2-p13.1*	Notch3	Cell signaling
HCHWA-D	*21q21*	Amyloid Beta A4	Unknown proteinase inhibitor
HCHWA-I	*20p11.2*	Cystatin C	

An example of how molecular technology has furthered our understanding of neurovascular disease is the use of microarrays. Lesions from patients with AVMs were analyzed with gene chips for the differential expression of genes important in angiogenesis. Endoglin and alk1 are proteins involved in familial AVM, hereditary hemorrhagic telangiectasia types 1 and 2 (HHT1 and HHT2), mentioned later in this chapter. Gene expression for *ENG* mRNA is upregulated in AVMs. Additionally, gene expression of *angiopoietin-1*, *Tie1*, and *PECAM1* mRNAs are downregulated in AVMs.[12] All in all, over 100 genes were differentially expressed by AVMs when compared with other CNS vascular lesions and normal controls. This wealth of information will enable physician–scientists to investigate the way in which this disease develops over the course of a patient's life.

Cerebral Cavernous Malformations

Cerebral cavernous malformations (CCM) are vascular lesions consisting of abnormal vascular spaces lined by a single layer of disorganized endothelium that can affect any part of the central nervous system's vasculature. These lesions do not contain any intervening neural parenchyma or identifiable mature vessel wall elements.[13] Furthermore, gaps exist between the endothelial cells, devoid of tight junctions that would normally create the BBB, allowing for the leakage of red blood cells into the surrounding brain parenchyma, leading to heavy hemosiderin deposits.[14] Lesions are typically confined to the CNS skin and retina. Ultrastructural analyses of these lesions show dilated, disorganized sinusoidal areas containing endothelial cell–lined walls, absent of smooth muscle components, composed of an amorphous material lacking organized collagen.[15]

This disease has been recognized to be a common clinical entity since the advent of magnetic resonance imaging (MRI), which demonstrates characteristic lesions of variable signal intensity surrounded by a dark ring attributable to hemosiderin.[16] Both MRI and autopsy studies suggest a prevalence of cavernous malformation of 0.5%, although the prevalence of symptomatic disease is much lower.[17–19]

Symptomatic patients typically present in the third through the fifth decades of life.[19] Treatment ranges from therapy with antiepileptic drugs in patients who have seizures to surgical excision of accessible lesions in patients who suffer from hemorrhage or intractable seizures.[20–22]

Since its initial description, CCM has been recognized to be a familial disorder.[23–25] Several large kindreds affected with CCM have been reported; all have shown patterns of transmission consistent with autosomal dominant inheritance, although the proportion of at-risk offspring of affected subjects developing clinical disease is often less than 50%, suggesting incomplete penetrance of the trait.[23] Incomplete clinical penetrance is further supported in several kindreds by the finding of clinically normal parents who have affected siblings, transmitting the trait to multiple offspring. Since these initial reports, 10 to 30% of patients with CCM have been shown to have one or more relatives with the disease,[26–28] leaving 70 to 90% of cases as sporadic. Ten to 20% of Caucasian patients with CCM have a first-degree relative with the disease; this proportion increases to 50% among Hispanic Americans, representing a 20- to 100-fold increase in risk versus the general population.[23] These CCM families with transmission suggesting autosomal dominant inheritance provide the opportunity to identify the underlying genetic cause(s) of CCM by positional cloning strategies.

Linkage of Cerebral Cavernous Malformations in Hispanic-American Families

In the absence of compelling candidate genes for CCM, a positional cloning approach has been taken to the identification of the CCM gene(s). This approach takes advantage of the development of dense genetic maps of the human genome and is pursued by genotyping selected markers evenly spaced at intervals across the autosomes. The inheritance of marker alleles is then compared with the inheritance of CCM. Hispanic-American patients have been shown to have a higher prevalence of familial disease, raising the possibility that this ethnic group represents a genetically homogeneous population. Hispanic-American CCM kindreds were genotyped initially in an attempt to localize the gene responsible for CCM, providing extremely strong evidence that a gene causing familial CCM (*CCM1* gene) is located in a small segment of chromosome *7q* (**Fig. 3–4**).[28,29] This evidence did not provide any indication of what the mutant gene was or how it acted to produce disease; however, it provided an essential first step in the positional cloning of this gene.

Founder Effect in Hispanic Cerebral Cavernous Malformations Cases

The above linkage findings are consistent with cavernous malformation in all Hispanic kindreds being due to mutation in the same gene but provide no indication of whether the same or independent mutations cause the disease in different kindreds. Familial cases are particularly evident among Hispanic Americans of Mexican descent, with over 50% of cases having another relative affected with CCM.[30] This disproportionate number of familial cases raises the possibility that a common mutation inherited from a shared ancestor (a founder mutation) accounts for the higher disease prevalence in this

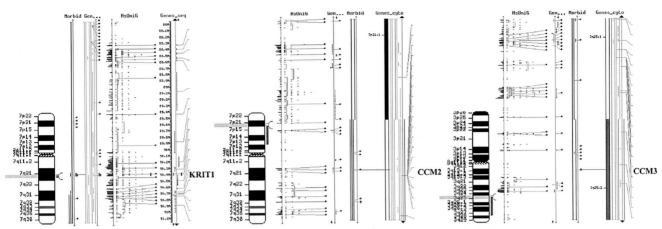

FIGURE 3–4 Graphic representation of the *CCM1*, *CCM2*, and *CCM3* intervals with respect to their physical chromosomal locations. For *CCM1*, note that the interval marked on the chromosome is small because the gene is known. The *CCM2* and *CCM3* intervals are large and contain many unique genes, some of which are identified (indicated in gray and light blue on the ideogram). The genotyping markers used to stratify the families identified are within the red bar marked on the chromosomes themselves.

group. To assess whether a founder mutation accounts for the high prevalence of familial disease among Hispanic Americans, the alleles of markers closely linked to the cavernous malformation gene in CCM cases from different Hispanic kindreds were compared. If all of these families have independent mutations in the same gene, these mutations will have occurred on unrelated chromosomes; consequently, alleles of genetic markers linked to the disease gene will show no greater similarity to one another in different kindreds than expected by chance, and marker alleles and cavernous malformation mutations are said to be in linkage equilibrium. Alternatively, if different families have all inherited the identical mutation from a common ancestor, alleles of markers closely linked to the disease will be identical to one another since they are all descending from the same ancestral chromosome. This analysis revealed that all Hispanic patients with familial CCM have inherited the same set of genetic markers, or haplotype, in the portion of *7q* linked to CCM.[31]

Among Hispanic Americans of Mexican descent, a founder mutation in *KRIT1* (*Q455X*) inherited from a common ancestor is responsible for *CCM1* in the majority of cases. A positive family history predicts nearly a 90% chance of having this founder mutation result in CCM. In apparently sporadic cases, 60% are shown to have this founder mutation (unpublished data). In most instances, sequencing data have shown nonsense point mutations, splice site, or frame shift mutants leading to premature stop codons, distributed throughout the *KRIT1* gene.

Mutations in the *KRIT1* gene could lead to a loss of function through a dominant-negative effect, haplo-insufficiency, or a two-hit model. All of the mutations identified to date encode a truncated KRIT1 protein; the process of nonsense-mediated mRNA decay is expected to lead to degradation of these aberrant transcripts such that the truncated gene products are never produced, making dominant-negative models unlikely. The two-hit model is much favored over the haplo-insufficiency mechanism for several reasons. In the two-hit model, patients with the inherited form of *CCM1* are born with one mutant *KRIT1* allele and one wild-type allele; they lose the second allele through a somatic mutation, ultimately leading to complete loss of *KRIT1* expression. Only the progeny of these cells develop into CCM1 lesions. In contrast, patients with the sporadic form of CCM are born with two wild-type copies of the *KRIT1* gene and have to acquire two independent somatic mutations to form CCM lesions. One result is that these sporadic cases tend to occur at older ages and have multiple CCM lesions much less frequently than their familial counterparts. Magnetic resonance imaging of patients with familial and sporadic CCM supports this hypothesis, as it has demonstrated a correlation between the number of lesions and family history as well as the age of the patient. Patients with the sporadic form of CCM usually have a single lesion, as opposed to the familial cases, where multiple lesions are common and patients come to clinical attention at earlier ages. Lack of correlation between the location of mutations within the *KRIT1* gene and clinical symptomatology is also consistent with the notion that loss of function of both alleles of *KRIT1* is necessary for disease phenotype.

These findings have clinical implications. For example, among Hispanic Americans of Mexican descent, nearly all familial cases and most sporadic cases will have CCM due to a single mutation inherited from a remote founder. As a result, at-risk relatives can be readily identified prospectively, providing opportunity for premorbid intervention. Further correlation of the spectrum of mutations in CCM with patient phenotype may permit identification of risk factors at the genomic level. Should molecular markers exist which identify patients at risk for hemorrhage, neurosurgeons will be able to select candidates for treatment with early surgical intervention more appropriately. Similarly, mutations causing a clinically less severe phenotype may allow for more expectant management. These genotype–phenotype correlation studies for different *CCM* loci are currently being investigated.

Disequilibrium Mapping

Knowledge of a founder cavernous malformation mutation in this population was used to refine the location of the disease gene. The founder chromosome had one specific allele at each marker locus. The span of this ancestral haplotype has been reduced in subsequent generations by recombination, with ancestral alleles of markers more closely linked to the mutation being retained and more distant marker alleles being exchanged for alleles that are representative of the general population. Consequently, identification of the minimum set of marker alleles shared among all patients inheriting the founder mutation can be used to define the location of the disease gene; this approach, called disequilibrium mapping, takes advantage of many more meiotic events than can be observed in individual families. This approach narrowed the interval that the *CCM1* gene was located to less than 500 kb, followed by physical mapping of the region. This information was then used to identify the genes localized to this region. Mutational screening of these genes as candidates for *CCM1* finally revealed that *Krit1* was mutated in families linked to *CCM1*.[32]

Functional Genomics

To date, we know little about the Krit1 protein. Krit1 was found initially through a yeast-2-hybrid screen using Krev1/Rap1A as bait.[33] Krev1 is a member of the Ras family of GTPases. In assays with Ras-activating proteins (GAP), it was found not to be activated by GAP but to be bound tightly to GAP, thereby competitively inhibiting GAP-mediated Ras-GTPase activity.[34] Thus, Krev1 acts as a tumor supressor gene in Ras signaling.

The interaction between Krit1 and Krev1 implicates potential importance of Ras signaling in angiogenesis and in the pathophysiology of CCM. The literature suggests that GAP proteins (like Ras) are phosphorylated in response to VEGF in cultured endothelial cells to stimulate proliferation and angiogenesis.[35] Thus, the Krit1 functional data and previous work done on Ras and angiogenic factors suggests a novel involvement of the Ras signal transduction pathway in vasculogenesis and potentially in CCM pathogenesis (**Fig. 3–5**).

Other investigations aimed at understanding the function of KRIT1 protein, using molecular genetic and yeast two-hybrid technologies (**Fig. 3–2**) have demonstrated that it encodes a microtubule-associated protein,[36] which also interacts with integrin cytoplasmic domain-associated protein 1α(ICAP-1α).[37,38] Furthermore, this interaction is mediated specifically by an N-terminal Krit1 NPXY amino acid sequence, a motif critical for ICAP-1 binding to β 1-integrin.[37] All of these results implicate Krit1 in focal cell adhesion. Under this model, loss—of—function mutations in Krit1 would have predictable consequences in endothelial cell morphology and performance during angiogenesis directed by β1-integrin signaling.

Future elucidation of the disease mechanisms underlying CCM will allow immediate clinical applications including genetic screening, prediction of penetrance and clinical sequelae, and novel strategies for therapeutic modification of lesion behavior. These studies represent a paradigm for dissection of molecular pathways, and the findings therein provide means for potential modification of a specific cause of hemorrhagic stroke.

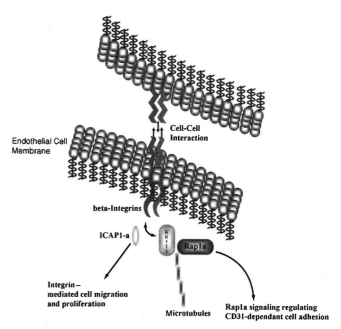

FIGURE 3–5 Illustrated in this figure is the manner by which wild-type KRIT1 is believed to play a role in the regulation of endothelial cell morphology, proliferation, and focal cell adhesion. Current data suggest that KRIT1 may sit at the crossroads between the cytoskeleton (microtubules), focal adhesion (integrins), and cell-cycle control (Rap1a and ICAP1 α).

Genetic Heterogeneity of CCM1, CCM2,
and CCM3 Genes

To test whether familial CCM in non-Hispanic families is caused by *Krit1* mutations, we have analyzed linkage in extended non-Hispanic CCM kindreds, comparing the inheritance of CCM to the inheritance of markers spanning the location of *CCM1* on *7q*. Results of this study showed that CCM was not caused by mutation in *CCM1* in these families[39] and that mutations in *Krit1* were responsible for only ~40% of these non-Hispanic kindreds.

These findings demonstrated genetic heterogeneity of cavernous malformation and revealed the presence of at least one additional CCM locus. Based on these results, another genome-wide linkage study on non-Hispanic kindreds uncovered two additional loci, *CCM2* on *7p* and *CCM3* on *3q*, which when mutated could cause cavernous malformation (**Fig. 3–4**).[40] The *CCM2* gene was eventually cloned and found to be *MGC4607*, an unknown gene flanked by markers *D7S478* and *D7S621*.[41,42] The *CCM3* locus was later cloned and found to have mutations in a gene known as programmed cell death 10 (*PDCD10*), also called "*TFAR15*," initially identified through a microarray screen during the induction of apoptosis in the *TF-1* premyeloid cell line.[43] The function of these two genes and their role in CCM development is still unknown. These findings have implications for the pathogenesis of CCM, indicating that mutations in these two additional genes can result in a CCM phenotype that is indistinguishable from *CCM1*, raising the possibility that the *CCM1, CCM2,* and *CCM3* gene products all act in a common physiologic pathway.

Hereditary Hemorrhagic Telangiectasia

The most progress toward the understanding of the underlying molecular pathology of arteriovenous malformations has resulted from the identification and dissection of the molecular genetics of hereditary hemorrhagic telangiectasia (HHT) or Rendu–Osler–Weber syndrome. Hereditary hemorrhagic telangiectasia is a Mendelian form of stroke signified by an autosomal dominant vascular dysplasia. Involvement of multiple tissues including the skin, mucosa, and viscera including the lung, liver, and brain leads to multiple telangiectases and arteriovenous malformations (AVMs). The criteria for a diagnosis of HHT are the presence of any two of the following: a pattern of autosomal dominance inheritance, telangiectases in the nasal mucosa, recurrent epistaxis, or visceral telangiectases.

The risk of intracranial hemorrhage among people with HHT is believed to be low, and furthermore, patients have a good functional outcome after hemorrhage. Hereditary hemorrhagic telangiectasia lesions within the CNS are mostly low-grade AVMs (Spetzler–Martin grade I or II) and are frequently multiple. About 7 to 12% of patients with HHT with have CNS lesions, and female patients are more often affected than male patients are. Much controversy exists as to whether or not patients with HHT should undergo frequent screening for CNS lesions. By comparison, pulmonary arteriovenous fistulae are a much more frequent cause of neurological symptoms in this population.

Hereditary hemorrhagic telangiectasia pathology was first described in the literature by Osler in 1901 as a "family form of recurring epistaxis, associated with multiple telangiectases of the skin and mucous membranes."[44] When lesions from this inherited disorder are examined histologically, there is no reported difference between mucosal and cutaneous telangiectases and those found in the viscera[45] or the neurovasculature.[46] Representative reconstructions from serial embedded structures have shown much of the pathogenesis of HHT. Based on the histopathology of telangiectasias from the skin and mucosa, it was argued that the earliest HHT lesions are focal dilations of postcapillary venules composed of prominent stress fibers and pericytes along the adlumenal border.[47] These telangiectasias enlarge as the AVMs develop. Once fully matured, they are evenly dilated, have multiple layers of smooth muscle often without an elastin component, and connect through one or more capillaries to dilated arterioles.[47] An associated perivascular mononucleocyte cell infiltrate is also seen during these maturation events; electron microscopy (EM) displayed that most of the infiltrating cells are lymphocytes or macrophages.[47]

Prior to recent extensive genetic linkage studies, it was estimated that the minimal penetrance of HHT in a heterogeneous population was 1:16,500.[48] Using microsatellite markers from polymorphic sequences, two distinct loci were found to show significant LOD scores for linkage of the disease genotype. The first gene, *HHT1*, was mapped to *9q34.1*[49]; a second group of families showed linkage to a second locus, *HHT2*, on *12q11-q14*.[50] Upon closer analysis, it was found that the gene coding for endoglin, a transforming growth factor β (TGF-β)-binding protein, was mutated in affected individuals with linkage to the *HHT1* locus.[51] This was the first locus for human disease based on a mutation in the TGF-β signaling complex. Within the *HHT2* locus on *12q11-q14*, loss-of-function mutations were found in the activin receptor-like kinase 1 gene, Acvrl1, a type I serine-threonine kinase receptor for the TGF-β superfamily of growth factors[52] expressed extensively in the endothelium with a likely role in vasculature repair or genesis. A third locus for HHT is suspected in a large family that excludes linkage to chromosome 9 or 12 with a distinct phenotype of HHT including angiodysplastic liver involvement.[53]

Expression studies of transformed cell lines using vector-delivered mutant endoglin have shown that when expressed, mutant endoglin doesn't ever make it to the cell's surface, as it essentially becomes "trapped" in the endoplasmic reticulum or the Golgi complex.[54] The mutant endoglin protein remains intracellular and, in most familial mutant forms, does not appear to act as a dominant-negative in vascular dysmorphism.[54] One mutation examined, a delta-GC frameshift, was able to dimerize with normal endoglin and acted in a dominant-negative fashion.[54] It can then be concluded that *HHT1*

mutations can act in either a dominant-negative or a haplo-insufficiency model. All of the HHT mutations in Acvrl1 shown to date have a deleterious effect on Acvrl1 signaling, leading to a disruption of the control of the quiescent state.[55] Both Acvrl1 and endoglin are required as receptor-partners for TGFβRI, TGFβRII, and TGFβRIII to maintain the balance between the positive and negative biphasic effect TGF-β signaling has on angiogenesis (**Fig. 3–6**).[56]

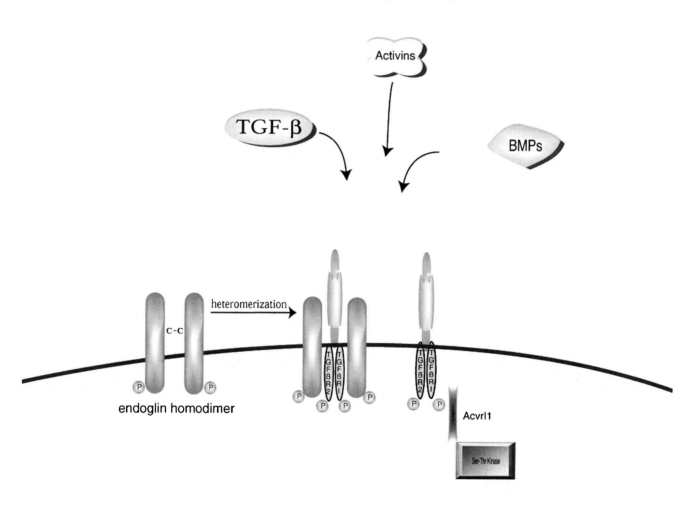

Effected Transcription Responses
  -endothelial re-modeling
  -vascular smooth muscle
   development
  -recrutiment and differentiation of
   mesenchymal cells
  -stabilization of interactions between
   vasculogenesis endothelial tubes and
   extracellular matrix

FIGURE 3–6 Endoglin- and Acvrl1- signaling TGF-β1 receptors can exist as either homodimers alone or as homodimers in concert with endoglin or Acvrl1. The endoglin homodimer, held together by cystein–cystein bonds, can dimerize with TGF-β1 receptors to modulate signaling with TGF-β. In a similar fashion, Acvrl1 can signal in response to TGF-β stimulation; however, this is only when complexed with TGF-β1 receptors. Loss of function of either endoglin or *Acvrl1* results in *HHT1* and *HHT2*, respectively. Mouse knockout studies have revealed that endoglin and Acvrl1 are important in vascular remodeling and development and differentiation between arterial and venous sides of circulation during embryogenesis.

Endoglin

Endoglin, a type III TGF-β receptor, is a member of a family of cell surface receptors that among the most densely expressed receptors across a given cell's surface.[57] Endoglin, specifically, is a membrane glycoprotein expressed in limited amounts in organ tissues but is found in high levels predominately in vascular endothelial cells and in hematopoietic cell types.[58] The endoglin gene codes for a 561–amino acid protein, including the cell localization signal peptide, multiple extracellular N- and O-linked glycosylation sites, and a 47–amino acid cytoplasmic domain that can vary in length due to alternative splicing events.[59] The native protein exists as a homodimer linked by multiple cystein–cystein bonds.[60]

Endoglin has been shown through immuno coprecipitation assays to interact with several molecules including TGF-β1 and TGF-β3, activin-A, BMP-7, and BMP-2.[60] (**Fig. 3–6**) When TGF-β is added to cultured vascular smooth muscle cells, an increase in endoglin expression occurs.[60] Endoglin readily binds to multiple cytokines, and in native quiescent blood vessels, vascular smooth muscle and endothelial cell proliferation are inhibited.[61] Binding of all three subtypes of TGF-β, TGF-β1, TGF-β2, and TGF-β3, and other extracellular signals is not the sole purpose of endoglin. It also alters the affinity of other receptors for TGF-β as it forms heterodimers with both the type I and type II TGF-β receptors (TGFβRI/II).[60]

One proposed model states that TGF-β can act as either a positive or negative regulator of angiogenesis; this biphasic effect of TGF-β receptor signaling in response to doses of TGF-β itself appears to be concentration dependant.[62] There may be multiple receptors for TGF-β on a cell's surface that have varying affinities, and modulation of these affinities involves heterodimerization with endoglin and interaction with Acvrl1. Because mutations in endoglin or *Acvrl1* causing an HHT phenotype can alter angiogenesis mechanisms through disruption of TGF-β signaling through either haplo-insufficiency or dominant-negative events, plausible support is lent to this theory of a delicate and necessary balance between negative and positive regulation of TGF-β.

Endoglin Knockout Mice

Li et al generated a targeting vector and subsequently used homologous recombination to disrupt the first two exons of endoglin. Heterozygotes showed no phenotype, but homozygous mutants (–/–) were generated, and it was found that no –/– mice survived past E11.5 (11.5 days after fertilization).[58] The –/– mice were three times smaller than the heterozygous and normal mice and exhibited a profound absence of vascular organization.

Interestingly, Flk-1, Flt-1, Tie1, and Tie2, in addition to TGF-β expression, were all undisrupted in intensity. This indicates that endothelial cell differentiation and primitive hematopoiesis from precursor cells are not developmental processes solely regulated by endoglin. Instead, the presence of an immature perineural vascular plexus in the –/– mice indicated that endoglin is responsible for endothelial modeling. In addition to a strictly vascular phenotype, the cardiac tube did not complete rotation, and the dorsal aortae, branchial arteries, intersomitic vessels, and carotid arteries were atretic and disorganized morphologically. The vascular structures showed markedly impaired smooth muscle cell maturation, as pericytes and vascular smooth muscle precursors were absent from supporting structures of the nascent capillary networks. The endoglin knockout phenotype correlates the histological findings of arterialized vessels throughout the telangiectatic vessel walls, leading to the hypothesis that mutant endoglin is not able to regulate endothelium and vascular smooth muscle cell proliferation and organization upon TGF-β signaling.

A second group of investigators generated a –/– knockout mouse that had a similar phenotype to that generated by Li et al The exception noted here was that some of the heterozygotes (+/–) generated from the 129/01a murine strain had signs of HHT such as telangiectases and epistaxis.[63] It can then be argued that there must be some epigenetic or modifying factors present in this strain, but not the other strain, that contribute to the disease mechanism for HHT.

Activin Receptor-Like Kinase

Activin receptor-like kinase, Acvrl1, much like endoglin, is an endothelial cell receptor for members of the TGF-β superfamily. While endoglin is argued to be required as a receptor–partner between negative and positive regulation of angiogenesis, Acvrl1 alternatively may signal through a second, independent cascade that does not involve TGF-β specifically due to the identification of a third, but unknown, ligand.[4] Acvrl1 indeed has some homology to the TGF–β type I receptor family. Acvrl1, when expressed at the cell surface alone, shows little or no activity in response to all TGF-β protein subtypes.[4] However, when bound as a chimeric heterodimer to the TGF-β type I receptor, Acvrl1 signaling activity markedly increases in response to TGF-β1 and TGF-β3, but not TGF-β2.[4] Potentially adding to the already established specificity of the Acvrl1/TGFβRI complex for either TGF-β1 or TGFβ3 (**Fig. 3–6**), activin A, BMP-1 and 7, and inhibin A cannot activate Acvrl1 signaling.[4] Additionally, the Acvrl1 complex with TGFβRI yields a 20% reduction in signal with TGF-β induction in comparison to TGFβRI signaling alone.[4]

Cellular signaling dependent upon heterodimer binding specificity with TGF-β type I receptors is a similar model to that of endoglin, lending further support to the notion that endoglin and Acvrl1 are in the same molecular and developmental pathway—each able to keep TGF-β angiogenic signaling in check. This would explain why families that show linkage to either the endoglin or *Acvrl1* loci have similar phenotypes. From these studies, it can be concluded that the quiescent state of mature, adult blood vessels is regulated by endogenous negative effectors, acting through endoglin and Acvrl1 signaling.

Homozygous Acvrl1 Knockout Mice

Similar to the methodology behind the endoglin knockout, a targeting vector was generated, and subsequently used through homologous recombination, to disrupt transcriptional and translational initiation of *Acvrl1*.[64] Up until E9.5, the homozygous mutant (−/−) mice appeared grossly normal, but by E9.5, the *Acvrl1* −/− mice had yolk sacks that failed to form distinct vitelline vessels and remained a meshwork of interconnected and homogenous endothelial tubes. Like the endoglin mice, no embryos survived past E11.5. At day 8.5, *Acvrl1* −/− mice showed primary arterial–venous (A-V) shunting of the central vascular tree with subsequent disruption of endothelial remodeling and vascular smooth muscle cell development. From this model, the process of angiogenesis and early vascular development can be broken down into a couple of distinct, but critical, processes. First, proteins like VEGF and other growth factors must differentiate the angioblasts and vascular stem cells into the endothelial tubes that form the vitelline capillary plexus of the yolk sac and the central vascular tree (**Fig. 3–3**).[65] Second, the assignment of AV identity must occur to create the mature circulatory system, a process dependent on Acvrl1.[64] Without the distinction between arterial and venous boundaries in the early embryo, A-V shunting will occur. Interestingly, in the haplo-insufficiency model of *HHT2*, Acvrl1 must continue to play a role in angiogenesis and vessel turnover through the remodeling of mature blood, again supporting theories about the formation of telangiectasias and AVMs.

Aneurysms

Another major cause of hemorrhagic neurovascular disease is cerebral aneurysm. The pathogenesis is likely to be multifactorial, with genetic factors playing a role in at least 7 to 20% of cases reported.[66] A genetic basis for aneurysms is actually supported by multiple lines of evidence. There are several documented families in the literature that have (1) aneurysm transmission through multiple generations, (2) a younger average age of rupture

for familial cases, (3) middle cerebral artery aneurysms as the most common type of aneurysm in familial cases where as seen in sporadic cases, aneurysms are seen distributed throughout the Circle of Willis, and (4) occurrence at the same site or a mirror site in sibling pairs and identical twins.[67] Several inherited disorders have cerebral aneurysms among their pathologies including polycystic kidney disease (PKD), Ehlers–Danlos syndrome type IV, and Marfan's syndrome.[67] In adult PKD, the prevalence of intracranial aneurysms is ~25% and is significantly higher in patients with PKD and a positive family history for cerebral aneurysm.[68] All of this data—when taken together and added to a screening protocol of patients at risk of inheriting a mutated allele—plays an important role in planning the surgical management of this disease.

Although there are a few documented families with inherited forms of intracranial aneurysms, little is known about the underlying molecular pathology and genetics of this disease. Even though a few preliminary studies have found some associations between allele inheritance and a proclivity for the development of intracranial aneurysm,[69] much work remains to be done in this area before scientific conclusions can be reached. Microarray and differential display technologies are currently being used to examine lesion samples. Some of the recent studies have shown that aneurysm tissue taken at autopsy demonstrates increased activity among proteolytic enzymes, specifically matrix metalloproteinases that contribute to focal degradation of the vascular extracellular matrix.[70] Extracellular matrix remodeling is commonly associated with cerebral aneurysms and may play a role in the formation or rupture of these lesions. Up to a 3-fold increase in a 72-kDa serum gelatinase protein (matrix metalloproteinase-2) is seen in the walls of aneurysm tissue.[71] The role and subsequent manipulation of these matrix metalloproteinases in the formation and rupture of intracranial aneurysms is an area of current research focus.

To date, several studies have used linkage approaches to identify loci contributing to intracranial aneurysms (IA) risk.[72–79] Sibling pair studies from Japanese and Finnish populations and a recent report of a consanguineous Dutch family have identified candidate intervals.[75,76] The only intervals from such studies that meet genome-wide evidence of significant linkage are *19q13.3* in the Finnish population,[80] *2p13* in the Dutch family,[81] and *1p34.3-p36.13* in a large family from West Virginia.[82]

The identification of causative aneurysm genes will shed light on the pathways leading to disease. Whether this loci or pathways will play a role in more common forms of disease remains to be determined. Genes leading to IA identified, may better define the pathophysiology and natural history of aneurysm formation and rupture, and thus contribute to improved diagnostic and therapeutic approaches to this disease.

Intraparenchymal Hemorrhage

The underlying molecular pathology behind intraparenchymal hemorrhage is often multifactorial. One familial monogenic form of intraparenchymal hemorrhage, hereditary cerebral hemorrhage with cortical amyloid angiopathy (HCHWA), was one of the first Mendelian forms of stroke to be characterized on the molecular level. Hereditary cerebral hemorrhage with cortical amyloid angiopathy is subcategorized into two subsets: those with the Dutch type (HCHWA-D) and those with the Icelandic type (HCHWA-I). Serial studies of these populations showed sclerosis and amyloid-like deposits in the small arteries and arterioles in the cortex and covering arachnoid.[83,84] The pathological vessels in these two diseases are often irregularly distributed and clustered in the cortex. It was originally noted that the deposits seen in the walls of the affected arteries was different from those seen in the Icelandic form of this disease in that the deposits resembled the β-amyloid plaques typically seen in Alzheimer's or Down's syndrome.[85]

The Icelandic type of HSHWA is caused by the L68Q mutation (a substitution at amino acid position 68 of a glutamine for a leucine) in the cystatin C gene, a proteinase inhibitor, on chromosome *20p11.2*.[86] Cystatin C is an abundant extracellular inhibitor of proteinases that was found to have reduced expression in atherosclerotic blood vessel walls and aneurysm lesions.[87] In HCHWA-I, the mutant form of this protein is deposited within the walls of the affected vessels and leads to the hemorrhagic stroke phenotype.[83]

The Dutch type of HSHWA is caused by the E693Q mutation (a substitution at amino acid position 693 of a glutamine for a glutamic acid) in the beta A4 amyloid precursor protein gene on *21q21*, a logical locus in light of the early observations.[88] The mechanism by which these proteins become amyloid disease deposits is an intense area of research. The deposits and plaques from β-amyloid proteins seen in HSHWA-D, Down's syndrome, and Alzheimer's disease have led to numerous publications on the nature of protein structure and folding dynamics. There are also numerous mouse knockout and knock-in models for this disease. What is unclear, however, is how a glutamine substitution in two separate proteins leads to an insoluble protein isoform and subsequent vascular neuropathologies. Additionally, it is uncertain how polymorphisms (even SNPs) in these genes might contribute to sporadic cases of this disease.

Ischemic Disease

After an ischemic insult to the CNS, many events follow which contribute to neuronal death. The length and severity of the insult coupled with proinflammatory responses and stresses to the cellular architecture, electrophysiology, and genetic elements all augment the mechanism by which the brain becomes injured. Simply stated, two types of damage to the neuron may occur after a stroke. Initially, an immediate cell death may occur, caused by any number of extracellular events. Subsequently, a delayed or apoptotic cell death will occur, initiated by the ischemic injury, whose effects come over the days and weeks to come. Research focused on the prevention of neuronal death after stroke has aimed at minimizing the damage incurred, starting with the prevention of injury during the ischemic event, halting the progression to apoptosis, and subsequent avoidance of reperfusion injury. By using murine models of stroke, immunohistochemistry, molecular genetic analysis, and differential display technologies, certain genes have emerged as therapeutic targets. Literally thousands of proteins have been identified for their potential ability to either protect neurons from hypoxia or exacerbate cell death and infarct size after stroke. Some of the genes found to be either protective or damaging are listed in **Table 3–2**.

The pathology of ischemic stroke is very complex. As was shown with the vascular malformation molecular pathology, there are two ways to approach a complex disease like ischemic stroke to dissect and understand the molecular pathways: (1) use the Mendelian forms of common disease to investigate disease loci and genes, and (2) investigate potentially important target molecules that may be subject to therapeutic manipulations. For the purposes of this chapter, we will use cerebral autosomal dominant arteriopathy with subcortical infarcts and leukoencephalopathy, or CADASIL, as an example of the former approach, and nitric oxide (NO) pathway studies as an example of the latter.

Cerebral Autosomal Dominant Arteriopathy with Subcortical Infarcts and Leukoencephalopathy

A strictly Mendelian form of ischemic stroke, CADASIL is an inherited disease that is characterized by reoccurring strokes seen on CT exams as multiple occlusive cerebrovascular infarcts.[89] Examination of pathology specimens reveals multiple small, deep infarcts of the white matter with arterial walls, which have a thickened elastic component and large deposits of a nonamyloid, granular, nonfibrinoid, eosinophilic substance in the tunica media.[90] Histologic examination reveals an angiopathy mainly affecting the small penetrating arteries between 100 to 400 μm in diameter that supply the white matter and basal ganglia.[91] Linkage to a 8-cM interval on the short arm of chromosome 19, specifically *19p13.2-p13.1*, was shown.[92] Subsequently, to much surprise, mutations in the *Notch3* gene were shown to

TABLE 3–2 Genes Found through Differential Display Analysis of Stroke Tissues

Exacerbating Infarct Damage	Protects CNS from Damage	Understood or Proposed Pathway
DNA methyltransferase GFAP-absence Caspase-9 Caspase-3,8 p53, p21 Bcl2 disruption Presenilin-1 disruption BAX Calcineurin NF-kappaB	Protein-disulfide isomerase Poly (ADP-ribose) polymerase Bcl2 Bcl-X-L XRCC1 E2F1	Apoptosis
NMDA receptor activation NOS Transcription factor interferon regulatory factor-1	Interleukin-6 SOD Aquaporin-4 deletion TGF-β1 HSP HSP-70 Ornithine decarboxylase Heme oxygenase-1 FGF-13 Glycine binding site agonists NAIP Il-1 receptor antagonist Adrenomedullin	Cytotoxicity and inflammation

cosegregate with the disease phenotype.[93] How the disruption of *Notch3* specifically can lead to a vasculo-pathic phenotype is still unclear. Future knockout studies will certainly shed some light on the genesis of this disease.

Nitric Oxide

An interesting family of genes that have emerged as a target for molecular therapy studies in the prevention of CNS damage because of BBB breakdown are the NO syn-thase genes, *iNOS, nNOS,* and *eNOS.* NO, an intercellular messenger synthesized by the NO synthase enzyme (NOS), has multiple functions is different tissues. In the immune response, NO allows macrophages to kill tumor cells and bacteria; in endothelial cells, NO is a potent vasodilator of blood vessels; in the CNS, NO is a putative neurotransmitter. One isoform of NOS, *nNOS,* is found almost exclusively in selected neurons and is selectively activated in specific brain areas associated with an ischemic event.[94] NO can then interact with superoxide to form peroxynitrite, a powerful oxidant that destroys neurons.[95] Interestingly, in both *iNOS* –/– and *nNOS* –/– mice, the ischemic damage to the brain after a stroke is greatly reduced, even up to 10 days after infarct, when compared with wild-type or heterozygous mice.[94] Conversely, *eNOS* –/– mice have greater infarct size after MCA occlusion.[96] The ability of *eNOS* to prevent platelet aggregation and clot formation, coupled with its vasody-namic effects, must serve to protect the brain from hemodynamic injury, while NO produced by *iNOS* and *nNOS* can be toxic to brain tissue. These studies suggest that selective inhibition of *iNOS* or *nNOS* after an ischemic event to the CNS may have therapeutic and protective benefit. Furthermore, they show how research into candidate genes can lead to better understanding of disease pathways and of treatment avenues for neurovas-cular disease.

■ Gene Therapy Techniques

There are numerous powerful techniques aimed at iden-tifying potential target molecules for therapies. Even though no molecular therapy is currently available, there is extensive research focused on therapies based on gene transfer or replacement and stem cell transplantation (**Table 3–3**).

Viruses, because of their innate ability to evade host defenses, transform cells, and subsequently replicate within cells, are being investigated for clinical use in gene delivery. The viruses currently being employed are small, efficient at gene replication and expression, and more often than not, invisible to the host's defense sys-tem. The main hindrance to scientific progression in this area is in the realm of transformation efficiency and speci-ficity. For a virus to be used effectively in a laboratory

TABLE 3–3 Gene and Stem Cell Therapies

Therapy	Means of Delivery	Target Disorder	Disadvantages
Vector-delivered Gene therapy	Local stereotactic injection of virus or virus-producing cells	Small tumors, neurodegenerative disorders	Can't treat metastatic disease, stroke, or dividing cells
	CSF injection sub-dural, sub-arachnoid, cisternal, or intra-ventricular	Can be used to treat acute phase of stroke, meningeal pathology, or metastatic disease to the meninges. Can avoid immune surveillance	Poor diffusion from CSF into CNS; can't be used for parenchymal pathology due to lack of diffusion.
	Intravenous or Intra-arterial infusions	CNS metastatic disease, global applications; stroke; vasospasm	Toxicity to CNS or viscera.
Liposomal gene transfer	I.A. infusions	Stroke; Vasospasm; Aneurysm	Transient in effect, not applicable for parenchymal pathology
Stem cell therapy	Vector modified, stereotactic injections	Neurodegenerative, ischemic, vascular repair; stroke.	May make inappropriate neurophysiological connections; neoplasia.

or clinical setting for gene delivery, its pathogenicity must first be controlled or eliminated, while retaining its ability to recombine and transfect cells. Five viral means of delivering genes to cells are currently being investigated, while two nonviral means are also being used. **Table 3–3** shows the different therapeutic avenues being traversed by the specific molecular targeting techniques.

There are many possibilities for virus-based therapies including the use of retroviruses. Retroviruses have either one or two copies of an RNA genome within a capsule and are capable of transforming only rapidly dividing cells. The ability of the virus to replicate is eliminated by creating strains that require a packaging cell line to produce the proper structural elements to surround the RNA and gene(s) of interest. In the case of brain neoplasms, retroviruses are currently being used to deliver genes that produce toxic metabolites or apoptotic signals.[97,98] The usefulness of this technique is evident in the fact that the majority of the adult brain contains postmitotic cells. In the case of neurovascular disorders, the mutant gene could be replaced within the remodeling endothelium or vascular smooth muscle cell (VSMC) layer. Lentiviruses, a subfamily of retroviruses, are also RNA viruses in that they contain an RNA genome. Lentiviruses are efficiently transfected and integrated into both dividing and nondividing cells, making their range of applications more broad than retroviruses. Lentiviral vectors based upon simian immunodeficiency virus (SIV) have been developed recently to avoid the risk of using HIV-related retroviruses or lentiviruses.

Adenoviruses, adenovirus-associated viruses, and herpes simplex viruses are other popular modes of gene delivery used in the laboratory for cell transplantation studies. These viruses contain a double-stranded DNA genome and can transform a wide variety of tissues, including postmitotic ones. Once transfected, these cells show a high-titer of virus gene expression.[99] Currently, these viruses are being developed in clinical trials to deliver correct copies of genes to cells with germline mutations such as the *CFTR* gene in cystic fibrosis. Again, double-stranded DNA gene delivery modalities are deficient in certain early, immediate-early, and other virulence-conferring genes and lack the means of self-replication. To restrict and maintain gene expression, endogenous tissue-specific proteins are required. Adenovirus-associated viruses are an interesting tool because of their small size and relative invisibility to the host's immune system. The compact nature of adenovirus-associated viruses is currently being exploited in trials to ascertain its ability to traverse small pores, such as those that confer the BBB, and deliver the gene of interest to tissues that would otherwise require stereotactic injections.

Two areas of nonviral gene delivery being investigated are through liposomal-fusion methods and through the use of simple, naked DNA. Under proper molar concentrations of salt within an aqueous solution, lipids can form spherical structures known as micelles or liposomes. Making use of the negative charge surrounding DNA, liposomes can be engineered to contain a vector or plasmid of choice and can be used to fuse with a target cell's membrane for delivery of the vector or plasmid. Although often used in the laboratory, the efficiency of this method in transforming cells is very low, and even lower still is the rate of plasmid integration into the cell's genome. Thus, this sort of gene delivery is often referred to as "transient transfection," which makes it useful for gene expression in small bursts. In the area of naked DNA gene delivery, companies have developed a system by which DNA can be covalently bound to gold dust particles, loaded into a "bullet," and blasted through a noble gas jet gun into senescent or dividing cells. Once within the aqueous environment of a cell's interior, the DNA releases from the nontoxic gold particles and can express the engineered gene of interest. This method is currently being used in laboratory trials in in vivo animal models.

Gene Delivery

There is a methodological roadblock that remains; that is, how to deliver the gene or molecule of interest to specific areas of the CNS. After a stroke or an aneurysm, stereotactic injections using minimally invasive techniques could be used to deliver encoded therapeutic and protective genes. Similarly, injections into the ventricle or intrathecally could enable global gene therapy delivery while avoiding the BBB. This approach was used in some animal models of gene therapy for stroke. In one study, gerbils were administered glial-derived neurotrophic factor (GDNF), packaged in an adenovirus vector, by injection into the lateral ventricles.[100] GDNF is a neuroprotectant, capable of preventing necrosis in the cerebral cortex after ischemia and delayed neuronal apoptosis in the hippocampal CA1 neurons.[100,101] In the gerbils injected with the virus, the transformation rate in the ependymal cells was high, and there were fewer necrotic and apoptotic cells than in the control animals.[100] Other studies seek to target the fibrinolytic t-PA/PAI-1 system. In mouse knockout models of t-PA and PAI-1, adenovirus was used to deliver human recombinant proteins to restore thrombolytic potential.[102] There is evidence to support the theory that brain injury after stroke or SAH is due to the downregulation of t-PA.[103]

■ Stem Cell Therapies

In recent years, advances have been made in the area of identification, manipulation, and subsequent transplantation of stem cells. Stem cells are undifferentiated and can divide, renew, and subsequently differentiate into any tissue of choice. For years, stem cells have been isolated from fetal tissue and differentiated into any number of tissues. Currently, a focus of laboratory research has been the identification and isolation of stem cells and tissue-specific progenitor cells from adult tissues. The potential of these cells in organ repair has presented physicians and scientists with numerous possibilities for disease treatments.

The classic dogma that injury to the mammalian brain, whether it is caused by stroke, hemorrhage, or ischemia, is irreversible due to an absence of cortical regenerative capacity has been challenged in the basic science literature. Within the past decade, studies have shown the presence of neuronal stem cell populations in the adult animal that display a limited regenerative potential.[104,105] Although much less is understood with respect to these progenitor populations in humans, recent studies also suggest the presence of precursor cell populations and continued neurogenesis in adult human brain[13,106,107] from proliferating neuronal progenitor/ stem cells.

In the adult human brain, neural stem cells (NSCs) are located mainly in the subventricular zone of the lateral ventricle (SVZ) and the dentate gyrus of the hippocampus, but they are also present on the surface of the third and fourth ventricles of the spinal cord central canal.[106,108] These cells can be readily cultured, expanded, and differentiated into many different CNS cell types. What remains to be determined is whether this cell found in the adult human brain is truly a totipotent stem cell, similar to cells isolated and characterized in the hematopoietic system, or whether the adult human brain contains multiple, different, pluripotent cells committed to specific lineages. Despite the possibility that these cells may display a restricted potential, investigations are underway to see whether these cells can still be expanded and used, for instance, in neuronal regeneration.

Recently, a subset of embryonic stem cells, namely Flk1-positive stem cells, were shown to be vascular progenitors in vitro and in vivo.[109] Endothelial cells arise from Flk1-positive cells within the mesoderm, which represent a distinct population from cells in the mesoderm that become pericytes and smooth muscle cells.[110] Using cell-sorting techniques, Flk1-positive stem cells were isolated and shown to differentiate into sheets of endothelial cells upon treatment with VEGF and to form vascular tubes.[109] *LacZ*-expressing Flk1-positive cells were injected into stage 16–17 chick embryos and were found to have the capacity to incorporate into the nascent embryonic vasculature.[109] These cells show the incredible possibilities available through stem cell research. The potential to repair or replace dysfunctional vascular beds with endothelium-forming stem cells holds great promise in the areas of ischemic stroke or vessel disease such as AVM, or CCM repair.

■ Conclusion

Recent years have seen a rapid growth and advancement in molecular biology, physiology, and genetic research techniques. Application of these techniques toward specific areas such as neurovascular disorders is now happening. Novel therapeutic targets, which stem from the piecing apart of molecular pathways involved in disease molecular pathogenesis, have been found, and they will continue to be discovered at an exponential rate. The wealth of information available within the databases and literature have made in silico genetic and molecular research as powerful as in vitro or in vivo studies. Additionally, progress in the treatment of neurovascular syndromes will be given a boost from the current stem cell–based and gene transfer/therapy–based technologies also happening. Continuation of focus in these two areas (discovery of molecular targets and manipulation or targeting methodologies) will lead to novel, efficacious therapies for neurovascular disorders.

Patients can only benefit from this knowledge. Screening of those suspected to have disease will occur in the clinic. Those found to harbor potentially devastating mutated alleles will be treated prophylactically with appropriately frequent screening protocols, surgery, endovascular drug or cell delivery, or a novel treatment soon to emerge from benchtop work.

■ References

1. Hedenfalk I, Duggan D, Chen Y, et al. Gene-expression profiles in hereditary breast cancer. N Engl J Med 2001;344:539–548
2. Millauer B, Wizigmann-Voos S, Schnurch H, et al. High affinity VEGF binding and developmental expression suggest Flk-1 as a major regulator of vasculogenesis and angiogenesis. Cell 1993;72:835–846
3. Hanahan D. Signaling vascular morphogenesis and maintenance. Science 1997;277:48–50
4. Lux A, Attisano L, Marchuk DA. Assignment of transforming growth factor beta1 and beta3 and a third new ligand to the type I receptor ALK-1. J Biol Chem 1999;274:9984–9992
5. Folkman J. New perspectives in clinical oncology from angiogenesis research. Eur J Cancer 1996;32A:2534–2539
6. Folkman J, D'Amore PA. Blood vessel formation: what is its molecular basis? Cell 1996;87:1153–1155
7. Battegay EJ. Angiogenesis: mechanistic insights, neovascular diseases, and therapeutic prospects. J Mol Med 1995;73:333–346
8. Vikkula M, Boon LM, Carraway KL, et al. Vascular dysmorphogenesis caused by an activating mutation in the receptor tyrosine kinase TIE2. Cell 1996;87:1181–1190
9. Bean WB. Vascular Spiders and Related Lesions of the Skin. Springfield, IL: Charles C. Thomas; 1958
10. Boon LM, Mulliken JB, Vikkula M, et al. Assignment of a locus for dominantly inherited venous malformations to chromosome 9p. Hum Mol Genet 1994;3:1583–1587
11. Hashimoto T, Lam T, Boudreau NJ, Bollen AW, Lawton MT, Young WL. Abnormal balance in the angiopoietin-tie2 system in human brain arteriovenous malformations. Circ Res 2001;89:111–113
12. Shenkar R, Elliott JP, Diener K, et al. Differential gene expression in human cerebrovascular malformations. Neurosurg 2003;52:465–477, 477–468,
13. Russell DS, Rubenstein LJ. Pathology of tumors of the nervous system. In: Baltimore: Williams and Wilkins; 1989:730–736
14. Clatterbuck RE, Eberhart CG, Crain BJ, Rigamonti D. Ultrastructural and immunocytochemical evidence that an incompetent blood-brain barrier is related to the pathophysiology of cavernous malformations. J Neurol Neurosurg Psychiatry 2001;71:188–192
15. Wong JH, Awad IA, Kim JH. Ultrastructural pathological features of cerebrovascular malformations: a preliminary report. Neurosurgery 2000;46:1454–1459
16. Perl J, Ross J. Diagnostic imaging of cavernous malformations. In: Awad IA, Barrow, D., eds. Cavernous Malformations. Park Ridge, NJ: AANS; 1993: 37–48
17. Del Curling O, Kelly DL, Elster AD, Craven TE. An analysis of the natural history of cavernous angiomas. J Neurosurg 1991;75:702–708
18. Otten P, Pizzolato GP, Rilliet B, Berney J. 131 cases of cavernous angioma (cavernomas) of the CNS, discovered by retrospective analysis of 24,535 autopsies. Neurochirurgie 1989;35:82–83
19. Robinson JR, Awad IA, Little JR. Natural history of the cavernous angioma. J Neurosurg 1991;75:709–714
20. Barrow D, Awad IA. Conceptual overview and management strategies. In: Awad IA, Barrow, D., eds. Cavernous Malformations. Park Ridge, NJ: AANS; 1993:205–213
21. Barrow D, Krisht A. Cavernous malformations and hemorrhageIn: Awad IA, Barrow, D., eds. Cavernous Malformations. Park Ridge, NJ: AANS; 1993:65–80
22. Robinson JR, Awad IA, Magdinec M, Paranandi L. Factors predisposing to clinical disability in patients with cavernous malformations of the brain. Neurosurg 1993; 32:730–735, 735–736
23. Hayman LA, Evans RA, Ferrell RE, Fahr LM, Ostrow P, Riccardi VM. Familial cavernous angiomas: natural history and genetic study over a 5-year period. Am J Med Genet 1982;11:147–160
24. Kidd HA, Cumings JN. Cerebral angiomata in an Icelandic family. Lancet 1947;I:747–748
25. Michael JC, Levin PM. Multiple telangiectases of brain: a discussion of hereditary factors in their development. Arch Neurol Psychiatr 1936;36:514–536
26. Bicknell JM, Carlow TJ, Kornfeld M, Stovring J, Turner P. Familial cavernous angiomas. Arch Neurol 1978;35:746–749
27. Dobyns WB, Michels VV, Groover RV, et al. Familial cavernous malformations of the central nervous system and retina. Ann Neurol 1987;21:578–583
28. Gunel M, Awad IA, Anson J, Lifton RP. Mapping a gene causing cerebral cavernous malformation to 7q11.2-q21. Proc Natl Acad Sci U S A 1995;92:6620–6624
29. Johnson EW, Iyer LM, Rich SS, et al. Refined localization of the cerebral cavernous malformation gene (CCM1) to a 4-cM interval of chromosome 7q contained in a well-defined YAC contig. Genome Res 1995;5:368–380
30. Rigamonti D, Hadley MN, Drayer BP, et al. Cerebral cavernous malformations. Incidence and familial occurrence. N Engl J Med 1988;319:343–347
31. Gunel M, Awad IA, Finberg K, et al. A founder mutation as a cause of cerebral cavernous malformation in Hispanic Americans. N Engl J Med 1996;334:946–951
32. Laberge-le Couteulx S, Jung HH, Labauge P, et al. Truncating mutations in CCM1, encoding KRIT1, cause hereditary cavernous angiomas. Nat Genet 1999;23:189–193
33. Serebriiskii I, Estojak J, Sonoda G, Testa JR, Golemis EA. Association of Krev-1/rapla with Krit1, a novel ankyrin repeat-containing protein encoded by a gene mapping to 7q21–22. Oncogene 1997;15:1043–1049
34. Frech M, John J, Pizon V, et al. Inhibition of GTPase activating protein stimulation of Ras-p21 GTPase by the Krev-1 gene product. Science 1990;249:169–171
35. Guo D, Jia Q, Song HY, Warren RS, Donner DB. Vascular endothelial cell growth factor promotes tyrosine phosphorylation of mediators

of signal transduction that contain SH2 domains. Association with endothelial cell proliferation. J Biol Chem 1995;270: 6729–6733

36. Gunel M, Laurans MS, Shin D, et al. KRIT1, a gene mutated in cerebral cavernous malformation, encodes a microtubule-associated protein. Proc Natl Acad Sci U S A 2002;99:10677–10682

37. Zawistowski JS, Serebrilskii IG, Lee MF, Golemis EA, Marchuk DA. KRIT1 association with the integrin-binding protein ICAP-1: a new direction in the elucidation of cerebral cavernous malformations (CCM1) pathogenesis. Hum Mol Genet 2002;11:389–396

38. Zhang J, Clatterbuck RE, Rigamonti D, Chang DD, Dietz HC. Interaction between krit1 and icap1alpha infers perturbation of integrin beta1-mediated angiogenesis in the pathogenesis of cerebral cavernous malformation. Hum Mol Genet 2001;10: 2953–2960

39. Gunel M, Awad IA, Finberg K, et al. Genetic heterogeneity of inherited cerebral cavernous malformation. Neurosurgery 1996; 38:1265–1271

40. Craig HD, Gunel M, Cepeda O, et al. Multilocus linkage identifies two new loci for a mendelian form of stroke, cerebral cavernous malformation, at 7p15–13 and 3q25.2–27. Hum Mol Genet 1998;7: 1851–1858

41. Denier C, Goutagny S, Labauge P, et al. Mutations within the MGC4607 gene cause cerebral cavernous malformations. Am J Hum Genet 2004;74:326–337

42. Liquori CL, Berg MJ, Siegel AM, et al. Mutations in a gene encoding a novel protein containing a phosphotyrosine-binding domain cause type 2 cerebral cavernous malformations. Am J Hum Genet 2003;73:1459–1464

43. Bergametti F, Denier C, Labauge P, et al. Mutations within the Programmed Cell Death 10 gene cause cerebral cavernous malformations. Am J Hum Genet 2005;76:42–51

44. Osler W. On a family form of recurring epistaxis, associated with multiple telangiectases of the skin and mucous membranes. Bull Johns Hopkins Hosp 1901;7:333–337

45. Winterbauer RH. Multiple telangiectasia, Raynaud's phenomenon, sclerodactyly and subcutaneous calcinosis: a syndrome mimicking hereditary hemorrhagic telangiectasia. Bull Johns Hopkins Hosp 1964;114:361–383

46. Rothbart D, Awad IA, Lee J, Kim J, Harbaugh R, Criscuolo GR. Expression of angiogenic factors and structural proteins in central nervous system vascular malformations. Neurosurg 1996;38: 915–924, 924–915

47. Braverman IM, Keh A, Jacobson BS. Ultrastructure and three-dimensional organization of the telangiectases of hereditary hemorrhagic telangiectasia. J Invest Dermatol 1990;95:422–427

48. Guttmacher AE, Marchuk DA, White RI Jr. Hereditary hemorrhagic telangiectasia. N Engl J Med 1995;333:918–924

49. McDonald MT, Papenberg KA, Ghosh S, et al. A disease locus for hereditary haemorrhagic telangiectasia maps to chromosome 9q33–34. Nat Genet 1994;6:197–204

50. Johnson DW, Berg JN, Gallione CJ, et al. A second locus for hereditary hemorrhagic telangiectasia maps to chromosome 12. Genome Res 1995;5:21–28

51. McAllister KA, Grogg KM, Johnson DW, et al. Endoglin, a TGF-beta binding protein of endothelial cells, is the gene for hereditary haemorrhagic telangiectasia type 1. Nat Genet 1994;8:345–351

52. ten Dijke P, Yamashita H, Ichijo H, et al. Characterization of type I receptors for transforming growth factor- beta and activin. Science 1994;264:101–104

53. Piantanida M, Buscarini E, Dellavecchia C, et al. Hereditary haemorrhagic telangiectasia with extensive liver involvement is not caused by either HHT1 or HHT2. J Med Genet 1996;33:441–443

54. Lux A, Gallione CJ, Marchuk DA. Expression analysis of endoglin missense and truncation mutations: insights into protein structure and disease mechanisms. Hum Mol Genet 2000;9:745–755

55. Berg JN, Gallione CJ, Stenzel TT, et al. The activin receptor-like kinase 1 gene: genomic structure and mutations in hereditary hemorrhagic telangiectasia type 2. Am J Hum Genet 1997;61: 60–67

56. Shovlin CL, Hughes JM, Scott J, Seidman CE, Seidman JG. Characterization of endoglin and identification of novel mutations in hereditary hemorrhagic telangiectasia. Am J Hum Genet 1997; 61:68–79

57. Massague J. Receptors for the TGF-β family. Cell 1992;June 26; 69(7):1067–1070

58. Li DY, Sorensen LK, Brooke BS, et al. Defective angiogenesis in mice lacking endoglin. Science 1999;284:1534–1537

59. Gougos A, Letarte M. Primary structure of endoglin, an RGD-containing glycoprotein of human endothelial cells. J Biol Chem 1990;265:8361–8364

60. Barbara NP, Wrana JL, Letarte M. Endoglin is an accessory protein that interacts with the signaling receptor complex of multiple members of the transforming growth factor-beta superfamily. J Biol Chem 1999;274:584–594

61. Cheifetz S, Bellon T, Cales C, et al. Endoglin is a component of the transforming growth factor-beta receptor system in human endothelial cells. J Biol Chem 1992;267:19027–19030

62. Pepper MS, Vassalli JD, Orci L, Montesano R. Biphasic effect of transforming growth factor-beta 1 on in vitro angiogenesis. Exp Cell Res 1993;204:356–363

63. Bourdeau A, Dumont DJ, Letarte M. A murine model of hereditary hemorrhagic telangiectasia. J Clin Invest 1999;104:1343–1351

64. Urness LD, Sorensen LK, Li DY. Arteriovenous malformations in mice lacking activin receptor-like kinase-1. Nat Genet 2000;26: 328–331

65. Pepper MS. Transforming growth factor-beta: vasculogenesis, angiogenesis, and vessel wall integrity. Cytokine Growth Factor Rev 1997;8:21–43

66. Schievink WI. Genetics of intracranial aneurysms. Neurosurg 1997;40:651–662, 662–653

67. ter Berg HW, Dippel DW, Limburg M, Schievink WI, van Gijn J. Familial intracranial aneurysms. A review. Stroke 1992;23: 1024–1030

68. Schievink WI, Torres VE, Piepgras DG, Wiebers DO. Saccular intracranial aneurysms in autosomal dominant polycystic kidney disease. J Am Soc Nephrol 1992;3:88–95

69. Keramatipour M, McConnell RS, Kirkpatrick P, Tebbs S, Furlong RA, Rubinsztein DC. The ACE I allele is associated with increased risk for ruptured intracranial aneurysms. J Med Genet 2000; 37:498–500

70. Bruno G, Todor R, Lewis I, Chyatte D. Vascular extracellular matrix remodeling in cerebral aneurysms. J Neurosurg 1998;89: 431–440

71. Todor DR, Lewis I, Bruno G, Chyatte D. Identification of a serum gelatinase associated with the occurrence of cerebral aneurysms as pro-matrix metalloproteinase-2. Stroke 1998;29:1580–1583

72. de Paepe A, van Landegem W, de Keyser F, de Reuck J. Association of multiple intracranial aneurysms and collagen type III deficiency. Clin Neurol Neurosurg 1988;90:53–56

73. Farnham JM, Camp NJ, Neuhausen SL, et al. Confirmation of chromosome 7q11 locus for predisposition to intracranial aneurysm. Hum Genet 2004;114:250–255

74. Kuivaniemi H, Prockop DJ, Wu Y, et al. al. e: Exclusion of mutations in the gene for type III collagen (COL3A1) as a common cause of intracranial aneurysms or cervical artery dissections: results from sequence analysis of the coding sequences of type III collagen from 55 unrelated patients. Neurology 1993;43: 2652–2658

75. Olson JM, Vongpunsawad S, Kuivaniemi H, et al. Search for intracranial aneurysm susceptibility gene(s) using Finnish families. BMC Med Genet 2002;3:7

76. Onda H, Kasuya H, Yoneyama T, et al. Genomewide-linkage and haplotype-association studies map intracranial aneurysm to chromosome 7q11. Am J Hum Genet 2001;69:804–819

77. Pope FM, Limburg M, Schievink WI. Familial cerebral aneurysms and type III collagen deficiency. J Neurosurg 1990;72:156–158

78. Takenaka K, Sakai H, Yamakawa H, et al. Polymorphism of the endoglin gene in patients with intracranial saccular aneurysms. J Neurosurg 1999;90:935–938

79. Yoneyama T, Kasuya H, Onda H, et al. Association of positional and functional candidate genes FGF1, FBN2, and LOX on 5q31 with intracranial aneurysm. J Hum Genet 2003;48:309–314

80. van der Voet M, Olson JM, Kuivaniemi H, et al. Intracranial aneurysms in Finnish families: confirmation of linkage and refinement of the interval to chromosome 19q13.3. Am J Hum Genet 2004;74:564–571

81. Roos YB, Pals G, Struycken PM, et al. Genome-wide linkage in a large Dutch consanguineous family maps a locus for intracranial aneurysms to chromosome 2p13. Stroke 2004;35:2276–2281

82. Nahed BV, Seker A, Guclu B, et al. Mapping a Mendelian form of intracranial aneurysm to 1p34.3-p36.13. Am J Hum Genet 2005;76:172–179

83. Jensson O, Gudmundsson G, Arnason A, et al. Hereditary cystatin C (gamma-trace) amyloid angiopathy of the CNS causing cerebral hemorrhage. Acta Neurol Scand 1987;76:102–114

84. Luyendijk W, Bots GT, Vegter-van der Vlis M, Went LN, Frangione B. Hereditary cerebral haemorrhage caused by cortical amyloid angiopathy. J Neurol Sci 1988;85:267–280

85. van Duinen SG, Castano EM, Prelli F, Bots GT, Luyendijk W, Frangione B. Hereditary cerebral hemorrhage with amyloidosis in patients of Dutch origin is related to Alzheimer disease. Proc Natl Acad Sci U S A 1987;84:5991–5994

86. Ghiso J, Jensson O, Frangione B. Amyloid fibrils in hereditary cerebral hemorrhage with amyloidosis of Icelandic type is a variant of gamma-trace basic protein (cystatin C). Proc Natl Acad Sci U S A 1986;83:2974–2978

87. Shi GP, Sukhova GK, Grubb A, et al. Cystatin C deficiency in human atherosclerosis and aortic aneurysms. J Clin Invest 1999;104:1191–1197

88. Levy E, Carman MD, Fernandez-Madrid IJ, et al. Mutation of the Alzheimer's disease amyloid gene in hereditary cerebral hemorrhage, Dutch type. Science 1990;248:1124–1126

89. Mas JL, Dilouya A, de Recondo J. A familial disorder with subcortical ischemic strokes, dementia, and leukoencephalopathy. Neurology 1992;42:1015–1019

90. Tournier-Lasserve E, Iba-Zizen MT, Romero N, Bousser MG. Autosomal dominant syndrome with strokelike episodes and leukoencephalopathy. Stroke 1991;22:1297–1302

91. Baudrimont M, Dubas F, Joutel A, Tournier-Lasserve E, Bousser MG. Autosomal dominant leukoencephalopathy and subcortical ischemic stroke. A clinicopathological study. Stroke 1993;24: 122–125

92. Dichgans M, Mayer M, Muller-Myhsok B, Straube A, Gasser T. Identification of a key recombinant narrows the CADASIL gene region to 8 cm and argues against allelism of CADASIL and familial hemiplegic migraine. Genomics 1996;32:151–154

93. Joutel A, Corpechot C, Ducros A, et al. Notch3 mutations in CADASIL, a hereditary adult-onset condition causing stroke and dementia. Nature 1996;383:707–710

94. Eliasson MJ, Huang Z, Ferrante RJ, et al. Neuronal nitric oxide synthase activation and peroxynitrite formation in ischemic stroke linked to neural damage. J Neurosci 1999;19:5910–5918

95. Gonzalez-Zulueta M, Ensz LM, Mukhina G, et al. Manganese superoxide dismutase protects nNOS neurons from NMDA and nitric oxide-mediated neurotoxicity. J Neurosci 1998;18: 2040–2055

96. Huang Z, Huang PL, Ma J, et al. Enlarged infarcts in endothelial nitric oxide synthase knockout mice are attenuated by nitro-L-arginine. J Cereb Blood Flow Metab 1996;16:981–987

97. Sandmair AM, Loimas S, Puranen P, et al. Thymidine kinase gene therapy for human malignant glioma, using replication-deficient retroviruses or adenoviruses. Hum Gene Ther 2000;11:2197–2205

98. Sandmair AM, Turunen M, Tyynela K, et al. Herpes simplex virus thymidine kinase gene therapy in experimental rat BT4C glioma model: effect of the percentage of thymidine kinase-positive glioma cells on treatment effect, survival time, and tissue reactions. Cancer Gene Ther 2000;7:413–421

99. Wilson JM. Adenoviruses as gene-delivery vehicles. N Engl J Med 1996;334:1185–1187

100. Yagi T, Jikihara I, Fukumura M, et al. Rescue of ischemic brain injury by adenoviral gene transfer of glial cell line-derived neurotrophic factor after transient global ischemia in gerbils. Brain Res 2000;885:273–282

101. Kitagawa H, Hayashi T, Mitsumoto Y, Koga N, Itoyama Y, Abe K. Reduction of ischemic brain injury by topical application of glial cell line-derived neurotrophic factor after permanent middle cerebral artery occlusion in rats. Stroke 1998;29:1417–1422

102. Carmeliet P, Schoonjans L, Kieckens L, et al. Physiological consequences of loss of plasminogen activator gene function in mice. Nature 1994;368:419–424

103. Zlokovic BV, Apuzzo ML. Cellular and molecular neurosurgery: pathways from concept to reality—part II: vector systems and delivery methodologies for gene therapy of the central nervous system. Neurosurgery 1997;40:805–812

104. Gould E, Tanapat P, McEwen BS, Flugge G, Fuchs E. Proliferation of granule cell precursors in the dentate gyrus of adult monkeys is diminished by stress. Proc Natl Acad Sci U S A 1998;95: 3168–3171

105. Kempermann G, Gage FH. Experience-dependent regulation of adult hippocampal neurogenesis: effects of long-term stimulation and stimulus withdrawal. Hippocampus 1999;9:321–332

106. Eriksson PS, Perfilieva E, Bjork-Eriksson T, et al. Neurogenesis in the adult human hippocampus. Nat Med 1998;4:1313–1317

107. Kukekov VG, Laywell ED, Suslov O, et al. Multipotent stem/progenitor cells with similar properties arise from two neurogenic regions of adult human brain. Exp Neurol 1999;156:333–344

108. Alonso G. Neuronal progenitor-like cells expressing polysialylated neural cell adhesion molecule are present on the ventricular surface of the adult rat brain and spinal cord. J Comp Neurol 1999;414:149–166

109. Yamashita J, Itoh H, Hirashima M, et al. Flk1-positive cells derived from embryonic stem cells serve as vascular progenitors. Nature 2000;408:92–96

110. Yamaguchi H, Azuma H, Shigekiyo T, Inoue H, Saito S. A novel missense mutation in the endoglin gene in hereditary hemorrhagic telangiectasia. Thromb Haemost 1997;77:243–247

4

Implications of Trends in the Marketplace for Neurovascular Diseases

CHARLES B. WILSON

Objectives: Upon completion of this chapter, the reader should be able to describe how government policy, insurance, industry, and an educated public will effect significant changes in neurosurgical practice over the next decade.

Accreditation: The AANS* is accredited by the Accreditation Council for Continuing Medical Education (ACCME) to sponsor continuing medical education for physicians.

Credit: The AANS designates this educational activity for a maximum of 15 credits in Category 1 credit toward the AMA Physician's Recognition Award. Each physician should claim only those hours of credit that he/she spent in the educational activity.

The Home Study Examination is online on the AANS Web site at: http://www.aans.org/education/books/controversy.asp

* The acronym AANS refers to both the American Association of Neurological Surgeons and the American Association of Neurosurgeons.

■ The Market

This market, as most markets, is defined by products, providers, intermediaries, financing, and consumers. *Products* are a range of services for the treatment and prevention of three major categories of neurovascular disease: cerebral aneurysms, arteriovenous malformations and fistulas, and cerebral ischemia. Excluding intracerebral hemorrhage, these three categories represent the market under consideration. *Providers* are surgeons (neurosurgeons and vascular surgeons), radiosurgeons, endovascular surgeons (neuro- and cardio-interventionists) and nonsurgeons (principally neurologists). Physicians who play a crucial role in preventing cerebrovascular occlusive disease by instituting measures to halt or reverse atherosclerosis and to control high blood pressure and cardiac arrhythmias are not customarily considered as providers. The *intermediaries* in this market are insurers and, less often, large employers who do direct contracting. *Consumers* in the strict sense are consumers if they are unaware of their disease; they are patients when they seek

care and may be either presymptomatic or symptomatic. For the sake of simplicity, both consumers and patients can be referred to as consumers because in whichever category they are or will be they consume services. *Financing* for the transaction between purchaser and provider has three sources—employer, government, and self—as either sole or joint payers.

The market for neurovascular disease, like most markets involving health and health care, is an imperfect market because of the asymmetry of product information. In the case of health care services, information belongs disproportionately in the hands of providers, and there is no safeguard against bias and self-interest based on financial and other considerations on the part of the provider. Today, the consumer and payer have sources of information that did not exist in the past, but much of it is difficult for the educated public to understand, and some that is understandable is incorrect. In this and every market, information is empowerment, and you need to think no further than *Consumer Reports* and Web-based sources of information in purchasing an automobile or a new computer. It is this dissonance between the public's ability to obtain information about every other industry and their inability to obtain information about the health care industry that has led to their insatiable desire to read, see, and hear anything about health from any accessible source.

■ Trends in the 2010s

Public Policy

A continuing tension will involve consumers, employers, government, and the health care industry over the conflicting goals of constraining costs and allowing access to expensive new technologies ranging from pharmaceuticals to keyhole cardiac surgery. In the short term, all new technology will inflate the cost of care, whereas in the long term the same technology may or may not lower the cost of care. As an example, an expensive pharmaceutical for the prevention of atherosclerosis, like many preventive measures, may be an added cost in the short term but a savings in the long term if one thinks of lifetime costs or population health. Any measure that reduces health care costs is likely to decrease the industry's investment in research and development of new technologies. The major cause of rising expenditures for health is the introduction of and use of new technologies, but unrestrained this inevitably leads to a rising proportion of the gross domestic product's going to the provision of health care services. Therefore, the public can demand either cost containment or unrestrained access to costly technology, but not both at the same time. This conflict will not be resolved by the introduction of some version of universal coverage because polls indicate that the political will to push for enabling legislation is lacking. Consequently, it is likely that over time Americans will choose to expend a larger proportion of their resources to obtain the benefits of improved health. Stated in another way, devoting 15% of the gross domestic product to health care, which we do today, is an arbitrary limit on spending: If those who can afford it are asked "Would you be willing to pay a higher proportion of your income for better health obtainable through access to newer technologies?" I believe that the majority would say "yes."

Insurance

The insurance products of today—HMO, PPO, point of service, fee-for-service—will survive in some form throughout the next decade. The major change will occur in employer-sponsored coverage, which will move steadily toward a defined dollar contribution to the employee rather than a defined benefit of all necessary health care. From the standpoint of employers, a defined contribution, paid directly to the employee to use in purchasing whatever insurance package the employee selects, limits the employer's financial outlay. The concept is attractive to many employees because of their freedom to choose the most suitable kind of insurance taking into consideration age, health risks, present state of health, and family, if any. In this circumstance, employees will be spending their own dollars and consequently will become more discriminating in their purchasing decisions for health and health care services.

Organization within the Industry

In the past 10 years, mergers, buy-outs, acquisitions, and alliances have characterized reorganization in every sector of the health care industry. The number of national insurers has declined at the same rate as the nation's large accounting firms, and for similar reasons—complementary strengths, scale economies, reach, and domination of specific markets. There is a reason that when Aetna and HealthNet make major decisions, the impact somewhere in the system is serious. Industries providing goods and services for the delivery of health care—pharmaceutical companies, device manufacturers, suppliers of disposable items, and group purchasing organizations—have merged for the same reasons. Hospitals have merged, joined systems or chains, created alliances or joint ventures, or, if not feeling particularly vulnerable in their geographic market, remained independent. The incentives range from securing a dominant position in a particular small or large region to obtaining access to capital and strategic leadership. Physicians began the process of consolidation by joining groups, either large or small group practices—a trend that began in the late 1980s and has escalated over the past few years. Simply stated, if a group becomes large enough, and especially if the most desired physicians join the group, in a given geographic area, whether a town, a city, a defined sector of a metropolis, or an even larger region, any insurer doing business in that area cannot go around this dominant group. As soon as a prospective purchaser learns that the best physicians, possibly his or her own physician, are not on the plan (and typically a close connection exists between best physicians and the best hospitals where they practice), the group has established a strong position in negotiating conditions, including reimbursement with the insurer. To state that the physician group "owns" this market is legally inaccurate, but in practice it is a reality. Unionization of physicians is another issue that will be played out over the coming decade, and anyone who predicts the outcome is likely to get it wrong.

The New Consumer

We are well into a period dominated by a new breed of consumers who have rewritten the rules of interaction in every major industry except health care, and over the past 3 years they have been forging new contracts with each component of the trillion-dollar industry that deals with their health. Half of the adults in this country qualify as new consumers—having education (at least 1 year of college), a disposable income providing purchasing discretion, and connection with the Internet. The core characteristic of the new consumers is their use of information for empowerment, which foreshadowed the role that the Internet would play in the power shift. This new consumer wants choice, involvement and control in making decisions about their health, diagnostic procedures and treatment, superior service, and information that is individually customized and understandable. They are bringing insurers, medical groups, physicians, and hospitals into the courtroom, and in effect they have dismantled key mechanisms for controlling the cost of health care. The more they know, the more they want the latest and best technology, often a new pharmaceutical or a new operative procedure, whether or not evidence supports its press releases and irrespective of appropriateness.

The impact of new consumers in the health care marketplace is clear. Within 5 years, more than one half of the population will have information on which to base choices about health plans, hospitals, physicians, and specific diagnostic and therapeutic interventions. Entities that understand their needs will win their approval, trust, and loyalty, while the remainder will long for the way things used to be. Consumers will require a new level of open accountability from the health care industry, and this means interacting with patients who know more about you and your practice than you know about them.

Marketing

Rules for marketing (advertising) have become liberal. Any verifiable statement is allowable, but whether conveyed to the public in a brochure or through a Web page, an unsubstantiated claim is subject to fraud and deceit claims. The rules are simple: don't speculate, don't exaggerate, and don't misrepresent the "best outcomes" of another institution or physician as the outcomes that you've obtained. Omission of attribution, or misattribution, if challenged, will be difficult to defend.

Today, several informational and marketing media can be used. Published reports in professional periodicals are invaluable, because the media covers significant reports and the public has a never-ending appetite for information about health care. Imagine the dollar value of a breakthrough clinical trial originating from your institution (department, center, or group) that appears in the *New England Journal of Medicine.* An invited article or expert interview can serve the same purpose. Today, the most used source of information is the Internet. Competing with

your peers in this and future markets for cerebrovascular services requires a well-designed and informative personal Web page unless you already have attained celebrity status and can survive on reputation alone.

What Americans Value in Health Care

The public's major means of education is through the media. Every poll indicates a high level of interest in anything dealing with health, health care, illness, diet, fitness, diseases, and revelations of error, negligence, or cover-up in the industry. You need think back no further than the deluge of publicity generated by the Institute of Medicine's report on medical errors—even the checkout clerk at your supermarket can quote a number for the resulting deaths and injuries. This story was not the work of a whistle-blower (although they seem to be everywhere), but a scholarly and thoughtful analysis by one of the nation's most prestigious and respected institutions. Anything that is newsworthy is aired, printed, and broadcast. It is not surprising that the public is abreast of trends, new technologies, and significant medical news originating from a number of professional sources. Today, physicians are not dealing with a naïve and entirely trusting public.

So, what do Americans want? Whatever it is, a diagnostic test or a therapy, they want to know about risks, and I mean *all* risks. As a rule, they prefer medical to surgical interventions, and a growing number prefer alternative approaches to biomedicine. One of the major movements has been the evolution of minimally invasive surgery (MIS), and I include endovascular surgery as surgery through a catheter. Similarly, radiosurgery is used as a surgical tool and belongs in the MIS category. "Evidence-based" and "outcomes" are becoming familiar terms. A potential patient who fails to inquire about a surgeon's volume of experience with a recommended procedure is exceptional in the region where I practice.

Whom do Americans trust for information and advice about health decisions? Friends and family members top the list, followed by the patient's personal physician. "Branded" sources of information—the Mayo Clinic, Johns Hopkins, and the AMA—have credibility, as do certain branches of the government—the NIH, Surgeon General, National Cancer Institute, and Centers for Disease Control and Prevention. There is an overwhelming mass of health information on the Internet, but the public is just as aware as the medical community that much of it is dead wrong or amounts to nothing more than flagrant advertising.

At the risk of overstating its importance, the public's skepticism, bordering on mistrust, of our current system of health care constitutes a powerful force in the public's relationship with every component of the industry. The new consumer wants accurate and comprehensive information for making decisions about health-related decisions. For physicians, this means profile and practice transparency. Hospitals will be forced or convinced to open their records on infection rates, mortality by procedure and surgeon, and some metric of medical errors. For insurers and suppliers, a *Consumer Guide* counterpart will be sufficient. This final movement toward accountability is inevitable and is underway today. To borrow a metaphor from the boxing ring, "We can run, but we can't hide."

As a final note, expect to see rapid growth of specialty hospitals, specialty units, and specialists who are more tightly focused on a limited area of their specialty. Americans have shown that they do not want a generalist when it is perfectly obvious to them, rightly or wrongly, that they need a specialist. Even more than any specialist, they want a specialist that knows a lot about their specific problem and has had a lot of experience—and success—treating it. A tour around many larger cities in the United States will uncover a proliferation of specialty units, embedded or freestanding, and this trend will continue throughout the coming decade. The principal reasons for this are the consumer's desire for specialized treatment by a whole team of specialist physicians, nurses, and ancillary personnel; the superior outcomes achieved by focus and driven by volume; and the observation by investors that "if you build it, they will come."

5

Neuroendovascular Diseases: Past, Present, and Future

DANIEL TUDEN AND JOSEPH M. FITZGERALD

Objectives: Upon completion of this chapter, the reader should be able to explain the current state of the endovascular industry and report how evolving endovascular technologies might impact aneurysm and ischemic stroke management in the future.

Accreditation: The AANS* is accredited by the Accreditation Council for Continuing Medical Education (ACCME) to sponsor continuing medical education for physicians.

Credit: The AANS designates this educational activity for a maximum of 15 credits in Category 1 credit toward the AMA Physician's Recognition Award. Each physician should claim only those hours of credit that he/she spent in the educational activity.

The Home Study Examination is online on the AANS Web site at: http://www.aans.org/education/books/controversy.asp

* The acronym AANS refers to both the American Association of Neurological Surgeons and the American Association of Neurosurgeons.

The field of neurointerventional medicine in the United States has experienced rapid growth over the past decade. In 2002, nearly 20,000 endovascular procedures were performed in the United States. This number is projected to increase to more than 50,000 over the next 5 years (**Fig. 5–1**).

Some of the same foundations that have revolutionized the field of interventional cardiology are the basis for the success of neuroendovascular procedures—a reliance on a technology-based, less-invasive approach to the treatment of a complex set of diseases. Technology generates solutions to clinical needs in a dynamic and

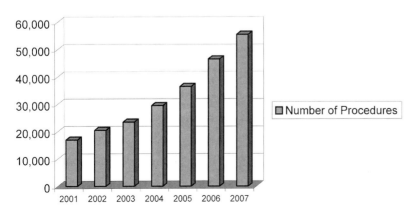

FIGURE 5–1 The projected growth rate in neuroendovascular procedures. From Boston Scientific Data and Estimates, Natick, MA. Reprinted by permission.

fast-paced fashion, and the less-invasive nature of the therapy permits lower rates of procedural morbidity, shorter lengths of stay, and quicker recovery times. Just as interventional cardiology has become the preferred procedural treatment for the heart, within the next 5 years neuroendovascular procedures will be used in the majority of all therapeutic neurovascular cases.

While the advantages of a technology-driven, less-invasive therapy are the main drivers of neuroendovascular therapy's success, several other factors have helped and will continue to help fuel its growth. First, enough physicians have attended neuroendovascular training programs to keep pace with the expanding number of procedures. Second, clinical data and research comparing surgical and neuroendovascular treatment of aneurysms has helped demonstrate some of the advantages of the less-invasive approach and persuaded patients and physicians to use the procedure. The next generation of research in this area is underway and could provide conclusive, level-one evidence that neuroendovascular therapy should be the front-line aneurysm treatment. In addition, this research and other research on the impact of hospital volume on aneurysm treatment outcomes could help centralize care into centers specializing in neuroendovascular therapy. Finally, the ischemic stroke market will be a significant accelerant of case growth. This market is large, presenting an urgent need for an effective treatment; and neuroendovascular approaches offer significant promise in this regard.

In this chapter we attempt to capture the current state of neuroendovascular treatments in the United States and project the possible development of this field in the next 5 years. Neuroendovascular procedures include the treatment of aneurysms, AVMs, ischemic disease and various embolization procedures for conditions like fistulas and menenginomas. We will focus on the two primary areas of growth—aneurysms and ischemic disease above the carotid bifurcation.

■ Market Infrastructure Supports the Neuroendovascular Market

Neuroendovascular approaches to vascular disease have made significant inroads against traditional surgical treatments. In 1996, there were fewer than 1000 endovascular aneurysm treatments in the United States. By 2004, that number had increased to over 11,000 cases (**Fig. 5–2**). Endovascular treatment of aneurysms now accounts for over 50% of treated cases, and overall there were ~18,000 neuroendovascular procedures in the United States in 2002.

Structurally the market has responded to the demand for neuroendovascular services. The number of physicians able to perform neuroendovascular procedures has increased substantially since 1995. Physician training should continue to keep pace with demand. The number of fellowship-trained neuroendovascular physicians practicing in the United States is projected to be 475 by 2007 (**Fig. 5–3**).

The number of hospitals with neuroendovascular services has dramatically increased over the past 8 years. The total number of hospitals performing neuroendovascular procedures (all types) will increase moderately in the next 5 years; it is likely that existing centers will be treating a much larger number of patients (**Fig. 5–4**). The creation of

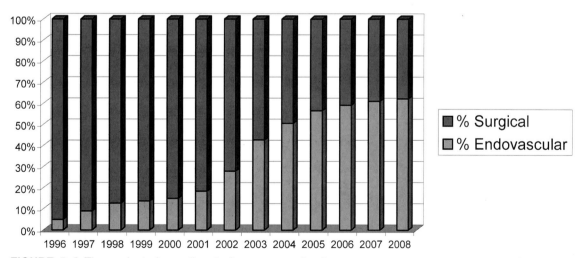

FIGURE 5–2 The projected growth rate in aneurysm treatments in the United States. From Boston Scientific Data and Estimates, Natick, MA. Reprinted by permission.

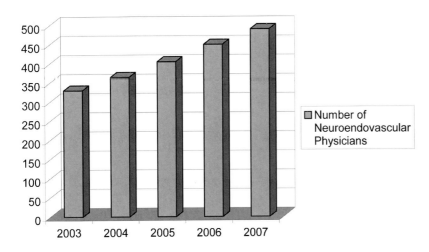

FIGURE 5–3 The projected growth rate in the number of neuroendovascular physicians. From Boston Scientific Data and Estimates, Natick, MA. Reprinted by permission.

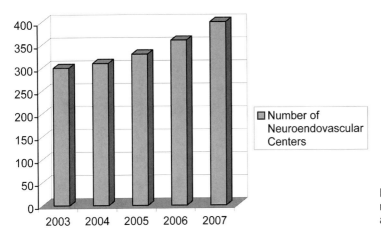

FIGURE 5–4 The projected growth rate in the number of neuroendovascular centers. From Boston Scientific Data and Estimates, Natick, MA. Reprinted by permission.

Neurovascular Centers of Excellence, focused on clinical excellence and protocol-driven patient care in all diagnostic and therapeutic approaches directed specifically at neurovascular diseases, will contribute to the centralization of cases at the best and biggest neurovascular centers.

■ Outcomes Research Demonstrates Clinical Profile

Endovascular therapy developed because of technology's ability to fit devices into small tubes and navigate them through the vasculature. This approach allows diseased vessels in the head to be accessed through a small incision in the groin. The trauma to patients is significantly less than that involved in a craniotomy—an advantage well understood by patients. Patients with unruptured aneurysms, who typically have time to consider treatment options, opt for endovascular therapy at a higher rate than do patients with ruptured aneurysms, who usually rely on the recommendation of the treating surgeon.

Research comparing the short-term outcomes of neuroendovascular treatment of aneurysms with surgical results has helped document what is intuitively obvious—that endovascular therapy should offer shorter lengths of stay, lower procedural morbidity, and shorter recovery time. Claiborne Johnston's research has played an important role in legitimizing the endovascular treatment of aneurysms. Johnston compared outcomes for surgical and endovascular cases at the University of California, San Francisco (UCSF), in a retrospective double-blind study of unruptured aneurysms. The study found significantly less morbidity and a much shorter recovery time for patients treated endovascularly.[1] A retrospective database analysis of unruptured aneurysms treated at university hospitals across the country found better outcomes associated with the endovascular approach.[2] Johnston conducted a similar database analysis of unruptured aneurysms in California and found significantly lower rates of morbidity for patients undergoing endovascular therapy.[3]

Although these studies have not provided level I evidence, the careful methods involved and the consistent findings demonstrating that neuroendovascular aneurysm treatment has less short-term morbidity have been extremely persuasive. It is has been conceded that this approach is superior to surgery in terms of procedural morbidity and patient recovery, and the debate has shifted to whether neuroendovascular treatment is durable as well.[3A]

■ Technological Innovation Expands Treatment Applications

The technological basis of endovascular therapy also generates benefits for physicians interested in "pushing the envelope" of treatment options. Technology often advances faster than human manual skills in treating difficult features of the human anatomy; technological innovations can compensate for skill limitations. The FDA clearance of Guglielmi Detachable Coils (GDC) in late 1995 opened the floodgates to a wave of technology development and innovation. Most of the early tools used in neuroendovascular treatments were borrowed technologies from either the interventional cardiology or peripheral vascular fields. In the past decade, numerous companies or divisions of larger companies have focused specifically on the design and development of tools for the neuroendovascular field. The major technological advancements over the past decade have been aimed at developing tools that overcome the tortuosity of the intracranial vasculature and developing coils suited for more difficult aneurysm morphologies in order to improve treatment efficacy.

The development of microguidewires with enhanced durability and steering ability has allowed physicians to reach intracranial vessels in a safe manner and to avoid multiple wire exchanges. The first decade of neuro interventional procedures saw rapid microguidewire development. Guidewires made of more durable materials, with better hydrophilic coatings and equipped with tips that could be more easily shaped, were introduced. Since then, newer materials and enhanced design and manufacturing techniques have improved these early technologies. Braided microcatheters and guiding catheters provide a level of support and luminal integrity that allows therapeutic tools to be delivered through microcatheters with internal lumens as small as 0.015 inches. The enhanced malleability of microcatheters has also added a level of stability not available in prior microcatheters.

Today's neuroendovascular physician can choose between more than 20 different varieties and makes of microcatheters and guidewires. In 2005, eight new guidewires and microcatheters were introduced into the U.S. market.

The detachable coil market has experienced major change and innovation over the past 5 years. At last count, there are seven different companies marketing endovascular coils to neuroendovascular physicians around the world. The major advancements in basic coil technology include softer coils, two-dimensional coils, three-dimensional or complex-shaped coils, stretch-resistant coils, ultrasoft stretch-resistant coils, and second-generation "coated" coils.

■ What Will Drive the Growth of Neuroendovascular Procedures?

The increase in neuroendovascular procedures has been meteoric, and the projections suggest that these procedures will soon become the first-line treatment for some diseases. **Figure 5–2** displays the estimate of penetration rates for endovascular treatment of aneurysms versus surgical treatment. Future projections include an assumption that endovascular aneurysm cases grow at 10%. This growth rate suggests that in 2008 endovascular aneurysms will represent about 60% of all treated intracranial aneurysms in the United States.

These projections may seem ambitious; however, the key elements to support this growth are already in place or are on the horizon. First, the physician and hospital infrastructure required to support this caseload is growing at a pace that will easily allow it to deliver these services. Second, technology is continuing to improve to meet unmet clinical needs. Third, accumulating clinical evidence combined with institutional changes in the delivery of care have the potential to change treatment and referral patterns so that care is concentrated in high-volume centers of excellence that offer endovascular services. Finally, it will be the implementation of neuroendovascular treatment in cases of ischemic stroke that will drive its growth as the treatment of choice.

■ Market Infrastructure Will Continue to Meet Demand

In simple terms a 70% penetration rate would result in 13,000 neuroendovascular treatments of intracranial aneurysms in 2008. The total projected case volume per hospital is given in **Figure 5–5**. The total aneurysm case volume per neuroendovascular physician is shown in **Figure 5–6**. Currently, there are ~400 practicing (mostly fellowship-trained) neuroendovascular specialists in the United States. In 2004, U.S. training centers produced 35 graduating fellows. Assuming the number of fellowship programs continues to grow in response to the demand for training, by 2007 there will be almost 500 fellowship-trained neuroendovascular specialists practicing in the United States; neuroendovascular physicians' caseloads then would average only 27 aneurysm cases per year.

■ Innovations Are Allowing More Aneurysms to Be Treated

Achieving 70% aneurysm penetration will require neuroendovascular therapy to treat a wider array of aneurysm morphologies.

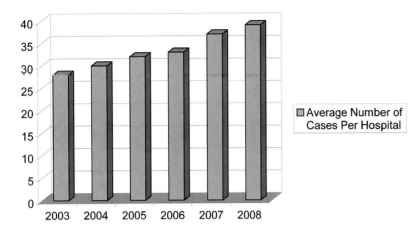

FIGURE 5–5 The projected growth rate in the number of endovascular aneurysm cases per U.S. center (300 neuroendovascular hospitals in 2003, growing to 340 in 2008).

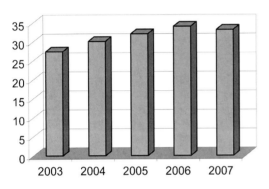

FIGURE 5–6 The projected growth rate in the average number of aneurysm procedures per physician. From Boston Scientific Data and Estimates, Natick, MA. Reprinted by permission.

Certain types of aneurysms are still problematic for the neuroendovascular approach. Aneurysms located in the middle cerebral arteries are difficult to access. Aneurysms with wide necks present the risk that coils could fall out of the aneurysm. Coils placed in giant aneurysms are prone to compacting, which allows the aneurysm to recannalize, putting the patient at a higher risk for hemorrhage.

While these morphologies present technical challenges, they do not provide an upper limit to the successful treatment of aneurysms. Specialists have begun placing stents across aneurysm necks to keep coils inside the dome; in 2002, the FDA approved the first stent specifically indicated for treating wide-neck aneurysms. Boston Scientific (Natick, MA) has introduced bioactive coils that generate tissue growth across the neck of the aneurysm in animal models and could help to reduce the risk of coil compaction. Other companies are working with coils that attempt to achieve the same goal by expanding to fill the space in the aneurysm. Some of the new catheters and guidewires will allow physicians to access previously unreachable aneurysms.

■ Evidence-Based Medicine May Centralize Treatment Patterns

Institutional factors are potentially a more serious barrier to the growth of neuroendovascular treatments.

Although there are easily enough neuroendovascular specialists to support 70% aneurysm penetration, getting these cases to these physicians is the issue. The treatment pattern for aneurysms, particularly ruptured aneurysms, is extremely decentralized. An 18-state study (representing 56% of the U.S. population) found that half of all patients with ruptured aneurysms presented in emergency rooms of hospitals that treated fewer than 19 such cases a year.[4] These emergency room cases were treated in 1000 hospitals, compared with the 84 highest volume hospitals, which treated 25% of the patients in those states. Because the availability of endovascular therapy is concentrated in a smaller number of high-volume centers, less than 25% of ruptured aneurysm patients present to hospitals that offer neuroendovascular therapy. Although there is some transfer of patients out of lower-volume hospitals, the majority of patients who present to these smaller-volume hospitals remain there.

Treatment and transfer patterns are governed by a web of factors, including insurance policies, hospital-to-hospital contracts, physician preference, and inertia. However, there is an increasing array of evidence strongly suggesting that this type of decentralized approach to treatment is not good for patients. The 18-state study found that hospitals in the lowest quartile, those treating 1–9 cases per year, have a 40% higher mortality rate than hospitals in the highest-volume quartile. A study in California on subarachnoid hemorrhage

(SAH) treatment found a similar disparity in outcomes between high- and low-volume hospitals. Studies looking at various aspects of aneurysm treatment from surgical treatment to the treatment of unruptured aneurysms have found the same strong relationship between higher volumes and significantly better outcomes.

The results of the International Subarachnoid Aneurysm Trial (ISAT) will play an important role in the centralization debate. The ISAT is the only multicenter, prospective randomized comparison of coiling and clipping. The study found that in patients with ruptured aneurysms suitable for either surgical or neuroendovascular treatment, endovascular therapy reduced the risk of being dead or disabled by 23.9% at one year. ISAT has also found that the large initial advantage for endovascular treatment appears to be durable. With over 6,000 patient years of follow-up beyond the first year, 2 of the surgical patients and 7 of the endovascular patients had rebled. If the reported rebleed rates remain constant, an endovascular patient would have to live for another 70 years after the procedure before the risks for surgery and endovascular treatment would be equal.[5]

Not surprisingly ISAT has had a significant impact on treatment patterns in countries that enrolled large numbers of patients in the trial such as England, Canada and Australia. ISAT also appears to have dramatically affected patient access to endovascular treatment in the United States despite the fact that only one center participated in the study. In 2003, the year after ISAT reported its results, the percentage of aneurysms treated endovascularly rather than surgically increased from 26% to 40%. ISAT and the reports surrounding it seem to have affected overall treatment patterns. The number of diagnosed aneurysms increased by 15% and the overall number of aneurysms treated by either surgery or endovascular therapy increased by over 40% suggesting that perhaps more patients were being referred to specialized centers where a higher percentage could be treated. The combined impact of more patients being diagnosed and receiving treatment with the shift toward endovascular therapy led to a more than doubling in endovascular aneurysm treatments from 3,910 in 2002 to 8,648 in 2003.[6] ISAT will continue to track patient outcomes, including long-term rebleed rates, and report on various findings through 2007.

The ISAT provides level I evidence that neuroendovascular therapy is the safer therapy, certainly in the short run, and probably in the long run as well. If the low long-term rebleed rates continue, the overall superiority of neuroendovascular therapy will be undeniable. Not only will the ISAT results hasten the conversion of patients from surgery to neuroendovascular treatment but they will provide a compelling rationale for moving patients to the smaller number of high-volume centers that offer front-line treatment.

Other research is likely to reinforce the direction toward centralized treatment of aneurysms in general and the use of neuroendovascular therapy in particular. The results of the International Study of Unruptured Intra-Cranial Aneurysms (ISUIA), reported in 2003, also found that patients receiving endovascular therapy were about 25% less likely to suffer procedural morality and morbidity compared to surgically treated patients despite the fact that the endovascular patients in ISUIA tended to be older and have higher risk aneurysms. UCSF is leading a study comparing long-term rebleed rates for surgical and endovascular patients at eight large neurovascular centers (UCSF; Stanford; University of Southern California; University of Texas Southwestern Medical Center at Dallas UTSW; Barrows; and University of California, Los Angeles; Methodist Hospital, Houston, Texas; The Mayo Clinic, Rochester, Minnesota). The CARAT study is tracking 1000 patients treated in 1996 and 1997 to determine the long-term durability of the two treatments.

■ The Accelerating Impact of Acute Ischemic Stroke

Despite the fact that there were 600,000 ischemic strokes in 2004, fewer than 2000 of those patients were treated endovascularly.[7] Ischemic stroke is the third leading cause of death and the leading cause of disability in the United States and neruoendovascular procedures offer promise for effectively treating strokes and preventing future ones. Preventing future strokes caused by intracranial atherosclerotic lesions is perhaps the most immediate opportunity. Patients who have suffered a stroke caused by accumulated plaque in brain arteries lack effective therapies and are at high risk for another stroke. A recent study published in the New England Journal of Medicine found that patients had a one year risk for another stroke of 12% regardless of the type of medical therapy they were given. The study also found that patients with severe stenoses ($\geq$70%) faced significantly more risk and had a one year stroke rate as high as 22.5%. About 90,000 ischemic events each year are caused by intracranial plaque and about 40% of these cases involve patients with severe stenoses that are at a high risk for another stroke.[8]

In 2005, Boston Scientific introduced the Wingspan Stent System and it is the only approved device available in the U.S. for treating intracranial atherosclerotic disease. In the 45 patient study submitted to the FDA, the device had a 97.3% procedural success rate and an ipsilateral stroke rate of 7% at six months. Currently, the device is approved under a Humanitarian Device Exemption (HDE). The indication is limited to patients who have failed medical therapy and the total number of treated cases cannot exceed 4,000 per year. However, there are plans to use the device in an NIH sponsored study and if the results are good, the next step would be a pivotal trial comparing Wingspan with medical therapy.

Acute stroke cases currently represent less than 5% of neuroendovascular cases. Given the severity of this disease, the lack of any pharmacological treatments beyond the 3-hour time window, and the availability of both endovascular tools and trained neuroendovascular specialists, the number of acute ischemic stroke patients treated with an endovascular approach will increase over the next 5 years. A key question is just how many of the 600,000 patients diagnosed with ischemic stroke each year will be treated in a neuroendovascular suite.

Dramatically increasing the number of acute stroke patients treated will require clinical trial success, significant changes in treatment patterns and referral rates, and changes in reimbursement within the United States.

Currently, there are more than five clinical trials being conducted in the United States that involve the neuroendovascular treatment of patients suffering from some form of thromboembolic or thrombotic acute ischemic stroke. In addition, multiple products are currently on the market that are used to address the problem of acute treatment of intracranial thrombosis or thromboembolic events. The use of retrieval devices, angioplasty balloons, stents, thrombectomy devices, thrombolytic infusion devices, and ultrasound delivery technologies is generating an entirely new procedural base and source of growth for neuroendovascular therapy.

For neuroendovascular therapy to capitalize on technological advances there will need to be significant changes in the institutional patterns of care as well as critical improvements in the reimbursement for treating stroke. Acute stroke treatment is even more decentralized than aneurysm repair. The 3-hour time window from symptom onset for delivering the only FDA-approved therapy for acute strokes severely limits the ability of smaller hospitals to transfer patients to large "stroke centers." Determining what constitutes a stroke center also is hardly straightforward. The lack of well-accepted treatment protocols and the paucity of clinically proven stroke therapies means that there is little visible differentiation between the types of care given at different hospitals.

Ischemic stroke treatment faces an additional barrier that could slow adoption of new treatments—the lack of adequate reimbursement for physicians or hospitals. Ischemic disease involves primarily the segment of the population that is receiving Medicare. While Medicare provides payment for stroke hospitalizations, there are no ICD-9 (International Classification of Diseases, Ninth

Revision) procedure codes describing stroke treatments that would enable the Diagnostic Related Groups' (DRG) system to supply higher payment for hospitals that provide affirmative treatment. A hospital that treats a patient with tissue plasminogen activator (TPA) receives no additional payment despite the drug's $5,000 price tag. Physicians fare even worse. There are only three approved neuroendovascular CPT (current procedural terminology) codes, and none for the treatment of ischemic disease. Medicare specifically prohibits payment for intracranial angioplasty.

■ Conclusion

The neuroendovascular specialty has made tremendous progress over the past decade, and a significant number of factors will drive its further development. The continued growth in the number of fellowship-trained neuroendovascular specialists, the adoption of neuroendovascular fellowship training by neurosurgeons and neurologists, changing referral and treatment patterns, and clinical-based evidence of neuroendovascular efficacy will be key factors behind this growth. But, as always, technology will play the key role.

■ References

1. Johnston SC, Wilson CB, Halbach VV, et al. Endovascular and surgical treatment of unruptured cerebral aneurysms: comparison of risks. Ann Neurol 2000;48:11–19
2. Johnston SC, Dudley RA, Gress DR, Ono L. Surgical and endovascular treatment of unruptured cerebral aneurysms at university hospitals. Neurology 1999;52:1799–1805
3. Johnston SC, Zhao S, Dudley RA, Berman MF, Gress DR. Treatment of unruptured cerebral aneurysms in California. Stroke 2001;32:597–605
3A. Harbaugh RM. Chairman's Message Fall 2002. Cerebrovascular News Online http://www.neurosurgery.org/Sections/newsletter.aspx?Section=CV&Issue=fall02. Accessed: December 19, 2005
4. Cross DT, Tirschwell DL, Clark MA, et al. Mortality following subarachnoid hemorrhage varies with hospital case volume in 19 states. J Neurosurg. Forthcoming
5. Molyneux, AJ, et al. International subarachnoid aneurysm trial (ISAT) if neurosurgical clipping versus endovascular coiling in 2143 patients with ruptured intracranial aneurysms: a randomized comparison of effect on survival, dependency, seizures, rebleeding, subgroups, and aneurysm location. Lancet 2005;366:808–817
6. Boston Scientific. BSC analysis based on HCUP (Healthcare Cost Utilization Project) data. 2002–2003
7. Chimowitz, R. 2003 American Stroke Association (doc 70-2249 5/03), Presentation
8. Chimowitz, M, et al. Comparison of warfarin and aspirin for symptomatic intracranial arterial stenosis. N Engl J Med 2005 Mar 31;352:13

Clinical Controversies

6

Unruptured Aneurysms: A Neurological Perspective

NERISSA U. KO AND DARYL R. GRESS

Objectives: Upon completion of this chapter, the reader should be able to describe the difficulties in deciding how best to manage a patient with an unruptured aneurysm, with observation, surgical clipping, or endovascular coiling.

Accreditation: The AANS* is accredited by the Accreditation Council for Continuing Medical Education (ACCME) to sponsor continuing medical education for physicians.

Credit: The AANS designates this educational activity for a maximum of 15 credits in Category 1 credit toward the AMA Physician's Recognition Award. Each physician should claim only those hours of credit that he/she spent in the educational activity.

The Home Study Examination is online on the AANS Web site at: http://www.aans.org/education/books/controversy.asp

* The acronym AANS refers to both the American Association of Neurological Surgeons and the American Association of Neurosurgeons.

The management of unruptured intracranial aneurysms (UIAs) has become more challenging for clinicians. In the past, all UIAs were considered for treatment to prevent the most devastating consequence of aneurysm rupture, subarachnoid hemorrhage (SAH). Because SAH is associated with an overall mortality of 50% and major morbidity of 30%,[1] significant treatment risks were often justified to prevent these poor outcomes. More recent data, however, suggest that risks of treatment are not without consequence, and the risk of aneurysm rupture may be lower than expected.

As our diagnostic imaging technology improves, the ability to detect incidental UIAs increases. To add to the complexity of designing rational treatment guidelines, individual patient characteristics as well as aneurysm characteristics may affect the natural history and alter the risks of intervention. The appropriate treatment for UIAs is also controversial, with endovascular coiling as an increasingly employed alternative to surgical clipping. Given all these issues, treatment decisions by a multidisciplinary team, comprising a vascular or intensive care neurologist, a vascular neurosurgeon, and a neurointerventionist is essential. Increasing evidence suggests that the availability and experience of surgeons and endovascular specialists factor into the risks and cost-effectiveness of treatment for these patients. Outcomes are also better at centers with higher volumes that provide the expertise of a multidisciplinary team.

The challenge facing clinicians today is balancing the risk of treatment designed to prevent SAH with the natural history risk of rupture. Clinicians need to be more careful in deciding which patient is appropriate for intervention. If local expertise is limited, transfer to an experienced center with a multidisciplinary team is recommended.

■ Epidemiology

Unruptured intracranial aneurysms are common, with a reported prevalence ranging from 0.2 to 8.9% of the general population. In a systematic review, retrospective autopsy studies reported the lowest rates and prospective angiography studies the highest rates, likely reflecting the different study designs and patient populations. For adults without specific risk factors, the estimated prevalence was 2.3%.[2] The majority of UIAs are asymptomatic and are incidentally discovered in evaluation for headaches and other neurological symptoms. Less than half of patients present with symptoms from compression of neighboring nerves or brain or from embolic events distal to the aneurysm site.[3,4] Detection of incidental UIAs has increased with improvement of noninvasive vascular imaging. Magnetic resonance angiography (MRA) and computed tomographic angiography (CTA) are used increasingly as alternatives to digital subtraction angiography (DSA) (the "gold standard"). However, they have difficulty detecting aneurysms less than 5 mm in size, which make up a third of all aneurysms.[5] Sensitivity for CTA and MRA was 76 to 98% and specificity was 85 to 100%, in a population with SAH, but this may be an overestimation of the accuracy of these techniques.[6] Given these limitations, screening with noninvasive measures for aneurysms is not cost-effective but may have a limited role in those with specific risk factors.[7]

Risk factors for the formation of intracranial aneurysms include two first-degree relatives with cerebral aneurysm, any first-degree relative with history of SAH, age greater than 50 years, female gender, smoking, cocaine use, and inherited disorders such as polycystic kidney disease.[2,8] Patient characteristics such as smoking, younger age, female gender, prior SAH, and hypertension have been associated with increased risk of aneurysm rupture. Active smoking status was associated with a relative risk (RR) of 1.46, increasing to RR 3.04 with time.[9] Smoking and female gender were also associated with increased risk of aneurysm growth and de novo aneurysm formation.[10]

Based on prior studies, risk of rupture may also be influenced by aneurysm characteristics such as location, morphology, and size. In retrospective reviews, location in the anterior circulation, size greater than 10 mm, and multiple aneurysms were associated with higher rupture rates.[9,11–14] Aneurysm size has been reported as the main predictor of risk of subsequent rupture in most natural history studies. Risk factors for increasing aneurysm size included multiple aneurysms, female gender, age over 70 years, and anterior communicating and basilar artery location.[12]

■ Natural History

Until recently, the natural history of UIAs has been based primarily on case reports and case series. Rupture rates have been estimated at 1 to 2% per year, varying widely from studies. The highest annual rupture rates of 3.2% are from a Japanese national hospital registry of 427 patients with 217 person years of follow-up.[15] The Helsinki study which reported 1.4% annual rupture rate benefited from longer follow-up times (2575 person years) without surgical selection but tended to represent a younger patient population in a single center.[10] Size was the biggest predictor of rupture, along with multiple aneurysms in younger patients.[9]

Our best data on the natural history of UIAs comes from the prospective multicenter International Study of Unruptured Intracranial Aneurysms (ISUIA), which involved 61 centers enrolling patients from 1991 to 1998 with nearly 1700 patients and 6544 person years of follow-up.[16] To date, this is the largest and most comprehensive natural history study on UIAs published. Both the retrospective and prospective arms of this study have generated much controversy because the reported rupture rates are much lower than expected, and the risks of treatment were not without consequence. In the retrospective arm of ISUIA, patients were divided into subgroups based on previous history of SAH. For aneurysms less than 10 mm, the annual rupture rate was 0.05% per year in Group I (no SAH) and 0.5% per year in Group II (with SAH).[17] In the prospective study, the overall incidence of aneurysm rupture was 0.8% per year with a mean follow-up time of 3.9 years. Risk of rupture was highest with aneurysms located in the posterior circulation and posterior communicating artery (RR 2.3), similar to findings in the retrospective study. Size greater than 7 mm in diameter, history of prior SAH, and younger age was also associated with an increased risk of rupture.[16]

The main limitation of ISUIA was lack of randomization. Patients were selected for treatment based on clinicians' preference. Treatment of selected patients introduces bias that could lead to underestimating the rupture rates. Symptomatic aneurysms tend to be underrepresented in most natural history studies, including ISUIA, because they are often preferentially treated. The most common symptoms were cranial neuropathies, ischemic changes from embolic events, and visual loss.[4] Nonetheless, ISUIA represents our best natural history data and suggests that treatment may not be justified in patients with small, asymptomatic aneurysms in the anterior circulation without prior history of SAH.

■ Treatment

The goal of treating UIAs is to reduce the risk of rupture and the devastating consequences of SAH. As with all treatment interventions, the risks of treatment should be balanced against the risk of rupture if UIAs are left untreated. The American Heart Association (AHA) Stroke Council recommends treatment for all symptomatic intradural aneurysms regardless of size, aneurysms in patients with prior SAH, and asymptomatic aneurysms greater than 10 mm.[18] In light of recent data, however, critical assessment of factors such as aneurysm size, location, and morphology; patient age and comorbidities; and experience of treating physicians must also be considered. Although many UIAs would be considered for treatment, conservative management may be a reasonable choice for some patients. For patients who do not undergo treatment, serial imaging along with risk factor modification with smoking cessation and control of hypertension is warranted. Serial imaging, typically with MRI or CT, within the first year after diagnosis can be reassuring to document stable aneurysm size, but it is likely not a reliable means to detect acute changes in aneurysm size associated with rupture.

Surgical Clipping

Once the decision to treat UIAs is made, the next dilemma is choosing the appropriate treatment modality, surgical clipping or endovascular coiling. Surgical clipping has been the mainstay of aneurysm treatment since the first successful clipping was performed by Walter Dandy in 1937. Microsurgical techniques have continued to evolve, but reported rates of surgical morbidity and mortality vary widely among case series. In the largest meta-analysis, consisting of 2460 cases with UIAs published in 61 reports, the mortality rate was 2.6% and the permanent morbidity rate was 10.9%.[19] The most-comprehensive data came from the ISUIA study of 1971 clipped patients with an average 4 year follow-up including functional and cognitive outcomes. At 1 year follow-up, mortality was 3.2% and neurological disability was 12%, with a combined surgical morbidity and mortality of 15.2%.[16] Risk factors for poor outcome in surgical patients included patient age greater than 50 years, aneurysm size greater than 12 mm, location in the posterior circulation, calcified or atherosclerotic aneurysms, and presence of symptoms.[16,19]

Endovascular Coiling

Since the development of the Guglielmi detachable coil, coil embolization has been used with increasing frequency. Early cases were often selected for endovascular treatment because of poor surgical risk. Recent technological advances may not be reflected in prior studies of outcomes after coil embolization. In a recent meta-analysis of 90 UIAs treated with coil embolization, annual mortality was reported as 1.4% with total procedural morbidity and mortality of 8.1%.[20] Endovascular coiling of 1811 aneurysms, both ruptured and unruptured, at a single center reported early mortality of 1.5% and morbidity of 5.3%.[21] The ISUIA study, which included 451 coiled patients with less than 4 years of follow-up, reported a mortality of 3.4% and total morbidity and mortality of 9.8% at 1 year, similar to surgically treated patients. Direct comparison of the two groups was not possible given lack of randomization and significant differences in patient age, aneurysm size, and location between treatment groups. Risk factors for endovascular coiling included larger aneurysms in the posterior circulation.[16]

Comparative Studies

Unfortunately, no randomized trials of treatment for UIAs have been performed to determine the indications for clipping versus coiling in this patient population. A small, randomized trial of 109 patients with ruptured aneurysms at a single center failed to show any significant differences in outcome after 3 months or 1 year.[22] The only other direct comparison between clipping and coiling is from the International Subarachnoid Aneurysm Trial (ISAT). The trial found a significant 23% reduction of relative risk (7% absolute risk reduction) in dependency or death at 1 year with endovascular treatment.[23] These trials included patients with ruptured aneurysms; hence, the results cannot be directly extrapolated to the UIA population.

In a retrospective cohort study using the National Inpatient Sample Data from 1996–2000, short-term outcomes were examined for patients with UIAs undergoing clipping versus coiling. There were far more patients clipped during this period, and clipped patients were slightly younger. There were no differences in mortality and discharge to long-term care; however, coiled patients were discharged home more frequently, had a shorter length of stay, lower hospital costs, and less neurological complications. This study was limited in determining long-term efficacy and functional outcomes.[24] In a cohort study of 2612 patients with UIAs treated at 70 university hospitals between 1994 and 1997, hospital death, and discharge to nursing home or rehabilitation center were more common in surgical- compared with endovascular-treated patients (18.5% vs. 10.6%, $p = 0.002$).[25] Similarly, a study of 2069 patients with UIAs in California treated between 1990 and 1998 reported significantly less adverse outcomes with endovascular compared with surgical treatment (10% vs. 25%, $p < 0.001$).[26] In a single-center cohort study, similar findings were reported including a longer follow-up of 3.9 years, suggesting persistent new symptoms or disability in surgical cases, 34% versus 8%, and a longer recovery period, 1 year versus 27 days for 50% return to normal.[27] These observational studies all consistently suggest that endovascular coiling is safer than surgical clipping for UIAs but are limited by the possibility that patient selection may be contributing to outcome differences.

Functional and Cognitive Outcomes

Few studies have reported functional and cognitive outcomes after treatment of UIAs. The ISUIA study looked at significant cognitive change pre- and post-treatment and found a 3 to 5% risk of disability for cognitive change alone, with little improvement between 1-month and 1-year follow-up measurements. The risks appeared to be somewhat higher in those treated by surgical rather than endovascular means, although again this study did not randomize treatment, and comparability is not certain.

In a recent prospective observational study of embolization and surgical clipping, surgical clipping was associated with short-term functional deficits that improved by 1 year, while coiled patients had no deficits in these areas. When outcome measures such as quality of life and mood are assessed, coil embolization also had more favorable outcomes, with surgery having a considerable but often reversible effect in the first 3 months postprocedure.[28] Coiled patients had significantly better short-term outcomes compared with clipped patients, particularly older patients greater than 65 years of age.[24]

Efficacy of Treatment

The primary goal of treatment of UIAs is to prevent aneurysm rupture and the devastating consequences of SAH. Rupture rates after aneurysm treatment may give us the best estimate of treatment efficacy. Unfortunately, many studies fail to report the duration of follow-up needed to calculate these rates. In a recent case series including both ruptured and unruptured aneurysms, the risk of hemorrhage after surgical clipping ranged from 0.2 to 1.5% per year.[29–31] Incomplete aneurysm occlusion was associated with increased risk of rupture.[31]

The main criticism of endovascular coiling has been the durability of treatment. In a Scientific Statement from the AHA, six studies of coil embolization of ruptured aneurysms had a combined rerupture rate of 0.9% per year. Coil embolization had generally higher rupture rates, ranging from 0.6 to 3.0% per year, when compared with surgical clipping.[32] Larger aneurysms and incompletely occluded aneurysms had more frequent aneurysm growth and increased risk of rupture after treatment.[33] A significant number of patients do not achieve complete occlusion after the first endovascular treatment, up to 50 to 78% in reported studies.[6,16,20] Long-term follow-up for durability of coiled patients will be important. Based on this limited evidence, both treatment modalities appear to reduce the risk of rebleeding, but surgical clipping may be more effective.

Treatment Experience

Higher-volume hospitals had fewer adverse outcomes than hospitals that treat a limited number of UIAs. Similarly, high-volume surgeons had significantly lower morbidity and modestly lower mortality rates.[34] The higher-volume centers had shorter lengths of stay and lower total hospital charges, suggesting better cost effectiveness of treatment.[35] In addition, the propensity for a hospital to use endovascular therapy was also associated with better outcomes. These studies suggest that selective referral of UIAs to centers with higher volume and with experienced neurosurgeons and interventional neuroradiologists could improve outcomes.[36]

■ Conclusion

The natural history of UIAs is better defined with the results of large cohort studies like ISUIA. The current literature exposes the complexity of decision-making for clinicians when presented with asymptomatic patients with UIAs. Treatment decisions, including medical observation, require balancing the risk of intervention with the natural history of risk of rupture for each individual patient. Clinicians must rely on judgment and expertise given the scarcity of evidence to help guide these decisions.

The choice of treatment modality, surgical clipping or endovascular coiling, should be individualized. Specific characteristics of the patient and the aneurysm influence the risks of treatment and the likelihood of complete obliteration of the aneurysm. Aneurysm location, size, and morphology often determine the best therapy. Selecting the best treatment modality requires incorporating information about the patient's age and medical condition, the aneurysm characteristics, and the technical ability of the practitioners. Given the absence of randomized trials in the treatment of UIAs, no specific recommendations can be made about the indications for surgical clipping and endovascular coiling. Direct comparison of treatments in the observational studies is limited by lack of randomization with differences in patient characteristics. A randomized trial is needed to define the best treatment for UIAs. The majority of evidence suggests that endovascular coiling is safer than surgical clipping; it should be considered preferentially in older patients with posterior circulation aneurysms. Surgical clipping may be a more durable treatment and be preferred by patients who desire a single treatment procedure, have wide-necked aneurysms, and have aneurysms arising in the middle cerebral artery.

Advances in imaging techniques that can evaluate aneurysm flow and hemodynamics, improvements in coiling with stents, microsurgical techniques, and combined surgical and endovascular treatments will likely improve outcomes for patients with UIAs. A multidisciplinary approach, with input from practitioners with the appropriate expertise, is probably the most reliable way to make the best treatment decisions. Patient outcomes are better at hospitals that offer both surgical clipping and endovascular therapy regardless of whether a patient is ultimately treated with surgery or coil embolization.

■ References

1. Hop JW, Rinkel GJ, Algra A, van Gijn J. Case-fatality rates and functional outcome after subarachnoid hemorrhage: a systematic review. Stroke 1997;28:660–664

2. Rinkel GJ, Djibuti M, Algra A, van Gijn J. Prevalence and risk of rupture of intracranial aneurysms: a systematic review. Stroke 1998;29:251–256

3. Qureshi AI, Mohammad Y, Yahia AM, et al. Ischemic events associated with unruptured intracranial aneurysms: multicenter clinical study and review of the literature. Neurosurgery 2000;46:282–289, 289–290

4. Friedman JA, Piepgras DG, Pichelmann MA, Hansen KK, Brown RD Jr, Wiebers DO. Small cerebral aneurysms presenting with symptoms other than rupture. Neurology 2001;57:1212–1216

5. White PM, Wardlaw JM. Unruptured intracranial aneurysms. J Neuroradiol 2003;30:336–350

6. Wardlaw JM, White PM. The detection and management of unruptured intracranial aneurysms. Brain 2000;123(Pt 2):205–221

7. Weir B. Unruptured intracranial aneurysms: A review. J Neurosurg 2002;96:3–42

8. King JT Jr. Epidemiology of aneurysmal subarachnoid hemorrhage. Neuroimaging Clin N Am 1997;7:659–668

9. Juvela S. Risk factors for multiple intracranial aneurysms. Stroke 2000;31:392–397

10. Juvela S. Natural history of unruptured intracranial aneurysms: risks for aneurysm formation, growth, and rupture. Acta Neurochir Suppl Suppl 2002;82:27–30

11. Wiebers DO, Whisnant JP, Sundt TM Jr, O'Fallon WM. The significance of unruptured intracranial saccular aneurysms. J Neurosurg 1987;66:23–29

12. Yonekura M. Small unruptured aneurysm verification (suave study, Japan)—interim report. Neurol Med Chir (Tokyo) 2004;44:213–214

13. Weir B, Disney L, Karrison T. Sizes of ruptured and unruptured aneurysms in relation to their sites and the ages of patients. J Neurosurg 2002;96:64–70

14. Ohashi Y, Horikoshi T, Sugita M, Yagishita T, Nukui H. Size of cerebral aneurysms and related factors in patients with subarachnoid hemorrhage. Surg Neurol 2004;61:239–245, 245–237

15. Tsukahara T, Murakami N, Sakurai Y, Yonekura M, Takahashi T, Inoue T. Treatment of unruptured cerebral aneurysms—a multicenter study of Japanese national hospitals. Acta Neurochir Suppl 2002;82:3–10

16. Wiebers DO, Whisnant JP, Huston J III, et al. Unruptured intracranial aneurysms: natural history, clinical outcome, and risks of surgical and endovascular treatment. Lancet 2003;362:103–110

17. Unruptured intracranial aneurysms—risk of rupture and risks of surgical intervention. International Study of Unruptured Intracranial Aneurysms Investigators. N Engl J Med 1998;339:1725–1733. Erratum in: N Engl J Med 1999 Mar 4;340(9):744

18. Bederson JB, Awad IA, Wiebers DO, et al. Recommendations for the management of patients with unruptured intracranial aneurysms: a statement for healthcare professionals from the stroke council of the american heart association. Stroke 2000;31: 2742–2750

19. Raaymakers TW, Rinkel GJ, Limburg M, Algra A. Mortality and morbidity of surgery for unruptured intracranial aneurysms: a meta-analysis. Stroke 1998;29:1531–1538

20. Brilstra EH, Rinkel GJ, van der Graaf Y, van Rooij WJ, Algra A. Treatment of intracranial aneurysms by embolization with coils: a systematic review. Stroke 1999;30:470–476

21. Henkes H, Fischer S, Weber W, et al. Endovascular coil occlusion of 1811 intracranial aneurysms: early angiographic and clinical results. Neurosurgery 2004;54:268–280, 280–265

22. Koivisto T, Vanninen R, Hurskainen H, Saari T, Hernesniemi J, Vapalahti M. Outcomes of early endovascular versus surgical treatment of ruptured cerebral aneurysms. A prospective randomized study. Stroke 2000;31:2369–2377

23. Molyneux A, Kerr R, Stratton I, et al. International Subarachnoid Aneurysm Trial (ISAT) of neurosurgical clipping versus endovascular coiling in 2143 patients with ruptured intracranial aneurysms: a randomised trial. Lancet 2002;360:1267–1274

24. Barker FG II, Amin-Hanjani S, Butler WE, et al. Age-dependent differences in short-term outcome after surgical or endovascular treatment of unruptured intracranial aneurysms in the United States, 1996–2000. Neurosurgery 2004;54:18–28 discussion 28–30

25. Johnston SC, Dudley RA, Gress DR, Ono L. Surgical and endovascular treatment of unruptured cerebral aneurysms at university hospitals. Neurology 1999;52:1799–1805

26. Johnston SC, Zhao S, Dudley RA, Berman MF, Gress DR. Treatment of unruptured cerebral aneurysms in California. Stroke 2001;32:597–605

27. Johnston SC, Wilson CB, Halbach VV, et al. Endovascular and surgical treatment of unruptured cerebral aneurysms: comparison of risks. Ann Neurol 2000;48:11–19

28. Brilstra EH, Rinkel GJ, van der Graaf Y, et al. Quality of life after treatment of unruptured intracranial aneurysms by neurosurgical clipping or by embolisation with coils. A prospective, observational study. Cerebrovasc Dis 2004;17:44–52

29. Yoshimoto T, Uchida K, Kaneko U, Kayama T, Suzuki J. An analysis of follow-up results of 1000 intracranial saccular aneurysms with definitive surgical treatment. J Neurosurg 1979; 50:152–157

30. Tsutsumi K, Ueki K, Usui M, Kwak S, Kirino T. Risk of recurrent subarachnoid hemorrhage after complete obliteration of cerebral aneurysms. Stroke 1998;29:2511–2513

31. David CA, Vishteh AG, Spetzler RF, Lemole M, Lawton MT, Partovi S. Late angiographic follow-up review of surgically treated aneurysms. J Neurosurg 1999;91:396–401

32. Johnston SC, Higashida RT, Barrow DL, et al. Recommendations for the endovascular treatment of intracranial aneurysms: a statement for healthcare professionals from the Committee on Cerebrovascular Imaging of the American Heart Association Council on Cardiovascular Radiology. Stroke 2002;33:2536–2544

33. Hayakawa M, Murayama Y, Duckwiler GR, Gobin YP, Guglielmi G, Vinuela F. Natural history of the neck remnant of a cerebral aneurysm treated with the guglielmi detachable coil system. J Neurosurg 2000;93:561–568

34. Barker FG II, Amin-Hanjani S, Butler WE, Ogilvy CS, Carter BS. In-hospital mortality and morbidity after surgical treatment of unruptured intracranial aneurysms in the United States, 1996–2000: the effect of hospital and surgeon volume. Neurosurgery 2003; 52:995–1007, 1007–1009

35. Hoh BL, Rabinov JD, Pryor JC, Carter BS, Barker FG II. In-hospital morbidity and mortality after endovascular treatment of unruptured intracranial aneurysms in the United States, 1996–2000: effect of hospital and physician volume. AJNR Am J Neuroradiol 2003; 24:1409–1420

36. Berman MF, Solomon RA, Mayer SA, Johnston SC, Yung PP. Impact of hospital-related factors on outcome after treatment of cerebral aneurysms. Stroke 2003;34:2200–2207

7

Unruptured Aneurysms: A Surgical Perspective

CHIRAG D. GANDHI, AMAN B. PATEL, AND JOSHUA B. BEDERSON

Objectives: Upon completion of this chapter, the reader should be able to identify the current indications for microsurgical clipping of unruptured aneurysms.

Accreditation: The AANS* is accredited by the Accreditation Council for Continuing Medical Education (ACCME) to sponsor continuing medical education for physicians.

Credit: The AANS designates this educational activity for a maximum of 15 credits in Category 1 credit toward the AMA Physician's Recognition Award. Each physician should claim only those hours of credit that he/she spent in the educational activity.

The Home Study Examination is online on the AANS Web site at: http://www.aans.org/education/books/controversy.asp

* The acronym AANS refers to both the American Association of Neurological Surgeons and the American Association of Neurosurgeons.

Although the last two decades have seen significant advances in the surgical and medical management of aneurysmal subarachnoid hemorrhage (SAH), the overall morbidity and mortality rates are as high as 40 to 50%.[1,2] Poor neurological outcomes after SAH are due to the effects of the initial hemorrhage, early rebleeding, and delayed cerebral ischemia. Prevention of SAH by surgical treatment of unruptured aneurysms is a definitive strategy by which to reduce poor outcomes. However, because all treatments carry at least some risk, there remains significant controversy as to the best treatment for unruptured intracranial aneurysms (UIAs). Autopsy studies have shown that the overall frequency of UIAs in the general population is ~1 to 5%.[3] The incidence of SAH is ~10 cases per 100,000 persons per year[4]; hence, it is likely that most intracranial aneurysms do not rupture. Detection of incidental intracranial aneurysms has increased recently because of improved diagnostic technology such as magnetic resonance imaging (MRI) and angiography, computerized tomography (CT) angiography, and digital subtraction angiography (which

remains the "gold standard" for diagnosis), making the management of UIAs a more common neurosurgical dilemma.

Various attempts have been made to establish rational treatment protocols for UIAs. Such protocols should take into account the risk of treatment as well as the risk of rupture of an UIA (its natural history). Studies have demonstrated that both the natural history of UIAs and the outcomes of treatment are strongly influenced by three factors: (1) patient characteristics such as previous SAH, age, and other medical comorbidities; (2) aneurysm characteristics such as size, location, and morphology[3]; and (3) management factors such as experience of the surgical team and treating hospital. These complex and interrelated factors have made evidence-based assessments of bleeding rate and treatment efficacy very difficult. In light of the lack of convincing prospective randomized studies comparing observation with treatment, UIAs are currently managed based on our best understanding of natural history versus risk of treatment.

■ The Natural History of Unruptured Aneurysms

Although the natural history of unruptured intracranial aneurysms has not been clearly defined, many retrospective cohort studies and clinical case reports have attempted to quantify both the patient and aneurysm factors that could modify the risk for rupture. A careful analysis of these factors can help clinical neuroscientists decide whether a particular aneurysm should be treated or observed.

Aneurysm characteristics such as size, location, and morphology influence the natural history of UIAs. A review of 945 patients found that ruptured aneurysms have a greater diameter than unruptured ones, 10.8 mm versus 7.8 mm.[5] Additionally, autopsy studies and retrospective reviews have found that aneurysms in certain locations such as the anterior communicating artery and pericallosal artery may be at a higher risk for rupture than other locations.[5,6] Morphological variations such as multilobulation and loculations may also increase the rupture risk.[7]

The natural history of patients with incidental aneurysms without prior SAH can be separated according to those that present with symptoms other than SAH (i.e., third cranial nerve palsy, headaches, orbital pain, seizures) and those that are truly incidental. In the 1969 Cooperative Aneurysm Study, 165 patients with symptomatic aneurysms were followed, and 79% of these aneurysms were treated surgically.[8] The remaining 34 cases were left untreated, and the natural course of the disease was studied. Of these remaining patients, 25% had a SAH at 3 months to 3 years. All of the aneurysms that hemorrhaged were 7 to 10 mm in diameter, and all were fatal. Aneurysms that were smaller than 7 mm did not bleed. Other studies have suggested that the risk of rupture is higher for symptomatic aneurysms with high mortality rates, although the magnitude of the reported increase in risk varies.[9–11] Very few studies following the natural history of this specific subgroup exist because they are selected for treatment. Aneurysms that present with symptoms of mass effect are likely to be larger. Nevertheless, the data suggest that symptomatic aneurysms have a higher rate of rupture that should be addressed somewhat urgently. Based on the recommendations of the Stroke Council, all intradural symptomatic UIAs should be considered for treatment, especially those that have recently increased in size.[12]

On the natural history of asymptomatic unruptured aneurysms, a recent study in Japan reported on 62 patients observed for more than 6 months to follow their saccular, nonthrombotic aneurysms. The aneurysms had been diagnosed on angiograms obtained for causes other than SAH.[13] Patients were followed for 6 months to

7 years; in seven patients SAH was documented on CT scans at a mean interval of 4.89 years. Six of the seven patients died from SAH, and the remaining patient suffered severe neurological deficit. Based on this, the cumulative risk for all aneurysms at 5 and 10 years were 7.5% and 22.5%, respectively. For aneurysms smaller than 10 mm, the 5- and 10-year rates were 4.5% and 13.9%, respectively; in aneurysms greater than 10 mm, the 5- and 10-year rates were 33.5% and 55.9%, respectively. These rates of aneurysm rupture are higher than other reports from North America. In a subset of the North American Carotid Endarterectomy trial, 66 patients (mean age of 66 years) were found to have unruptured, noncavernous sinus, intracranial aneurysms, and only one of the follow-up group of 58 patients suffered a SAH.[14] Although both studies have similar patient demographics, the rate of aneurysm rupture was significantly less in the North American study.

In another review by Weibers et al, 130 patients were followed for 8.3 years, during which time 15 patients suffered a SAH.[11] All 15 ruptured aneurysms were greater than 10 mm in diameter. The 102 aneurysms measuring less than 10 mm remained unruptured. The subsequent analysis determined that size was the only predictor of aneurysm rupture. However, 10 aneurysms were 8 to 9 mm, and 36 aneurysms were 6 to 9 mm; 10 mm could not definitively be established as the critical size for rupture. This finding promoted the further investigation of the influence of size on bleeding risk.

The International Study of Unruptured Intracranial Aneurysms (ISUIA) is the largest and most comprehensive natural history study of unruptured intracranial aneurysms conducted with a large number of patients. The study also allows for statistical significance and the analysis of secondary subgroups.[15] The preliminary report from this continuing study has generated much controversy and raises questions about conclusions drawn from prior studies in regards to the natural history and the indications for surgery in patients with UIAs. The retrospective component of the ISUIA evaluated natural history and included 1449 patients divided into two groups—patients with and without a prior history of SAH from a different treated aneurysm. Group I consisted of 727 patients with no history of SAH who were followed for an average of 7.5 years. Rates of rupture for aneurysms less than 10 mm they were 0.05% per year, for those greater than 10 mm they were 1% per year, and for those greater than 25 mm the rate of rupture was 6% in the first year. Predictors of rupture were increasing size and location, specifically at the basilar tip, posterior cerebral or vertebrobasilar distribution, or the origin of the posterior communicating artery.

Patients with a history of SAH from a different aneurysm were designated as Group 2 in the ISUIA. In Group 2, aneurysm size alone was not a predictor of rupture rate. Basilar tip location was the only predictor among these patients. In patients with aneurysms less than 10 mm, the risk of rupture was 11 times higher in patients with prior SAH than in patients without SAH (0.5% vs. 0.05% per year). In aneurysms greater than 10 mm, the rate was found to be equal between the two groups. The presence of multiple intracranial aneurysms was not a predictive factor for future rupture even though unruptured aneurysms in Group 2 were more likely to bleed.

The rate of rupture found in the ISUIA is significantly lower than prior reports of 1 to 2% per year.[13,16] Critics of the ISUIA argue that the retrospective portion of the study is invalid because it excludes those patients who are more likely to undergo treatment rather than conservative management, specifically younger patients. Additionally, the inclusion of intracavernous and proximal carotid artery aneurysms, which are much less likely to bleed, may have contributed to the lower rupture rate in this study. Critics also note that although the reported mortality rate of SAH is ~45%, the rate in the ISUIA study was 83%. This fact could be a result of wide confidence intervals or may reflect selection bias by having a larger number of older, medically frail patients who were not eligible for treatment. Additionally, the retrospective branch of the study had a variety of inclusion and exclusion criteria that some argue introduce further bias. Although the results of this study did not clearly support treatment of Group 1 patients with UIAs less than 10 mm in diameter, these conclusions have been challenged because of the criteria for inclusion in the study as discussed above.

Other studies have found that the rate of rupture in patients with prior SAH is higher than stated in the ISUIA study. Juvela et al retrospectively examined the natural history and the predictive risk factors for aneurysm rupture in 142 patients, 131 of whom had a prior SAH.[10] Median follow-up was 19.7 years, and the overall annual incidence of bleeding was 1.3% with a rate of 2.6% in symptomatic aneurysms and 1% in incidental aneurysms. Increasing size, age at diagnosis (inversely), and cigarette smoking were significant predictors of outcome. They assert that surgery should be considered in young and middle-age patients; smoking cessation may be an alternative in the elderly. However, the small number of cases weakened the statistical power of the study.

Various studies have concluded that most spontaneous SAHs are as a result of aneurysms that are 7 to 10 mm in diameter.[8,11] However, the ISUIA suggested that 10 mm is the critical size for rupture. This disagreement suggests that either there are a significantly higher number of 7 to 10 mm aneurysms, there is a decrease in aneurysm size at rupture, or that aneurysms that are more likely to rupture will do so at a smaller critical diameter. No clear evidence exists for any single theory.

Current evidence in natural history studies suggests that the risk of aneurysmal rupture increases with aneurysm size and the clinical presentation of the patient (previous SAH from different aneurysm, symptomatic vs. asymptomatic). Additionally, the risk is also likely influenced by location.[17] Existing studies reflect at least some bias in patient selection, and many lack statistical power because of limited patient cohorts. Many others have suggested that a prospective, randomized study comparing conservative management and intervention would be helpful. Although such a study would be very appealing, it remains impractical. It would require years of follow-up, and because of low rupture rates, a vast number of patients would need to be enrolled to permit adequate statistical analysis and stratification for specific risk factors.

Recent reviews suggest that aneurysms are more prevalent and much less likely to rupture in older individuals,[5,12] and that females are more likely to bleed.[9] The natural history of UIAs is also modified by environmental factors such as cigarette smoking. Weir et al found that ~3500 patients from five prospective studies of aneurysm rupture had smoking rates 2.5 times higher than the expected rates based on European and U.S. national surveys.[18] In another long-term study in Finland, active smoking status at the time of diagnosis was a significant risk factor for subsequent aneurysm rupture with a risk ratio of 1.46.[16] Active smoking as a time-dependent covariant was the most important risk factor for rupture, with a risk ratio of 3.04. Based on these results, the authors conclude that the cessation of smoking may be a good alternative to surgery in some older patients.

The discussion above suggests that treatment over observation should be considered in several scenarios. These are outlined in a recent review published by the American Heart Association's Stroke Council.[12] The AHA recommendations include a few keys points. The higher risk of treatment and shorter life expectancy of older individuals favors observation in the oldest patients with the smallest asymptomatic aneurysms. In other words, patient age is perhaps the most important factor in recommending treatment versus conservative management. For example, we would recommend treatment of even small aneurysms (i.e., 5 to 9 mm) in young patients, while even large aneurysms (i.e., >9 mm) might be treated conservatively in older individuals. Symptomatic intradural aneurysms of all sizes should be considered for treatment, especially those with new symptoms that should be treated with relative urgency. Coexisting aneurysms of any size in patients with prior SAH from another aneurysm should be considered for treatment. Asymptomatic aneurysms greater than 10 mm in size merit strong consideration for treatment. Special consideration for aneurysm treatment should be given for any young patients, patients with aneurysms with daughter sac formation or other unique hemodynamic factors, and patients with a family history of aneurysms or SAH.

■ Treatment of Unruptured Intracranial Aneurysms

The second controversy in the management of unruptured intracranial aneurysms concerns surgical clipping versus endovascular coiling. Microsurgical clipping has long been considered the *gold standard*, and a larger body of literature exists quantifying its efficacy with UIAs. However, endovascular techniques are rapidly advancing and now need to be closely considered by neurosurgeons. The optimal technique is the one that balances both acceptable morbidity and high efficacy. Traditionally, advocates for clipping have questioned the efficacy of coiling for unruptured aneurysms and advocates of coiling have pointed to the higher surgical morbidity and mortality rates. Unfortunately, no clear prospective studies exist to support either surgery or coiling and management continues to be based primarily on retrospective literature.

Several studies have estimated the surgical morbidity and mortality rate of elective treatment of UIAs to be 0 to 4% and 0 to 7.2%, respectively.[19–22] The morbidity rates for giant aneurysms have been shown to be as high as 20%, with size as the key predictor of outcome. King et al in a meta-analysis combined 28 previous studies and in 733 patients found the overall mortality and morbidity rate to be 1% and 4.1%, respectively.[23]

Although data suggest that both the mortality and morbidity rates may be higher than previously reported, the inclusion criteria of these studies remain controversial. Raaymakers et al in a meta-analysis of 2460 patients from 61 studies reported a mortality rate of 2.6% and a morbidity rate of 10.9%.[24] The higher rates maybe a result of inclusion of more symptomatic and larger aneurysms. Similar rates for morbidity and mortality were also supported by the prospective branch of the ISUIA study in which 1172 patients with newly diagnosed unruptured aneurysms were followed.[15] Similar to the retrospective arm, patients were divided into two groups consisting of those without a prior history of SAH (Group 1 with 961 patients) and those with a prior history of SAH from a different aneurysm that had been successfully repaired (Group 2 with 211 patients). Within Group 1, 83% of patients underwent surgery, and the remaining patients were treated by endovascular coiling, with a resulting 1-month and 1-year mortality of 2.3% and 3.8%, respectively. Similarly, in Group 2, 94% of patients were treated surgically with a 1-month and 1-year mortality rate of 0% and 1%, respectively. Both groups

were found to have a morbidity of ~12%. This is significantly higher than previously reported morbidity rates, which the ISUIA investigators attributed to more validated measures of neurological assessment, but their critics attributed to inadequate study design.

The surgical risks are modified by a variety of risk factors that include patient and aneurysm characteristics. Increasing age was found to be the only predictor of poor outcome in the prospective arm of ISUIA study, with combined morbidity and mortality rates doubling among the older age groups; 6.5% for patients younger than 45, 14.4% for patients 45 to 64, and 32% for patients older than 65 years of age.[15] These results should be considered in older patients who have a shorter risk period but a higher surgical morbidity. Any other presurgical comorbidities may also affect the outcome. In the ISUIA, it remains unclear whether a cohort with similar comorbid conditions managed conservatively might not also have a similar decrease in the Rankin score.

There is evidence to suggest that aneurysm size influences surgical risk, with larger aneurysms having greater surgical risks than smaller ones.[19,20,25] Additionally, both aneurysm morphology and location have been found to affect outcomes secondary to the need for greater microsurgical expertise. Those with atherosclerotic or calcified walls are considered to pose a significant risk for ischemic complications, as shown in one study in which among six patients, there was a 50% rate of ischemic complication following clipping.[26] Partially thrombosed vessels may be a source of emboli if not treated with great care. Additionally, large, poorly defined aneurysms, those located in the posterior fossa, those involving major vessel bifurcations, those partially located in the cavernous sinus, or ones originating from the basilar artery have been associated with worse outcomes.[3,24,27] The results, however, are inconsistent; other studies have found that location is only important in the case of giant aneurysms[20] and that surgical risk may be no higher in posterior circulation UIAs.[28]

Unruptured aneurysms presenting with symptoms of mass effect or cerebral ischemia also carry a greater surgical morbidity as compared with asymptomatic aneurysms.[20,25] Symptoms can be effectively treated in many cases to help relieve the mass effect and are considered an indication for intervention in appropriately healthy patients.[27]

Surgical clipping is associated with low rates of postoperative aneurysm rupture and has traditionally been considered highly efficacious. However, the results are not absolute, as shown by studies that have considered both the incidence of residual aneurysm necks and subsequent rates of SAH following clipping. David et al evaluated 102 patients with 160 surgically treated aneurysms with late angiographic follow-up at a mean of 4.4 years postsurgery.[29] Of 135 clipped aneurysms that initially demonstrated no residual necks, 1.5% later exhibited recurrence. Of the 12 aneurysms with known residual necks, 25% enlarged during the follow-up period. Among the 102 patients, one SAH developed, resulting in a risk of hemorrhage of 1.9% per year. Eight new aneurysms were also found in six patients, resulting in a de novo aneurysm-formation rate of 1.8%. This data confirm the long-term efficacy of clipping with an aneurysm obliteration rate of 98.5%. However, even with surgery, residual aneurysm necks do occur and pose a risk for SAH.

In another study, 115 patients with unruptured aneurysms were surgically treated and followed for a median of 8.8 years.[21] Four patients suffered SAH, two from de novo aneurysms, one from regrowth of a clipped aneurysm, and one from rupture of a wrapped aneurysm. The cumulative risk for SAH after treatment was 1.4% at 10 years, which is low but requires consideration.

Surgical experience of both the surgeon and the hospital may affect postoperative outcomes. At the Cleveland Clinic, 449 aneurysms in 366 patients were clipped by 10 different surgeons.[30] At the 6-month follow-up there was found to be a statistically significant relationship between the surgeon and patient outcome. Similarly, there is thought to be a direct relationship between the volume of craniotomies per year for aneurysms at an institution and better outcomes. Hospitals that performed 10 or more per year had an overall mortality rate of 5.3%, and those with fewer than 10 craniotomies per year had a mortality rate of 11.2%.[31] When assessing patients for treatment of unruptured aneurysms, it is of paramount importance for the individual surgeon to realize their technical capabilities and treat patients accordingly.

Over the past decade, endovascular coiling has been increasingly utilized in both the initial and adjunctive management of UIAs. With improvements in technology and technique, the complication rates have been steadily declining and the treatment results steadily improving. In a systematic review of 48 studies with 1383 patients from 1990 to 1997, the permanent complication rate was 3.7%,[32] and mortality rates were from 0.05 to 1%.[33,34] However, despite the low morbidity rate the incomplete obliteration rate has been found to be as high as 46%.[32] Based on such high recanalization rates and the low rates of UIA rupture, critics suggest that endovascular coiling may not alter the natural history of UIAs.

There are multiple factors that make the utility of embolization treatment difficult to assess. Current studies that compare coiling versus surgery are not randomized; furthermore, they compare unequal patient groups. For example, the initial patient population undergoing endovascular treatment was traditionally older and more medically frail. Alternatively, a patient with a posterior fossa giant aneurysm randomized to a surgical group would certainly face higher risks for morbidity. The rapid advances in endovascular therapies make it difficult to standardize techniques within a given study.

The safety of endovascular treatment was reviewed in recent retrospective studies by Johnston et al, who demonstrated that coiling of UIAs resulted in lower rates of morbidity and mortality when compared with surgery.[34,35] Although the safety of coiling has been demonstrated, its efficacy still requires further investigation. In a single institutional review of 42 unruptured aneurysms, Wanke et al reported a complete or near complete occlusion in 34 of 38 patients.[36] Similarly, a larger review of 115 patients with a 120 aneurysms located in a variety of locations and with varying sizes and morphology reported a 91% rate of complete or near complete aneurysm obliteration.[37] However, angiographic follow-up in this study revealed that 32% of the patients with a small neck remnant demonstrated recanalization. This suggests that an aneurysm that undergoes *complete* obliteration has a much better long-term outcome than one that undergoes only *near complete* obliteration. Some critics even argue that near complete obliteration may not change the natural history. In the follow-up study by Hayakawa et al the incompletely embolized aneurysms were further scrutinized for rates of progressive thrombosis and rates of recanalization.[38] The overall progressive thrombosis rate was 25%, with higher rates in small aneurysms with small necks. The overall recanalization rate was 49%; with large and giant aneurysms, the rate approached 90%. This suggests that although small aneurysms with small necks and, in some cases, wide necks can be successfully treated with endovascular coiling, larger aneurysms may not be adequately secured with this treatment and may need to be considered for surgery.

The University of California, Los Angeles (UCLA)-based interventional group discussed above published a study of their 11-year experience with aneurysm coiling in which they reviewed 818 patients harboring 916 aneurysms.[39] The patients were divided into Group A, which was the initial 5 years' experience, with 230 patients harboring 251 aneurysms, and Group B, which was the later 6 years' experience, with 588 patients harboring 665 aneurysms. The rate of complete embolization was higher in Group B than in Group A (56.8% vs. 50.2%), and the rates of recanalization were lower in Group B than in Group A (17.2% vs. 26.1%). As in previous studies, the rate of recanalization was related to the size of the aneurysm dome and neck. Additionally, the overall rate of aneurysm rupture was 1.6%, but within the past 5 years, that rate had fallen to 0.5%. This study demonstrates that both the efficacy and safety of aneurysm embolization have improved significantly over the past decade but that recanalization remains a major limitation of this technique. Recent advances in embolization technology including neurostents and bioactive coils may improve on the problems of aneurysm recanalization seen with traditional platinum coils, but these studies arc still pending. Based upon the studies detailed above, the appropriate treatment option requires an adequate assessment of various characteristics, the most important of which is the morphology of the aneurysm. Consideration should also include the location and size of the aneurysm as well as the age and medical condition of the patient.

At present our understanding of the natural history of unruptured aneurysms and the indications for their treatment are based upon studies limited by a variety of statistical weaknesses. The current literature on the natural history of UIAs offers evidence to consider surgical treatment over observation in some specific circumstances. These include symptomatic intradural aneurysms, coexisting aneurysms in patients with prior SAH from another aneurysm, and asymptomatic aneurysms greater than 10 mm in diameter. Surgical treatment should also be considered for all young patients regardless of aneurysm size or symptoms because of their longer period of risk. In addition, significant controversy persists in the question of clipping versus coiling. Despite the lower morbidity and mortality rates with coiling, current studies continue to demonstrate the long-term efficacy of surgery in contrast to the high rates of subtotal obliteration with endovascular coiling. This debate will undoubtedly persist; however, it should be clarified as our endovascular experience grows and as the factors that affect the natural history of UIAs are better elucidated.

■ References

1. Broderick JP, Brott T, Tomsick T, Miller R, Huster G. Intracerebral hemorrhage more than twice as common as subarachnoid hemorrhage. J Neurosurg 1993;78:188–191
2. Fogelholm R, Hernesniemi J, Vapalahti M. Impact of early surgery on outcome after aneurysmal subarachnoid hemorrhage. A population-based study. Stroke 1993;24:1649–1654
3. Weir B. Unruptured intracranial aneurysms: a review. J Neurosurg 2002;96:3–42
4. Ingall TJ, Whisnant JP, Wiebers DO, O'Fallon WM. Has there been a decline in subarachnoid hemorrhage mortality? Stroke 1989;20:718–724
5. Weir B, Disney L, Karrison T. Sizes of ruptured and unruptured aneurysms in relation to their sites and the ages of patients. J Neurosurg 2002;96:64–70
6. Inagawa T, Hirano A. Autopsy study of unruptured incidental intracranial aneurysms. Surg Neurol 1990;34:361–365
7. Asari S, Ohmoto T. Natural history and risk factors of unruptured cerebral aneurysms. Clin Neurol Neurosurg 1993;95:205–214
8. Locksley HB. Natural history of subarachnoid hemorrhage, intracranial aneurysms and arteriovenous malformations. J Neurosurg 1966;25:321–368
9. Rinkel GJ, Djibuti M, Algra A, van Gijn J. Prevalence and risk of rupture of intracranial aneurysms: a systematic review. Stroke 1998;29:251–256
10. Juvela S, Porras M, Heiskanen O. Natural history of unruptured intracranial aneurysms: a long-term follow-up study. J Neurosurg 1993;79:174–182
11. Wiebers DO, Whisnant JP, Sundt TM Jr, O'Fallon WM. The significance of unruptured intracranial saccular aneurysms. J Neurosurg 1987;66:23–29
12. Bederson JB, Awad IA, Wiebers DO, et al. Recommendations for the management of patients with unruptured intracranial aneurysms: a statement for healthcare professionals from the Stroke Council of the American Heart Association. Circulation 2000;102:2300–2308
13. Tsutsumi K, Ueki K, Morita A, Kirino T. Risk of rupture from incidental cerebral aneurysms. J Neurosurg 2000;93:550–553
14. Kappelle LJ, Eliasziw M, Fox AJ, Barnett HJ. Small, unruptured intracranial aneurysms and management of symptomatic carotid artery stenosis. North American Symptomatic Carotid Endarterectomy Trial Group. Neurology 2000;55:307–309
15. Unruptured intracranial aneurysms—risk of rupture and risks of surgical intervention. International Study of Unruptured Intracranial Aneurysms Investigators. N Engl J Med 1998;339:1725–1733
16. Juvela S, Porras M, Poussa K. Natural history of unruptured intracranial aneurysms: probability of and risk factors for aneurysm rupture. J Neurosurg 2000;93:379–387
17. Brennan JW, Schwartz ML. Unruptured intracranial aneurysms: appraisal of the literature and suggested recommendations for surgery, using evidence-based medicine criteria. Neurosurgery 2000;47:1359–1371, discussion 1352–1371
18. Weir BK, Kongable GL, Kassell NF, et al. Cigarette smoking as a cause of aneurysmal subarachnoid hemorrhage and risk for vasospasm: a report of the Cooperative Aneurysm Study. J Neurosurg 1998;89:405–411
19. Khanna RK, Malik GM, Qureshi N. Predicting outcome following surgical treatment of unruptured intracranial aneurysms: a proposed grading system. J Neurosurg 1996;84:49–54
20. Solomon RA, Fink ME, Pile-Spellman J. Surgical management of unruptured intracranial aneurysms. J Neurosurg 1994;80:440–446
21. Tsutsumi K, Ueki K, Usui M, Kwak S, Kirino T. Risk of subarachnoid hemorrhage after surgical treatment of unruptured cerebral aneurysms. Stroke 1999;30:1181–1184
22. Deruty R, Pelissou-Guyotat I, Mottolese C, Amat D. Management of unruptured cerebral aneurysms. Neurol Res 1996;18:39–44
23. King JT Jr, Berlin JA, Flamm ES. Morbidity and mortality from elective surgery for asymptomatic, unruptured, intracranial aneurysms: a meta-analysis. J Neurosurg 1994;81:837–842
24. Raaymakers TW, Rinkel GJ, Limburg M, Algra A. Mortality and morbidity of surgery for unruptured intracranial aneurysms: a meta-analysis. Stroke 1998;29:1531–1538
25. Wirth FP, Laws ER Jr, Piepgras D, Scott RM. Surgical treatment of incidental intracranial aneurysms. Neurosurgery 1983;12:507–511
26. Ohno K, Arai T, Isotani E, Nariai T, Hirakawa K. Ischaemic complication following obliteration of unruptured cerebral aneurysms with atherosclerotic or calcified neck. Acta Neurochir (Wien) 1999;141:699–705 discussion 705–696
27. Lawton MT, Daspit CP, Spetzler RF. Technical aspects and recent trends in the management of large and giant midbasilar artery aneurysms. Neurosurgery 1997;41:513–520, discussion 511–520
28. Rice BJ, Peerless SJ, Drake CG. Surgical treatment of unruptured aneurysms of the posterior circulation. J Neurosurg 1990;73:165–173
29. David CA, Vishteh AG, Spetzler RF, et al. Late angiographic follow-up review of surgically treated aneurysms. J Neurosurg 1999;91:396–401

30. Chyatte D, Porterfield R. Functional outcome after repair of unruptured intracranial aneurysms. J Neurosurg 2001;94: 417–421

31. Solomon RA, Mayer SA, Tarmey JJ. Relationship between the volume of craniotomies for cerebral aneurysm performed at New York state hospitals and in-hospital mortality. Stroke 1996;27: 13–17

32. Brilstra EH, Rinkel GJ, van der Graaf Y, van Rooij WJ, Algra A. Treatment of intracranial aneurysms by embolization with coils: a systematic review. Stroke 1999;30:470–476

33. Wardlaw JM, White PM. The detection and management of unruptured intracranial aneurysms. Brain 2000;123(Pt 2):205–221

34. Johnston SC, Zhao S, Dudley RA, Berman MF, Gress DR. Treatment of unruptured cerebral aneurysms in California. Stroke 2001;32:597–605

35. Johnston SC, Wilson CB, Halbach VV, et al. Endovascular and surgical treatment of unruptured cerebral aneurysms: comparison of risks. Ann Neurol 2000;48:11–19

36. Wanke I, Doerfler A, Dietrich U, et al. Endovascular treatment of unruptured intracranial aneurysms. AJNR Am J Neuroradiol 2002;23:756–761

37. Murayama Y, Vinuela F, Duckwiler GR, Gobin YP, Guglielmi G. Embolization of incidental cerebral aneurysms by using the Guglielmi detachable coil system. J Neurosurg 1999;90:207–214

38. Hayakawa M, Murayama Y, Duckwiler GR, et al. Natural history of the neck remnant of a cerebral aneurysm treated with the Guglielmi detachable coil system. J Neurosurg 2000;93:561–568

39. Murayama Y, Nien YL, Duckwiler G, et al. Guglielmi detachable coil embolization of cerebral aneurysms: 11 years' experience. J Neurosurg 2003;98:959–966

8

Surgical Treatment of Anterior Circulation Aneurysms

G. EDWARD VATES, GANESH SHANKAR AND ARTHUR L. DAY

Objectives: Upon completion of this chapter, the reader should be able to summarize the microsurgical techniques utilized in the treatment of internal carotid artery, middle cerebral artery, and anterior cerebral artery aneurysms, as well as the results that can be expected with these techniques.

Accreditation: The AANS* is accredited by the Accreditation Council for Continuing Medical Education (ACCME) to sponsor continuing medical education for physicians.

Credit: The AANS designates this educational activity for a maximum of 15 credits in Category 1 credit toward the AMA Physician's Recognition Award. Each physician should claim only those hours of credit that he/she spent in the educational activity.

The Home Study Examination is online on the AANS Web site at: http://www.aans.org/education/books/controversy.asp

* The acronym AANS refers to both the American Association of Neurological Surgeons and the American Association of Neurosurgeons.

Saccular or berry aneurysms display several anatomic characteristics (i.e., shape, relationship to their artery of origin) that distinguish them from other types of intracranial aneurysms (**Fig. 8–1**).[1,2] Saccular aneurysms typically (1) arise at bifurcations, usually just distal to a branch from a large parent vessel (i.e., internal carotid-posterior communicating [PComArt] junction), (2) arise along a curve of the parent vessel, (3) point in the direction that flow would have proceeded had the curve not been present, (4) are associated with a specific set of perforators, and (5) are best managed surgically with a specific clip type. In this chapter we address the surgical issues associated with saccular aneurysms that arise within the anterior circulation beyond the carotid artery exit from the cavernous sinus. We include internal carotid, anterior cerebral and middle cerebral artery lesions, both ruptured and unruptured.

■ Decision-Making

Each patient has a unique set of anatomical and clinical factors that affect the physician's choice of therapy. The principle anatomical factors that influence treatment of an anterior circulation aneurysm include aneurysm size, location, shape, intraluminal thrombus, and associated calcification. Other clinical factors to be considered include the presence of aneurysm rupture, patient age, general preexisting medical and neurological status, Hunt and Hess grade following subarachnoid hemorrhage (SAH), and other less-quantitative measures that suggest the patient's ability to tolerate the physiological stress of either open surgical or endovascular treatment.

More than 90% of all intracranial aneurysms arise on or near the circle of Willis, the vast majority from the anterior circulation.[3] Several large clinical series suggest

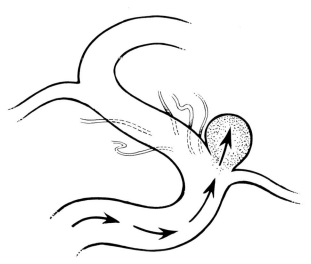

FIGURE 8–1 Intracranial saccular aneurysms generally: (1) arise at a branching site along the parent artery, (2) arise along the outside (convex) surface of a bend in the parent artery, (3) project in the direction of flow (arrows) that the parent artery would have if the bend had not been present, and (4) are associated with a specific set of perforators. Aneurysms at specific sites are usually best obliterated with a specific clip type that conforms to the lesion's shape, size, and anatomical relationships to the parent vessel, its branches, and adjacent structures.

a slight preponderance of aneurysms on the anterior cerebral artery/anterior communicating artery complex (**Table 8–1**), followed closely by the internal carotid artery (ICA). Autopsy series (which logically include a higher number of asymptomatic incidentally discovered aneurysms) suggest that middle cerebral artery aneurysms are actually the most common location.[3] More recent clinical series suggest that the factors involved in aneurysm formation are different from the factors that promote rupture.[4,5]

Aneurysm location and rupture risks appear to be influenced by sex and age. Overall, aneurysms are more common in women than men.[3,6,7] In children, the male:female ratio at time of presentation is 3:2, in young adults 1:1, and in older adults 2:3.[8] In women, the most common aneurysm site, either ruptured or unruptured,

is the supraclinoid ICA (66% and 40%, respectively). In men, the most common site for a ruptured aneurysm is the anterior communicating artery complex (44%), but for unruptured aneurysms it is the supraclinoid ICA (34%). Women are much more likely to develop ophthalmic segment (3.3 to 1) or communicating segment (2.1 to 1) aneurysms compared with men, but men are more likely to develop aneurysms of the anterior communicating artery complex (1.4 to 1). Aneurysms can occur at any time in life but are rare in children and adolescents. They are most common in 50 and 60 year olds.[3,6,9,10] Multiple aneurysms are found in 20 to 30% of patients with aneurysmal SAH.[11–16] Factors associated with increased risk of formation of multiple aneurysms include hypertension, smoking, female sex, and age.[13,14,17,18]

▪ Natural History and Conservative Management

The Unruptured Aneurysm

The International Study of Unruptured Intracranial Aneurysms Reports

Because of the widespread use and increasing sensitivity of imaging technology, a growing number of patients are diagnosed with unruptured, asymptomatic intracranial aneurysms. How these patients should be counseled is a hotly debated issue, prompted largely by the results of the International Study of Unruptured Intracranial Aneurysms (ISUIA).[5,14] Patients harboring unruptured aneurysms have a potentially devastating condition, but the decision to treat the asymptomatic lesion requires a careful comparison of the risks of rupture to those associated with intervention. The ISUIA was a combined retrospective and prospective study, published in two parts, primarily designed to address the relationship of aneurysm size to risk of rupture.[5,14] The retrospective data from the first report showed that aneurysm rupture risk depended on the size and location of the aneurysm and the presence or absence of a previously ruptured

Table 8–1 Aneurysm Distribution by Location

Parent Vessel	Cooperative Study[86] (n = 2630)	Fox[3] (n = 3110)	Yasargil[67] (n = 1012)	Cooperative Study[6,32] (n = 3521)	ISAT[81] (n = 2143)	ISUIA[5] (n = 3375)	Weighted Averages (n = 12349)
ICA	41	37	31.5	30	22	36	*33.5*
ACA	34	30.7	40.7	39	51	15	*35.7*
MCA	20	13.4	18.2	22	14	35	*19.1*
BA/VA	3.8	13.5	9.6	7	2.7	14	*7.9*

Abbreviations: ISAT, International Subarachnoid Aneurysm Trial; ISUIA, International Study of Unruptured Intracranial Aneurysms; ICA, internal carotid artery; ACA, anterior cerebral artery complex; MCA, middle cerebral artery; BA/VA basilar and vertebral artery complex.

aneurysm elsewhere. The goal of the prospective arm of the study was to determine the natural history of unruptured aneurysms and the morbidity and mortality associated with treatment. Size and location were the most important variables in predicting annual incidence of SAH, although the incremental size categories were changed. Age was not a significant factor in the risk of rupture, and a history of SAH had no effect on rupture rates except in the smallest size category.

Based on the findings from the retrospective study, the determined critical size of the "dangerous" unruptured aneurysm was set at 10 mm, unless there was a history of prior SAH from an aneurysm elsewhere, or the lesion arose from a posterior circulation or PComArt location.[19] With the publication of the prospective natural history data, the minimum size for treatment was lowered to 7 mm. These findings and treatment recommendations struck many as flawed, biased, and not representative of those commonly seen by practicing neurosurgeons. Nonetheless, these studies emphasize that the rupture risk from incidental aneurysms, while still undefined, is likely significantly lower than previously portrayed, particularly at certain locations. The studies also indicate that morbidity, mortality, and efficacy rates differ for the intervention and the practitioner. Therefore, treatment options for each individual patient must be carefully weighed and compared with the natural history of unruptured aneurysms left untreated.

The Ruptured Aneurysm

Subarachnoid Hemorrhage

The incidence of aneurysmal SAH varies from 6 to 26 per 100,000 population per year; Finland and Japan report the highest values.[20-30] Women outnumber men by a ratio of 1.6:1 in most large series,[31,32] although men predominate before age 50.[33] In the United States, the peak age for aneurysm rupture is between 40 and 60 years.[6,31,32,34-36] The annual incidence rate increases from 3 per 100,000 population in 30 year olds to 30 per 100,000 in 60 year olds.[21,24,26-28] For survivors of the acute hemorrhage, the untreated lesion carries a mortality rate during the first 2 weeks of 20 to 30%, with an additional morbidity rate of ~20%.[32,35,36] Rebleeding is a major cause of this early morbidity and mortality; the risk of rebleeding during the first 2 weeks is ~20% and increases to 33% at 1 month and 50% at 6 months.[32,36-39] The mortality rate for the untreated lesion is ~50% during the first year following rupture. The risk of rebleeding diminishes thereafter (estimated 3% annually); the mortality rate associated with second hemorrhage is 40 to 50%.[7,37] Up to 25 to 35% of patients are found dead after the initial hemorrhage.[6,7,18,32,40] Warning signs are reported in 15 to 60% of cases and may be attributed to

minor hemorrhage (or "sentinel leak"), aneurysmal expansion, or ischemia.[41-43] Half of these events occur within a week of the eventual SAH, and 90% within 6 weeks of SAH.[41,44] The obvious consequence of missing the warning event is a missed opportunity to prevent a neurologically devastating hemorrhage.

■ Treatment Risks, Indications, and Contraindications

When considering the treatment options of a particular aneurysm, several general anatomical factors should be analyzed. Saccular aneurysms typically have a narrower "neck" and a broader, rounded fundus. A small, narrow-necked aneurysm is amenable to both surgical and endovascular obliteration. Such shapes are particularly favorable for endovascular treatment, because the narrow neck makes it easier to pack the aneurysm fundus with a dense coil mass without coil prolapse into the parent artery or associated branch vessel. When the aneurysm neck is broad compared with the maximal diameter of the aneurysm, however, endovascular intervention is less likely to be curative, as the broad neck makes dense packing of the aneurysm difficult and coil prolapse into the parent artery or associated branch vessel more likely. New stent and balloon-assist techniques increase the endovascular obliteration rate for these lesions, but such techniques are also more hazardous than coiling alone, and open surgical reconstruction becomes preferable in some instances. Most large or giant aneurysms (10 to 25 mm or >25 mm, respectively) are currently better treated surgically. The durability of endovascular techniques is poor, often due to progressive compaction of the coil mass within the fundus of an aneurysm caused by arterial pressure waves that enter through a relatively large arterial orifice at the neck of the lesion. Larger lesions with intraluminal thrombus are very prone to this phenomenon; when managed by endovascular methods, retreatment is commonly required.

Anterior circulation aneurysms are generally associated with characteristic sets of very small perforating vessels, and recognition of the associated perforating arteries is critical to successful treatment. Surgical obliteration must spare these perforators to avoid a potentially devastating neurological injury. In certain locations (e.g., superior projecting anterior communicating artery aneurysms), the dissection and identification of these perforators are more difficult, and endovascular treatment may be preferred if other features of the aneurysm are also favorable to endovascular occlusion. Some aneurysms compress adjacent neural structures (e.g., optic or oculomotor nerves) or rupture to produce potential life-threatening increased intracranial pressure from an associated intraparenchymal hematoma. In these instances, endovascular techniques may obliterate the aneurysm, but mass effect is not eliminated; open surgical treatment is often preferable.

The Unruptured Aneurysm

In the ISUIA data, the 30-day morbidity and mortality associated with open surgical treatment of unruptured aneurysms (with or without a prior history of SAH) was 11% and 13.7%, respectively. Endovascular treatment showed morbidity and mortality at 7% and 9.3% for the same groups. The 1-year morbidity and mortality after open surgical treatment declined to 10.1% and 11.6%, and to 7.1% and 9.8% for endovascular treatment, respectively. Significant treatment risk factors associated with poor outcome were age > 50, aneurysm size >12 mm, and posterior circulation location. The natural history and results of treatment, however, are far from homogenous, with variations present depending on location, aneurysm morphology, patient characteristics, and experience of the treatment team. The decision to treat an unruptured aneurysm as well as how to treat an individual lesion should be made by a physician who is aware of the treatment options and their risks, compared with the available data about the risk of rupture without treatment. Clearly, the ISUIA data confirms that age is a significant risk factor for surgery; any patient over 65 years of age with an unruptured aneurysm should be given strong considerations for endovascular treatment when treatment is considered.

The Ruptured Aneurysm

Physicians traditionally assign a clinical grade to patients presenting with ruptured saccular aneurysms, using the Hunt and Hess grading system that heavily emphasizes level of consciousness at time of presentation (**Table 8–2**). A major limitation, however, is that the scale was devised before the advent of computerized tomography (CT) scanning; therefore, it does not differentiate between altered states of consciousness due to systemic derangement, hydrocephalus, or hemorrhage extent.[45–47]

A clinical grade calculated after maximal cardiopulmonary resuscitation and intracranial pressure (ICP) control with a ventriculostomy is actually a better predictor of ultimate outcome.

Aneurysmal SAH patients are generally divided into good (Hunt and Hess grades I, II, and III) and poor (Hunt and Hess grades IV and V) clinical grades.[48] Following the results of the International Study on the Timing of Aneurysm Surgery (ISTAS), early surgery is now the standard of care for most patients.[6,32,49] This standard has been reinforced by studies demonstrating that in good-grade patients (Hunt and Hess grades I to III), the combination of early surgery, calcium antagonists, and hypervolemic–hypertensive therapy can reduce overall management mortality to 10% or less, with good outcomes in 75% or more of those who survive.[50–53]

However, approximately 20 to 40% of patients with aneurysmal SAH fall in the poor grades; the association between poor outcome and poor clinical grade following SAH is clear.[48,54,55] Data suggest that 35 to 50% of poor-grade patients have a reasonable neurological outcome with aggressive therapy, particularly if the determination of clinical grade is made before the insertion of a ventriculostomy.[48,54–56] The initial clinical and radiographic findings are frequently inaccurate predictors of outcome; hence, aggressive treatment is warranted until the likelihood of irreversible brain injury is clarified. The brain of the high-grade SAH patient is often swollen and congested with bloody cerebrospinal fluid (CSF) throughout the subarachnoid space, and such a "tight" brain does not tolerate surgical manipulation or retraction well. Poor-grade patients, therefore, are generally best treated with ventriculostomy and endovascular intervention in most instances, unless a large, life-threatening clot is contributing to the obtundation. Radiographic evidence of permanent injury incompatible with functional survival (e.g., a large hematoma in the dominant basal ganglia), sustained elevated ICP greater than 50 mm Hg, or poor or absent intracranial filling of large or critical vascular territories on angiography are contraindications to surgical or endovascular treatment of any type.

■ Treatment Strategies

Diagnostic Evaluation

When SAH is suspected, evaluation should include a clinical history, general physical and neurological examination, routine laboratory studies (electrocardiography, electrolytes, complete blood count, coagulation tests), CT scan (lumbar puncture if the CT scan is negative), and some type of procedure demonstrating the

---

Table 8–2 Clinical Grading of Subarachnoid Hemorrhage*

Grade	Condition
I	Asymptomatic or with mild headache
II	Moderate or severe headache, nuchal rigidity
III	Confusion, drowsiness, or mold focal deficit (discounting third nerve palsy)
IV	Stupor or hemiparesis, early decerebrate rigidity
V	Deep coma, extensor posturing

*According to the Hunt and Hess scale.[46]

details of the intracranial vessels (computed tomographic angiography [CTA], magnetic resonance angiography [MRA], or four-vessel cerebral angiography). A CT scan is the first diagnostic test to be ordered when bleeding is suspected, as hemorrhage can be detected in ~95% of patients with aneurysm rupture if the study is obtained within 24 hours.[57,58] The distribution of blood suggests the aneurysm site in most cases and allows accurate predictions of the risk of subsequent vasospasm. A CT scan also clarifies associated conditions such as intracranial hematoma, edema, and hydrocephalus. It can also be extremely useful in clarifying the exact anatomical relation of the aneurysm to the skull base or the presence of thrombus or calcification within the aneurysm or parent vessel. A negative CT scan does not rule out SAH, and if the history is highly suggestive of an aneurysmal hemorrhage, lumbar puncture is mandatory. Evidence of hemorrhage in the CSF (xanthochromia) persists for 1 to 2 weeks, depending on the severity of the hemorrhage.

High-quality four-vessel angiography remains unsurpassed for diagnosis and surgical planning. Preoperative angiographic studies determine several key features: (1) the aneurysm's presence, location, size, shape, and relationship to parent and adjacent arteries; (2) the presence and distribution of vasospasm; (3) displacement of adjacent vessels suggesting mass effect from hematoma or partial thrombosis of an aneurysmal sac; and (4) the presence of other aneurysms or other vascular abnormalities. As many as 20 to 30% of patients have multiple aneurysms; therefore, a complete four-vessel study should be performed unless the patient's condition dictates otherwise. Computerized tomographic angiography (CTA) is rapidly gaining ground as an adjunct or even an alternative to conventional arteriography. While potentially not as sensitive as conventional angiography for the detection of small aneurysms, this technology is noninvasive and often quicker to obtain, making it more valuable in the patient acutely declining from an intraparenchymal hematoma who needs urgent intervention.[59] For patients with unruptured aneurysms, CTA and MRA combined with CT and magnetic resonance imaging (MRI) are excellent screening tests, and transfemoral arteriography may not be required when study quality is excellent, thereby sparing exposure to the risks of arteriography.

Treatment Options: Preoperative Assessment, Management, and Timing of Surgical Intervention

Unruptured asymptomatic anterior circulation aneurysms are treated electively, combining the preferences and schedules of both the patient and physician. Symptomatic lesions, however, are treated much more urgently, as the recent change in clinical status (i.e., recent oculomotor nerve dysfunction associated with an enlarging PComArt aneurysm) is often a harbinger of an upcoming hemorrhage. Our algorithm for the perioperative management of ruptured anterior circulation aneurysms is outlined in **Figure 8–2**. Initial management

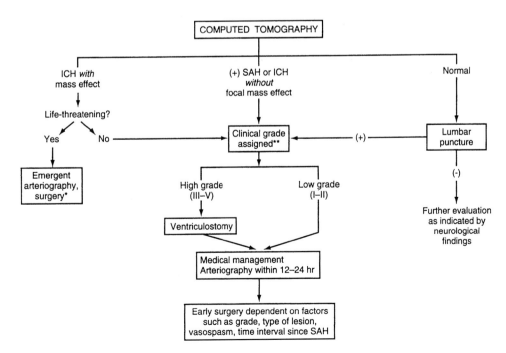

FIGURE 8–2 Algorithm for evaluation and management of anterior circulation aneurysms.

is focused on the conditions that could be acutely fatal or cause permanent injury, including hypoxia (from seizures, respiratory depression, and cardiovascular dysfunction) and increased intracranial pressure (from hydrocephalus and/or hematoma). Good-grade patients (Hunt and Hess grades I to III) harboring lesions judged to be best-treated surgically are treated within 24 hours after admission, unless other major clinical problems (i.e., myocardial dysfunction, pneumonia, etc.) or severe angiographic vasospasm are evident. In our opinion, all grade III or higher patients should have an immediate ventriculostomy, followed by intervention (either open surgical or endovascular) within 24 to 48 hours unless a life-threatening clot requires emergent evacuation. Great care is taken to prevent hypovolemia and hypotension in the perioperative period, especially during the interval of highest vasospasm incidence (4 to 10 days after SAH).

■ Treatment Techniques

General Operative Techniques: Single and Multimodal

Surgical approach to anterior circulation aneurysms is best performed through a pterional craniotomy. The details of the general surgical technique have been described previously. What follow here are some recent observations regarding site-specific nuances that affect surgical approach and that may sway the decision process away from open surgical clipping and toward endovascular therapy.

Site-Specific: Single and Multimodal

Proximal (Paraclinoid) Internal Carotid Artery Aneurysms (Clinoidal and Ophthalmic Segments)

Anatomy, Terminology, and Aneurysm Variants
Ophthalmic segment aneurysms occur as three variants: ophthalmic artery, superior hypophyseal, and dorsal carotid wall (**Fig. 8–3**). Ophthalmic artery aneurysms originate just beyond the takeoff of the ophthalmic artery and point dorsomedially toward the lateral half of the optic nerve.[60–63] Superior hypophyseal artery aneurysms arise from the inferomedial surface of the ophthalmic segment and have no relationship to the ophthalmic artery origin.[61–63] One (parasellar) variant burrows inferiorly and medially toward and below the diaphragma sella, expanding into the "carotid cave." When small, this variant is covered by parasellar dura, and its risk of SAH is extremely low. Once these lesions reach a size or projection sufficient to extend medially into the suprasellar space above the diaphragma sella (suprasellar variant), hemorrhage risks increase.[61–63]

The dorsal variant is the least common type and arises along the dorsal ICA surface well distal to the ophthalmic artery origin. Some appear to be pure hemodynamically induced saccular lesions, while others are blister-like and may represent dissections.[60–63] Ophthalmic segment aneurysms are very common, perhaps the most common aneurysm found in women. Most are small and asymptomatic, and hemorrhage risks are lower than for aneurysms arising elsewhere. Symptomatic lesions present in roughly equal proportions between visual symptoms and SAH; those presenting with visual deficits are usually giant (≥ 25 mm).

Clinoidal segment aneurysms are divided into the anterolateral and medial variants[64] (**Fig. 8–4**). The former arises from the anterolateral surface of the clinoidal segment as it ascends between the carotid-oculomotor membrane (COM) and the dural ring (DR) medial to the anterior clinoid process (ACP). The hemodynamic vector on this ICA portion promotes a superomedial projection that can erode into or through the optic strut and ACP, compressing the ipsilateral optic nerve within the optic canal or secondarily reaching the subarachnoid space.[61] The medial variant projects medially, below the diaphragma sella, into the pituitary fossa.[61] Larger lesions can cause pituitary dysfunction or eventually expand into the subarachnoid space or sphenoid sinus.

Careful interpretation of radiographic studies, including CT and MRI scans as well as cerebral arteriography, is required for an accurate differentiation between subtypes of clinoidal and ophthalmic segment aneurysms. The indications for intervention vary among paraclinoid aneurysm subtypes (e.g., small clinoidal segment lesions are not treated as aggressively as most ophthalmic segment aneurysms), as several variants have extremely low hemorrhage risks at that size. In addition, surgical technique differs between aneurysm variants (e.g., exposure of the cervical internal carotid artery, degree of clinoid removal), and each has specific problem areas of the exposure required for safe clip obliteration. A ruptured ophthalmic segment aneurysm usually produces hemorrhage within the chiasmatic and parasellar cisterns or, rarely, a focal clot within the orbitofrontale gyrus; because of the medial projection, bleeding is sometimes more prominent contralateral to the origin of the aneurysm.[61,63] Intraluminal thrombosis or calcification must be clarified, as well as the bony anatomy of the anterior clinoid process (e.g., demonstrable erosion of the anterior clinoid process or optic strut suggests an anterolateral variant clinoidal segment aneurysm). An MRI scan can provide anatomical information about the aneurysms relation to the optic nerves or pituitary gland.[65]

Four-vessel transfemoral cerebral arteriography is very helpful in defining the anatomic characteristics of lesions in this region and in defining other aneurysms

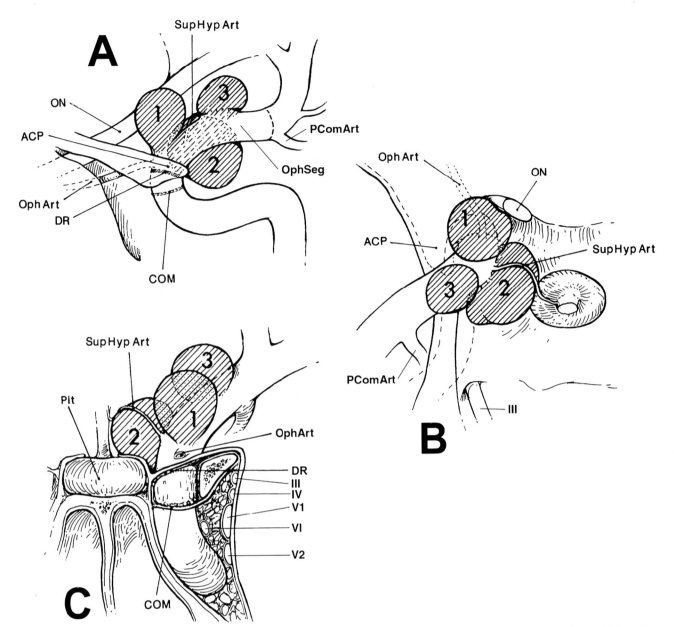

FIGURE 8–3 Ophthalmic segment aneurysms: **(A)** Lateral view. **(B)** Dorsal view. **(C)** Anteroposterior (AP) view. Ophthalmic artery (OphArt) aneurysms (hatched area 1) arise from the dorsomedial internal carotid artery surface just distal to the takeoff of the OphArt. SupHypArt aneurysms (hatched area 2) arise from the medial or inferomedial ICA surface distal to the OphArt in close association with the medially projecting superior hypophyseal perforators. Dorsal variant aneurysms (hatched area 3) are uncommon, usually purely hemodynamic lesions that arise from the dorsal ICA surface well distal to the OphArt origin and well apart from the optic apparatus. ACP, anterior clinoid process; AN, aneurysm; CN VI, abducens nerve; COM, carotid-oculomotor membrane; III, oculomotor nerve, IV, trochlear nerve; ON, optic nerve; PcomArt, posterior communicating artery; Pit, pituitary gland; V1, first division of the trigeminal nerve; V2, second division of the trigeminal nerve.

elsewhere in the circulation. Multiplicity is common; up to 50% of patients with a paraclinoid aneurysm will have at least one other aneurysm elsewhere, often in the contralateral paraclinoid region. Even when combined with three-dimensional reconstructions, however, the precise type of aneurysm can be difficult to differentiate (i.e., small medial variant clinoidal segment vs. parasellar variant superior hypophyseal lesions). The cervical carotid artery should be inspected for atherosclerotic disease that would make temporary clamping treacherous. The superficial temporal artery should be inspected for its possible use as a bypass conduit. Ophthalmic artery aneurysms arise from the dorsal surface of the internal carotid artery, above the posterior bend and just

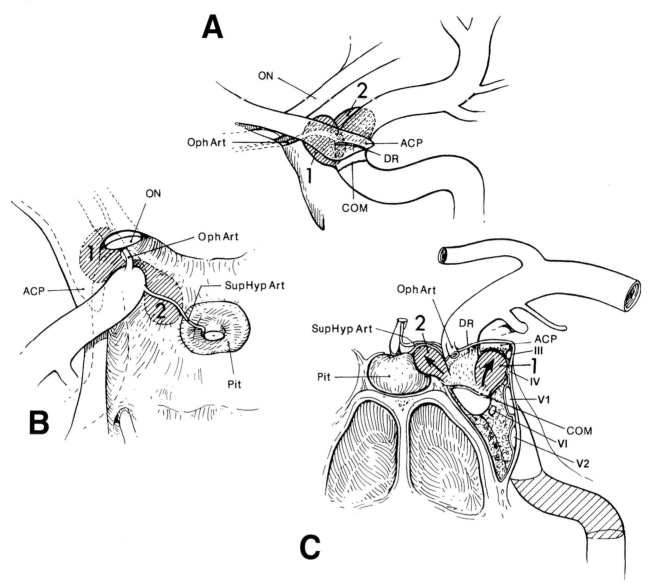

FIGURE 8–4 Clinoidal segment (ClinSeg) aneurysms schematic. **(A)** Lateral view. **(B)** Dorsal view. **(C)** Anteroposterior (AP) view. Aneurysm types (hatched areas): 1 = anterolateral variant; 2 = medial variant. Anterolateral variant ClinSeg aneurysms (hatched area 1) arise from the anterolateral bend of the ClinSeg and project dorsolaterally toward the anterior clinoid process (ACP), whereas medial variant ClinSeg aneurysms (hatched area 2) arise from the medial surface of the ClinSeg and project into the sella, below the diaphragma sella. Small ClinSeg aneurysms (<1 cm) typically remain interdural below the subarachnoid space, but larger lesions (~1 cm) may breach the overlying dura to enter the subarachnoid space. COM, carotid-oculomotor membrane; DR, dural ring; III, oculomotor nerve; IV, trochlear nerve; ON, optic nerve; OphArt, ophthalmic artery; Pit, pituitary gland; SupHypArt, superior hypophyseal artery; V1, first division of the trigeminal nerve; V2, second division of the trigeminal nerve; VI, abducens nerve.

distal to the origin of the ophthalmic artery (**Fig. 8–5**). Superior hypophyseal artery aneurysms arise from the inferior or inferomedial surface of the carotid artery and project medially or posterior-medially toward and above the sella. Dorsal carotid wall aneurysms project superiorly, similar to ophthalmic artery aneurysms, but they originate from a portion of the carotid artery distinctly separate from the origin of the ophthalmic artery. Clinoidal segment aneurysms appear as a "double density" overlying

the anterior ascending vertical segment of the ICA (**Fig. 8–6**). On antero-posterior (AP) projection, the anterolateral variant projects laterally toward or through the anterior clinoid process, whereas the medial variant projects off the medial ICA surface into the pituitary fossa below the diaphragma sella. Enlargement into the subarachnoid space is often accompanied by an angiographic "waist" that marks the point where the aneurysm traverses the dura to enter the subarachnoid space.[66]

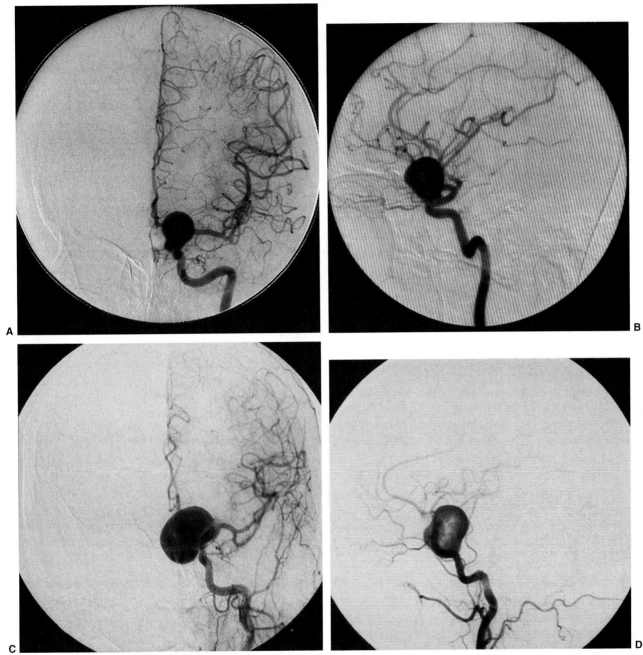

FIGURE 8–5 (A) Ophthalmic artery (OphArt) aneurysm: arteriogram (anterior–posterior view). **(B)** OphArt aneurysm: arteriogram (lateral view). Notice the aneurysm origin just distal to the OphArt origin, closing the carotid siphon, and remaining ipsilateral, tethered from further medial growth by the supero- medially displaced optic nerve. **(C)** Superior hypophyseal artery (SupHypArt) aneurysm: arteriogram (anteroposterior view). **(D)** SupHypArt aneurysm: arteriogram (lateral view). Notice the giant aneurysm projecting medially into the suprasellar space.

Specific Management

Broad-based, ophthalmic segment aneurysms are poorer candidates for complete endovascular obliteration unless a stent is added. Others carry a very low hemorrhage risk, and observation is often preferable, especially for older patients with small asymptomatic clinoidal (both variants) and parasellar variant superior hypophyseal ICA lesions. Thus, for those lesions that require treatment because of hemorrhage or neurological symptoms, surgical treatment in experienced hands is the safest and most secure way. This usually requires advanced surgical techniques, including anterior clinoidectomy, cervical carotid exposure and aneurysm trapping, and suction decompression of the aneurysm.

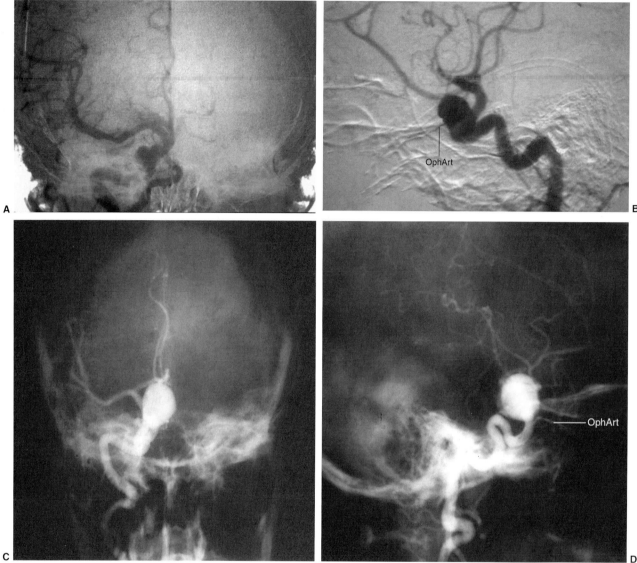

FIGURE 8–6 (A) Anterolateral variant clinoidal segment (ClinSeg) aneurysm: arteriogram (anteroposterior view). **(B)** Anterolateral variant ClinSeg aneurysm: arteriogram (lateral view). Notice the double density of the aneurysm origin from the clinoidal segment below the plane of the ophthalmic artery and the superolateral projection toward and through the anterior clinoid process. **(C)** Medial variant ClinSeg aneurysm: arteriogram (anteroposterior view). **(D)** Medial variant ClinSeg aneurysm: arteriogram (lateral view). Notice the similar double density of the aneurysm origin below the ophthalmic artery but with its projection medial to the internal carotid artery into the cell.

Distal Internal Carotid Artery Aneurysms

Distal ICA aneurysms are those arising beyond the ophthalmic segment PComArt, anterior choroidal (AChorArt), and ICA bifurcation lesions.

Anatomy, Terminology, and Aneurysm Variants

The communicating segment of the ICA begins with the takeoff of the PComArt and ends at the origin of the AChorArt. The PComArt originates from the posteromedial surface of the internal carotid artery, projects medially and inferiorly and penetrates the membrane of Lilliequist before joining the posterior cerebral artery (PCA) immediately lateral to the terminal basilar artery bifurcation. Several large thalamoperforators originate from the communicating segment, and these vessels often run near the PComArt through much of its course and may be adherent to the aneurysm wall. The typical PComArt aneurysm forms just distal to the origin of the PComArt and points posteriorly, slightly inferiorly, and slightly laterally (**Fig. 8–7**). There are two distinct subtypes defined by the degree of inferior or lateral projections: (1) posteroinferior lesions point medial to the tentorial incisura and may compress the oculomotor

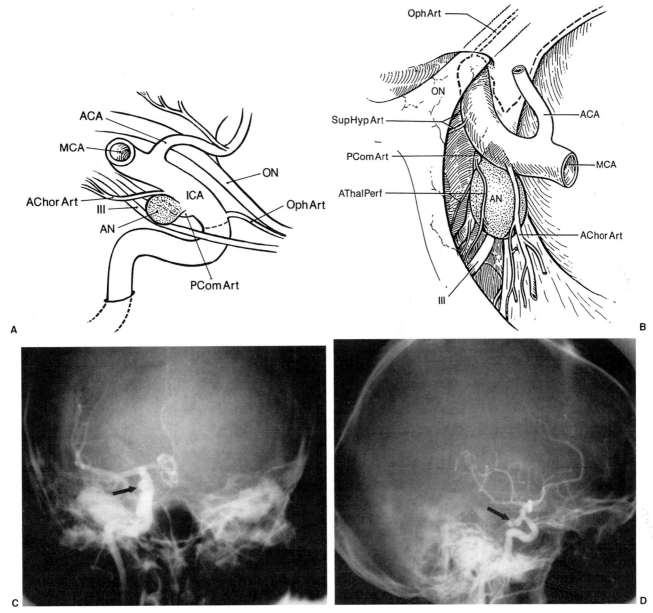

FIGURE 8–7 Posterior communicating artery aneurysm. Lateral **(A)** and dorsal **(B)** views (schematic). The aneurysm originates just beyond the posterior communicating artery and typically projects posteriorly, slightly laterally, and inferiorly, toward the oculomotor nerve. The posterior communicating artery courses medial to the aneurysm ("tethering" the aneurysm from medial expansion) and gives off small branches (the anterior thalamoperforating arteries) that may adhere to the medial aneurysm surface. **(C)** Anteroposterior and **(D)** lateral views on arteriography. Note the typical bilobed posterior communicating artery aneurysm (arrow) pointing posteriorly and slightly laterally and inferiorly off the posterior carotid artery wall. The dent separating the proximal from distal lobe invariably marks the compressed oculomotor nerve. ICA, internal carotid artery; MCA, middle cerebral artery; ACA, anterior cerebral artery; OphArt, ophthalmic artery; SupHypArt, superior hypophyseal arteries; PComArt, posterior communicating artery; AChorArt, nterior choroidal artery; AThalPerf, anterior thallamoperforating arteries; III, oculomotor nerve; AN, aneurysm.

nerve, and (2) laterally pointing lesions go above the tentorium and often densely adhere to the medial temporal lobe. Traditionally, PComArt aneurysms represent the most common type of anterior circulation aneurysm found in women, although the frequency of asymptomatic paraclinoid lesions is becoming increasingly recognized.[3,7,67] PComArt aneurysms typically present when small; they produce retro-orbital headaches, oculomotor nerve deficits (invariably involving the pupil), or SAH.[5]

The choroidal segment starts at the takeoff of the AChorArt, ends, and has similar hemodynamic factors as the communicating segment. The AChorArt typically arises several millimeters distal and lateral to the PComArt and swings posteriorly, following the optic tract and giving off branches to the tract, uncus, portions of the amygdala, and the anterior hippocampus before entering the choroidal fissure. The typical AChorArt aneurysm can be difficult to distinguish from a laterally projecting PComArt aneurysm. Internal carotid artery bifurcation aneurysms typically project upward toward and into the anterior perforated substance (**Fig. 8–8**). Lenticulostriate

perforating arteries rising nearby are always displaced posteriorly; they are often adherent to the aneurysm sac. An intracerebral hemorrhage from lesions in this location closely resembles a hypertensive basal ganglionic hemorrhage, both clinically and radiographically.[3,7,9,67]

Specific Management

In our experience, distal ICA aneurysms are potential candidates for either surgical or endovascular obliteration because they frequently have a small neck and are in

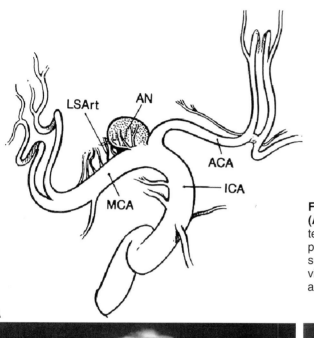

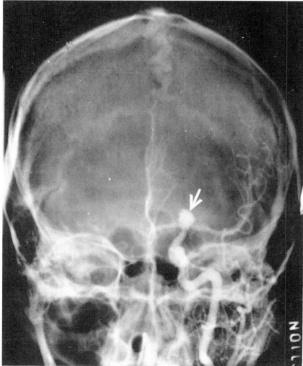

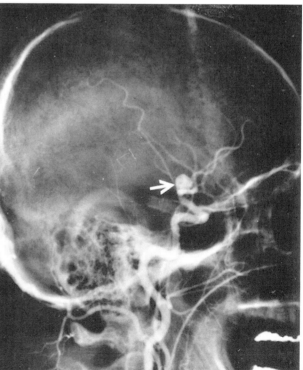

FIGURE 8–8 An internal carotid bifurcation aneurysm. **(A)** Frontal view (schematic). The aneurysm originates at the terminal carotid bifurcation, and the direction of flow generally projects the lesion superiorly toward the anterior perforated substance. **(B, C)** Arteriogram (anteroposterior and lateral views). Note the superior projection of the aneurysm (arrow) as a direct extension of the termination of the internal carotid artery.

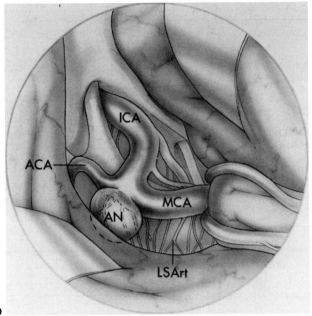
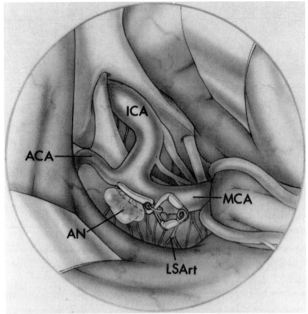

D

E

FIGURE 8–8 (continued) (D) Initial operative view, right pterional approach. The lenticulostriate arteries typically originate from the posterior-superior surface of the parent vessels, and the aneurysm arises more anteriorly. These perforating vessels are frequently adherent to the posterior or lateral aneurysm wall and must be separated from the aneurysm's base. (E) Final operative view, clipping. A gentle curved clip has been placed parallel to the anterior cerebral-middle cerebral axis, with the deep (posterior) blade closely applied to the posterior neck of the aneurysm to spare the lenticulostriate vessels. ICA, internal carotid artery; MCA, middle cerebral artery; ACA, anterior cerebral artery; LSArt, lenticulostriate arteries; AN, aneurysm.

readily accessible portions of the artery. As with lesions elsewhere, if the neck is broad or the aneurysm is large or giant, open surgery is preferred because the likelihood of complete endovascular obliteration is small. Aneurysms causing cranial nerve compression (i.e., optic tract or third nerve) or mass effect from an associated intraparenchymal hematoma are best treated by open occlusion and decompression.

Middle Cerebral Artery Aneurysms

Anatomy, Terminology, Aneurysm Variants

The middle cerebral artery (MCA) starts at the terminal bifurcation of the internal carotid artery and supplies the lateral two thirds of the cerebral hemisphere (**Fig. 8–9**). The M_1 segment travels laterally and parallel to the sphenoid ridge until it crosses the limen insulae, then takes a right-angle turn posteriorly and superiorly at the genu to enter the insular compartment of the deep sylvian fissure as the M_2 segment. Saccular MCA aneurysms arise in three distinct regions: (1) typical bifurcation—at the genu at the end of the M_1 segment, (2) distal—beyond the genu from the M_2 segment, and (3) proximal—M1 segment prior to the genu. Typical bifurcation lesions are by far the most common type and originate as a direct extension of the main trunk and project laterally, anteriorly, and slightly inferiorly between and beyond the branches at the genu, typically into the superior temporal gyrus. Distal aneurysms are rare and usually arise within the context of an elongated prebifurcation segment that does not bifurcate until reaching the deep insular compartment of the sylvian fissure. Most point laterally, superiorly, and somewhat posteriorly toward the inferior frontal lobe operculum. Proximal aneurysms are further subdivided into the M_1 branch from which they arise: (1) lenticulostriate—combined with an exaggerated bend in the M1 prebifurcation segment; (2) early (or anterior) temporal artery; and (3) short MCA prebifurcation segment (with correspondingly long postbifurcation trunks straddling the aneurysm). MCA aneurysms may present with hemorrhage, temporal lobe seizures, or ischemic stroke due to intra-aneurysmal thrombosis and embolism.[9] The CT SAH pattern is usually limited to the ipsilateral sylvian fissure; intraparenchymal hemorrhage usually occurs into the superior temporal gyrus, especially the typical bifurcation lesions.[3]

Specific Management

The majority of MCA aneurysms exhibit anatomy unfavorable for complete endovascular obliteration, and most lesions are currently best treated with open

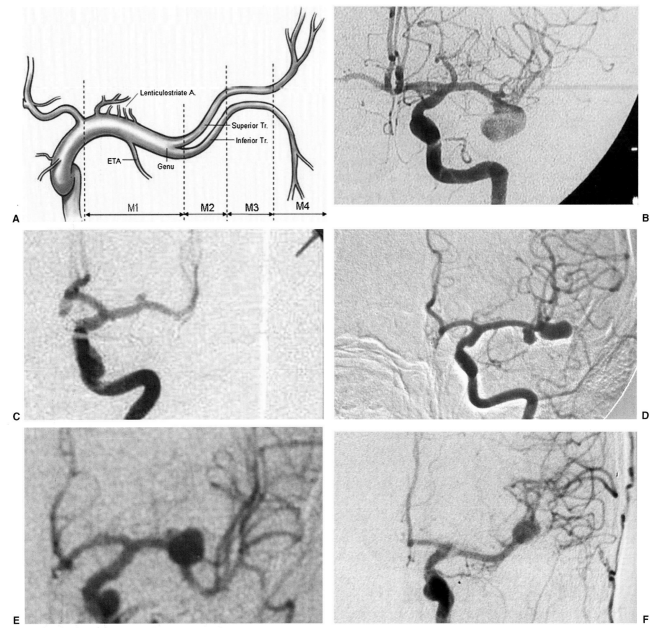

FIGURE 8–9 (A) Drawing showing MCA anatomy terminology. The M1 is the segment between the internal carotid artery bifurcation and the genu at the inferior border of the insula; M2 are the segments that run in the deep insular compartment of the sylvian fissure, including the superior and inferior trunks; M3 are the segments and branches that traverse the opercular surface of the sylvian fissure to reach the cortical surface; and M4 are the cortical surface branches. **(B)** Typical MCA bifurcation aneurysm: arteriogram (anteroposterior view). Notice how the aneurysm projects inferiorly and laterally into the superior temporal gyrus. **(C)** Lenticulostriate artery aneurysm: arteriogram (anteroposterior view). Notice how the aneurysm arises at a bend the M1 segment makes under the inferior frontal lobe in the region of the anterior perforated substance, where lenticulostriate branches enter the brain. **(D)** Typical MCA bifurcation aneurysm with an adjacent early temporal artery aneurysm more proximal on the M1 segment: arteriogram (anteroposterior view). **(E)** Short prebifurcation segment MCA aneurysm: arteriogram (anteroposterior view). Note how the foreshortened M1 segment places the bifurcation and associated aneurysm under the frontal lobe and not in the sylvian fissure. **(F)** Distal M2 segment MCA aneurysm: arteriogram (anteroposterior view). Unlike the short prebifurcation segment MCA aneurysm, this aneurysm is located in the sylvian fissure between the insula and the operculum because the MCA bifurcation occurs after the genu. ETA, early or anterior temporal artery; Tr, trunk.

microsurgical intervention. Special care should be taken during planning of the approach to preserve the dominant branch of the superficial temporal artery as a possible bypass donor vessel if needed. Typical MCA bifurcation aneurysms are easily approached through a standard pterional craniotomy, but proximal MCA aneurysms are situated under the insula and have a much more intimate association with the lenticulostriate vessels, making exposure and clipping more difficult. Greater resection of the sphenoid wing is required to provide a subfrontal trajectory. A fronto-orbital osteotomy may be added to give an even better viewing angle. Temporary clipping under barbiturate protection is particularly useful in treating these aneurysms because premature rupture risks disastrous perforator injury. Likewise, excessively long clips should be avoided to spare all perforators from inadvertent occlusion.

Distal MCA aneurysms usually lie completely within the insular compartment of the sylvian fissure and have no relationship to lenticulostriate vessels. The aneurysm often projects more superiorly, making any intracerebral hemorrhage more likely to be in the frontal lobe. When exposing distal lesions, the surgeon must note which trunk harbors the aneurysm, and then must work on the "safe" side of the fissure away from the aneurysm until proximal control is assured. The more peripheral middle cerebral branches and their aneurysms are usually smaller, and miniclips are therefore more appropriate so that the weight of the clip does not torque or kink the parent vessel.

Proximal Anterior Cerebral Aneurysms

Anatomy, Terminology, and Aneurysm Variants

The proximal anterior cerebral artery (A_1) begins at the terminal internal carotid artery bifurcation and proceeds medially and anteriorly over the optic chiasm to the interhemispheric fissure, where it joins its contralateral mate at the anterior communicating artery. Almost all aneurysms from this segment arise in association with the anterior communicating artery (AComArt). Aneurysms of the proximal anterior cerebral and anterior communicating arteries are the most common aneurysms in men (accounting for 40 to 50% in different series) and are some of the most challenging in terms of anatomy.[3,7,67] Most anterior communicating artery aneurysms are associated with a dominant A_1 segment and hypoplasia of the contralateral A_1, and consequently point toward the hemisphere contralateral to the dominant A_1 as a continuation of the direction of flow (**Fig. 8–10**). Variability in the number and size of the anterior communicating artery region is common. Perforators originating from the proximal anterior cerebral artery and the anterior communicating artery supply the fornix, optic chiasm, anterior hypothalamus,

anterior limb of the internal capsule, and other portions of the septal region. The distal anterior cerebral artery (A_2) begins at the anterior communicating artery and runs within the interhemispheric fissure to supply the medial third of the cerebral hemispheres and the corpus callosum. Usually, the A_2 segments of each hemisphere are equally sized; variations in this pattern include an unpaired (azygous) A_2 or a duplicated A_2, giving rise to three distal anterior cerebral arteries. The recurrent artery of Heubner typically originates from A_2 just beyond the communicating artery and courses laterally parallel to the course of the ipsilateral A_1 to supply the anterior parts of the caudate, globus pallidus, and internal capsule.

Specific Management

AComArt aneurysms can be divided into two types based on their direction of projection: (1) anterior/inferior—extending below the plane of the ascending A_2 vessels as seen on a lateral view angiogram, and (2) superior/posterior—projecting between or behind the two A_2 vessels (**Fig. 8–10**). The first type often adheres to the top of the visual system and produces hemorrhage patterns confined to the basal subarachnoid space or contralateral inferior frontal lobe and gyrus rectus. The inferior projection of the first type makes early visualization of the contralateral A_1 segment during surgery more difficult; it is best approached surgically from the side of the dominant A_1. However, surgical treatment of these aneurysms is more straightforward because the aneurysm fundus is usually free of any relationship to important septal perforators coming off the AComArt; for this reason, inferiorly projecting AComArt aneurysms are usually best treated surgically. In contrast, the fundus of the superior projecting lesion is embedded in the interhemispheric fissure. The aneurysm is completely hidden by the overlying gyrus rectus.[68] The septal perforators are typically plastered to the posterior wall of these lesions, and the contralateral A_2 is obscured by the aneurysm fundus. Consequently, adequate visualization of all the relevant anatomy and careful clip placement require much more extensive skull base resection, greater frontal lobe retraction, and more resection of the gyrus rectus. Therefore, endovascular treatment may be more advantageous for this type, but there are instances when aneurysm morphology may preclude endovascular obliteration, making surgery necessary.

Distal Anterior Cerebral Aneurysms

Anatomy, Terminology, Aneurysm Variants

In the typical case, two distal anterior cerebral arteries (also known as the A_2, postcommunicating, or pericallosal arteries) course dorsally from the anterior communicating complex and then arch within the midline

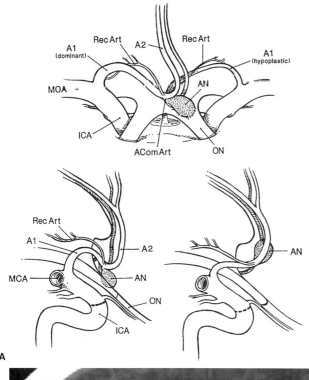

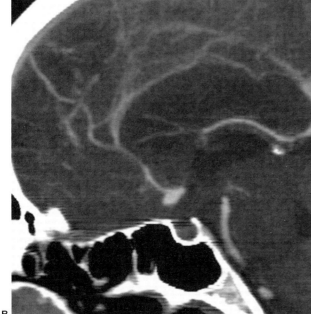

FIGURE 8–10 Anterior communicating artery aneurysms. **(A)** Frontal (top figure) and lateral (lower left and right figures) views (schematic). Many anterior communicating aneurysms arise in association with a hypoplastic A1 segment and project as a direct extension of the dominant A1 toward the contralateral frontal lobe (top figure). If the aneurysm is also directed inferiorly (lower-left figure), the fundus is often attached to the contralateral optic nerve, an attachment that makes exposure from the nondominant (hypoplastic) A1 side hazardous for premature rupture as the frontal lobe is elevated. If the lesion projects more superiorly (lower-right figure), expansion occurs between the two frontal lobes within the interhemispheric fissure, and the aneurysm will not be visible at the initial subfrontal exposure without some gyrus rectus removal. **(B)** Lateral CT angiogram reconstruction, demonstrating an inferiorly projecting anterior communicating artery aneurysm and its relationship to the optic chiasm and planum sphenoidale. **(C)** Lateral three-dimensional arteriogram of the same aneurysm demonstrating how an inferiorly projecting aneurysm lies below the A2 segments.

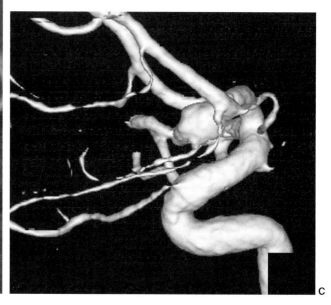

pericallosal sulcus deep within the interhemispheric fissure, parallel and adjacent to the genu and body of the corpus callosum (**Fig. 8–11**).[69] The callosomarginal artery arises from the pericallosal artery near the genu and runs within the cingulate sulcus, giving off several major cortical branches to the medial cerebral hemisphere. Almost all distal anterior cerebral aneurysms are saccular. Trauma can cause aneurysms in the region of the falx cerebri, and any aneurysm distal to the callosomarginal artery origin could be infectious.[3,7,67,70] Less common, distal aneurysms arise at the bifurcation of an azygous A_2 segment where it divides to form two pericallosal arteries.

Specific Management

The treatment of distal anterior cerebral artery aneurysms is generally surgical. Endovascular obliteration can be achieved in some cases, although the anatomy of the

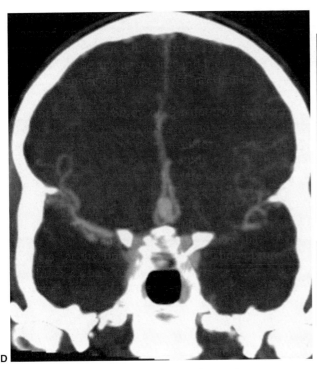

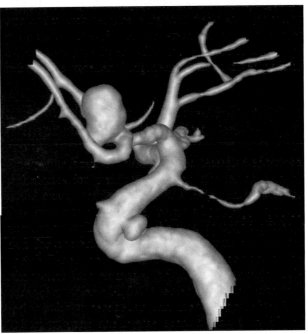

FIGURE 8–10 (continued) **(D)** Anterior CT angiogram reconstruction, demonstrating a superiorly projecting anterior communicating artery aneurysm and its position within the interhemispheric fissure. **(E)** Lateral three-dimensional arteriogram of the same aneurysm, showing how a superiorly projecting aneurysm resides between or behind the A2 segments.

anterior communicating complex and the size and distance of the pericallosal vessels usually make safe catheter navigation difficult.

■ Complications, Morbidity and Mortality

Once an intracranial aneurysm is suspected, the decision to treat rests on an analysis that primarily includes the risks associated with the natural history of the lesion, the risks of the proposed treatment, and the benefits derived from that procedure. Our current knowledge about the natural history of unruptured aneurysms is improving, but the specific predictability for an individual aneurysm patient may always be problematic. Simply put, the consequences of hemorrhage are devastating, and even if the likelihood of bleeding is very low, many patients handle that possibility poorly, despite the best reassurances by their treating physician. Certainly, the natural history is dependent on the patient's age and general health, which directly determine life expectancy and cumulative lifetime risk from hemorrhage. Surgical risks are also greatly influenced by these factors. Advanced age, especially when associated with significant cardiovascular, respiratory, or other systemic disease, increases the likelihood of perioperative complications and reduces

the patient's ability to recover from surgically related neurological and systemic injury.[71–73]

Increasing aneurysm size also clearly affects the natural history and surgical risks of the unruptured lesion. Large and giant aneurysms are not only more likely to bleed but are also much more likely to have associated arteriosclerosis or calcification, thereby increasing the difficulty of surgical repair without incurring additional neurologic deficits.[5,72–75] Not surprisingly, increased volume and experience can promote the expertise of the surgical team, resulting in better outcomes, lower costs of treatment, and shorter lengths of stay. Because a small uncomplicated and unruptured anterior circulation aneurysm can usually be repaired with a low combined perioperative morbidity and mortality if treated by an experienced microvascular surgeon (**Table 8–3**), surgical treatment is generally advised for patients in good health and who have longer life expectancies. Added risk factors increase the operative risks, and the choices of no treatment or endovascular intervention should be considered more strongly. Aneurysm location is also a clear factor in the natural history and the recommendations for treatment. Aneurysms arising in the paraclinoid region have a much lower risk of rupture than do PComArt lesions. Superiorly projecting AComArt aneurysms are more difficult to treat surgically than those projecting anteriorly and inferiorly are.

Table 8–3 Surgical Morbidity and Mortality for Unruptured Aneurysms

Series	Year	No. of patients	No. of aneurysms		Morbidity (%)		Mortality (%)
Salazar[87]	1980	29	38		3.3		0
Wirth et al[73]	1986	107	119		6.5		0
Eskesen et al[88]	1987	Sympt: 27	Sympt: 30		15		4
		Incid: 21	Incid: 23				
Inagawa et al[89]	1992	52	52		6		0
Solomon et al[72]	1994	202	Sympt: 113	*Size*	*Early*	*Late*	
			Incid: 34	<7	3	0	0
			Other: 55	7–10	7	2	0
				11–25	8	3	3
				>25	16	10	10
Nakagawa and Hashi[90]	1994	20	20		0		0
ISUIA[5]*	2003	1917	2884		9.8		2.3

*Includes patients with posterior circulation aneurysms. ISUIA, International Study of Unruptured Intracranial Aneurysms.

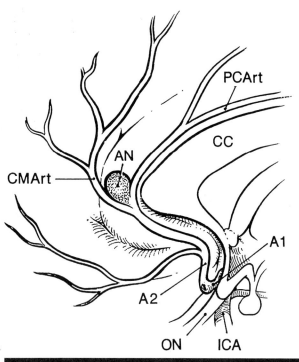

A

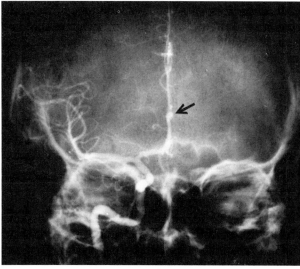

B

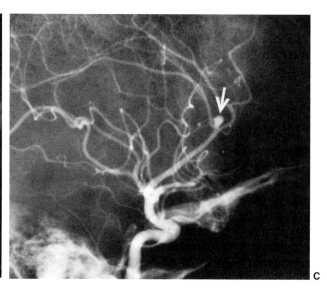

C

FIGURE 8–11 Distal anterior cerebral artery aneurysm. **(A)** Lateral view (schematic). Many distal anterior cerebral artery aneurysms arise at the bifurcation between the pericallosal and callosomarginal arteries, a point that is variable but often occurs near the genu of the corpus callosum. **(B, C)** Arteriogram (anteroposterior and lateral views). Note the origin of the aneurysm (arrow) at the bifurcation of the pericallosal and callosomarginal arteries. The studies should be carefully inspected for the exact site of aneurysm origin relative to the genu of the corpus callosus and its relationship to the coronal suture.

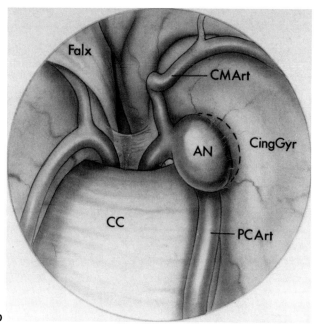

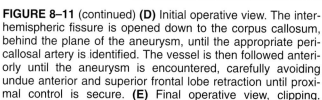

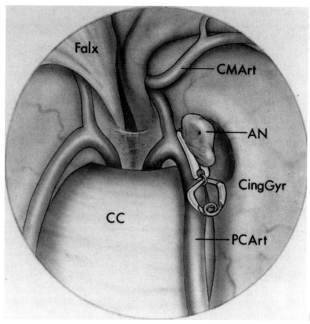

FIGURE 8–11 (continued) **(D)** Initial operative view. The inter-hemispheric fissure is opened down to the corpus callosum, behind the plane of the aneurysm, until the appropriate peri-callosal artery is identified. The vessel is then followed anteri-orly until the aneurysm is encountered, carefully avoiding undue anterior and superior frontal lobe retraction until proxi-mal control is secure. **(E)** Final operative view, clipping.

Without disturbing the aneurysm's attachment to the Falx or medial frontal lobe (dotted line), a straight or gentle curved clip is placed across the aneurysm neck parallel to the superior surface of the pericallosal artery. ICA, internal carotid artery; CMArt, callosomarginal artery; PCArt, pericallosal artery; CC, corpus callosum; Falx, falx cerebri; ON, optic nerve; CingGyr, cingulate gyrus; AN, aneurysm.

The security and certainty of a long-term "cure" is also a major factor in the decision-making process. In the ISUIA study, the complete occlusion rate in endovascu-larly treated aneurysms was only 50% at 1 year. In contrast, more than 90% of aneurysms undergoing surgical clip occlusion are completely obliterated at surgery.[76–78] Therefore, any assessment of comparative efficacy must include not only immediate morbidity and mortality but also long-term outcome and durability of treatment over at least 5 to 10 years. In general, endovascular therapy is preferable for patients with anterior circulation aneurysms where concerns about durability are over-shadowed by the less-invasive attractiveness of endovascu-lar obliteration, or where the specific aneurysm anatomy or other clinical factors makes a surgical approach signif-icantly riskier.

Unlike unruptured aneurysms, for which acute risks are generally low and decisions are elective, the ruptured saccular intracranial aneurysm is a dramatic intracranial catastrophe, associated with very high morbidity and mortality. The management and surgical outcomes for several large clinical series are included in **Table 8–4**. These results include patients of all clinical grades pre-senting at random time intervals after hemorrhage. Good outcome rates (and mortality) generally parallel the preoperative clinical grade, averaging 79% (9%) in grade I and II patients, 58% (19%) in grade III patients,

33% (35%) in grade IV patients, and 14% (45%) in grade V patients.[6,32] Early, aggressive intervention has clearly improved the outcome for patients in grades IV and V.[48,56,79] Surgical complications, such as intraoperative aneurysm rupture, major vessel occlusions, cerebral con-tusion, or intracerebral hemorrhage, are associated with ~10% of the morbidity and mortality after SAH.[6,32,56,80] There does not appear to be a greater incidence of sur-gical complications associated with higher patient grade, but it is not known whether the effects of a surgical com-plication in a poor-grade patient may have a greater impact than in a good-grade patient.

Recently, the International Subarachnoid Aneurysm Trial (ISAT) reported the results of its randomized trial of endovascular coiling versus surgical clipping for rup-tured intracranial aneurysms.[81] Like the ISUIA trial, the results of ISAT have been hotly debated. To be enrolled and randomized in the study, the patient had to be in a clinical state that "justified" treatment, and the aneurysm had to be equally suitable for endovascular or open sur-gical obliteration, or there had to be uncertainty as to which treatment was best. The authors reported a rela-tive risk reduction of 22.6% at 1 year with endovascular treatment compared with surgery, and an absolute risk reduction of 6.9%. Based on this, they concluded that endovascular treatment was superior to surgical aneurysm treatment in patients of good grade with small

Table 8–4 Management and Surgical Results for Ruptured Aneurysms

Clinical Series	Number of Patients	Management		Surgical	
		Morbidity (%)	Mortality (%)	Morbidity (%)	Mortality (%)
Yoshimoto et al[91]	1000	n/a	n/a	8.4	6.4
Sundt et al[92]	722	All grades: 10	17	12	4
		GI: 3	6	2	2
		GII: 16	11	7	4
Ropper et al[93]	112	20	11	n/a	n/a
Ljunggren et al[51]	251	39	19	20	5
Rosenorn et al[94]	1076	24	45.5	36	23
Disney et al[95]	437	1968–1977: 24	47	18	19
		1978–1985: 23	38	14	11
Chyatte et al[96]	244	13	23	14	15
Ohman et al[97]	216	AS: 3	6	3	6
		IS: 16	6	16	1.5
		LS: 7	13	8	4.7
Kassell et al[6,32]	3521	16	26	18	14
Lee[98]	780	n/a	n/a	2.7	4
Saveland et al[99]	325	23	21	24	10.4
Krupp et al[100]	131	All grades: 25	13	27.5	5
		GI, 2: 10	n/a	11	n/a
		GIII: 26	n/a	28	n/a
		GIV, V: 63	43	69	14
ISAT					

ISAT, International Subarachnoid Aneurysm Trial.

anterior circulation aneurysms. The authors expressed caution that the durability of endovascular treatment remains unproven in this study. To the authors' caution, we add the following concerns. First, the population of patients treated in this study is not representative of the patients seen in our practice; almost none of the patients in ISAT had posterior circulation aneurysms, the great majority of lesions were <10 mm, and the vast majority of patients were good-grade patients. In addition, the surgical results, while obtained at relatively high-volume centers located, for the most part, in the United Kingdom, are probably not representative of the results that could be obtained at centers in the United States because the number of aneurysms treated per surgeon and the surgical expertise, while not discussed, was probably not equivalent to the high-volume practices seen at major referral centers in the United States. In fact, the study states "it was deemed inappropriate to demand, as a prerequisite to being a participating centre, outcomes figures from individual operators for managing patients."[81] In addition, the authors do not describe in sufficient detail why the vast majority of patients were not randomized to this study, other than to say that sufficient "equipoise" did not exist for the treatment of these patients.

■ Therapeutic Efficacy and Follow-up

The main goals of aneurysm surgery are to isolate the aneurysm lumen from the circulation and to preserve the parent and branch vessels, without producing a new irreversible injury to brain tissue. Overall, more than 90% of aneurysms clipped surgically are completely obliterated. Although the durability of this repair is frequently assumed to be high, most patients do not undergo follow-up angiography except in the immediate postsurgical period. Several studies indicate that vessel occlusion or aneurysm remnants can be found on 5% of postoperative angiograms.[78,82–84] The impact of these remnants, often left because of parent vessel atherosclerotic changes, is likely much safer than those left by incomplete endovascular obliteration, in which the opening into the aneurysm is not narrowed by a clip. At our institution, intraoperative selective arteriography is used for all cases, as recent studies suggest that even experienced microvascular surgeons cannot always determine which cases need intraoperative angiography based on operative findings alone.[85] Treatment failure and incomplete aneurysm obliteration are also more likely when the surgical exposure is inadequate; hence, we strongly advocate the routine use of skull-base approaches to create a generous surgical corridor through which the aneurysm and all relevant vascular and brain anatomy can be readily seen without significant brain retraction.

■ Future Developments and Research

Improvements in the diagnosis and treatment of intracranial aneurysms will surely continue, for both surgical and endovascular methodologies. Genetic screening will potentially allow physicians to predict who is likely to develop an aneurysm. Noninvasive screening procedures such as MRA and CTA, combined with three-dimensional reconstructions, will become more refined, eliminating the need for and risks of diagnostic arteriography other than for exceptional cases. Clinical trials will further clarify the varying risks of aneurysms at specific locations, thereby reducing risks and apprehension for many patients, in particular with proximal ICA lesions. The field of proteomics may allow clinicians to identify markers in the CSF or circulating bloodstream that predict and anticipate vasospasm risks before clinical decline is evident. Pharmacologic manipulation of the inflammatory component of vasospasm may also reduce its incidence and severity.

From a surgical standpoint, many if not most of these cases should ideally be done by an individual with special expertise and a broad experience in microvascular and skull base neurosurgery, at a center that handles sufficient volumes so that critical care, endovascular, and nursing experience is high quality and available around the clock. Routine use of internal hypothermia, intraoperative arteriography and monitoring, and intraoperative visualization with fluorescein-like agents injected into the venous system to confirm patency of perforators hold promise for further reducing operative risks.

The operating room of the future may actually lay within the radiology suite, even for open surgical procedures. The endovascular capabilities delivered in such a unit, combined with direct visualization of the pathology, may amplify the capacity to treat complex lesions through simultaneous interactions between surgical and endovascular techniques. For instance, a clip could be directly applied to a broad-based aneurysm to narrow its neck, followed by endovascular coiling of the residual, with a perfect result confirmed in the operative room by the highest quality of neuroimaging.

■ Conclusion

Surgery occupies a critical position in the treatment of intracranial aneurysms. Methods of complete aneurysm obliteration have been refined over many years, and the durability is excellent. Since the introduction of endovascular methods, however, many of the "simple" aneurysms can be best treated by these techniques. This outcome is as it should be—we are all searching for the same result—the safest, least-invasive method for protecting the individual from the consequences (real and psychological) of continued aneurysmal growth and/or hemorrhage. This goal requires a team effort between endovascular and open microsurgical vascular specialists, who work together to select the best treatment for the individual patient in front of them, without regard to "territorial" or financial incentives.

■ References

1. Rhoton AL Jr. Anatomic foundations of aneurysm surgery (honored guest lecture). Clin Neurosurg 1994;41:289–324
2. Rhoton AL Jr. Anatomy of saccular aneurysms. Surg Neurol 1980; 14:59–66
3. Fox JL. Intracranial Aneurysms. New York: Springer-Verlag; 1983, Vol 1
4. Unruptured intracranial aneurysms—risk of rupture and risks of surgical intervention. International Study of Unruptured Intracranial Aneurysms Investigators. N Engl J Med 1998;339: 1725–1733
5. Wiebers DO, Whisnant JP, Huston J III, et al. Unruptured intracranial aneurysms: natural history, clinical outcome, and risks of surgical and endovascular treatment. Lancet 2003;362:103–110
6. Kassell NF, Torner JC, Jane JA, et al. The International Cooperative Study on the Timing of Aneurysm Surgery. Part 2: Surgical results. J Neurosurg 1990;73:37–47
7. Weir B. Aneurysms Affecting the Nervous System. Baltimore: Williams & Wilkins; 1987
8. Stehbens WE. Pathology of the Cerebral Blood Vessels. St. Louis: C.V. Mosby; 1972:351–470
9. Day AL, Morcos JJ, Revilla F. Management of aneurysms of the anterior circulation. In: Youmans JR, ed. Neurological Surgery. Philadelphia: W.B. Saunders; 1996: Vol 2, 1272–1309
10. Sahs AL, Perret G, Locksley HB, et al. Preliminary remarks on subarachnoid hemorrhage. J Neurosurg 1966;24:782–788
11. Andrews RJ, Spiegel PK. Intracranial aneurysms. Age, sex, blood pressure, and multiplicity in an unselected series of patients. J Neurosurg 1979;51:27–32
12. Cervoni L, Delfini R, Santoro A, et al. Multiple intracranial aneurysms: surgical treatment and outcome. Acta Neurochir (Wien) 1993;124:66–70
13. Ellamushi HE, Grieve JP, Jager HR, et al. Risk factors for the formation of multiple intracranial aneurysms. J Neurosurg 2001; 94:728–732
14. Investigators ISoUIA. Unruptured intracranial aneurysms—risk of rupture and risks of surgical intervention. N Engl J Med 1998; 339:1725–1733
15. Nehls DG, Flom RA, Carter LP, et al. Multiple intracranial aneurysms: determining the site of rupture. J Neurosurg 1985;63: 342–348
16. Ostergaard JR, Hog E. Incidence of multiple intracranial aneurysms. Influence of arterial hypertension and gender. J Neurosurg 1985;63:49–55
17. Juvela S. Risk factors for multiple intracranial aneurysms. Stroke 2000;31:392–397
18. Weir B. Unruptured intracranial aneurysms: a review. J Neurosurg 2002;96:3–42
19. Bederson JB, Awad IA, Wiebers DO, et al. Recommendations for the management of patients with unruptured intracranial aneurysms: a statement for healthcare professionals from the Stroke Council of the American Heart Association. Circulation 2000;102:2300–2308
20. Broderick JP, Brott T, Tomsick T, et al. The risk of subarachnoid and intracerebral hemorrhages in blacks as compared with whites. N Engl J Med 1992;326:733–736
21. Inagawa T. Trends in incidence and case fatality rates of aneurysmal subarachnoid hemorrhage in Izumo City, Japan, between 1980–1989 and 1990–1998. Stroke 2001;32:1499–1507
22. Inagawa T, Aoki H, Ishikawa S, et al. Aneurysmal subarachnoid hemorrhage in Izumo City and Shimane Prefecture of Japan. Seasonal variation. Hiroshima J Med Sci 1988;37:17–18
23. Ingall TJ, Whisnant JP, Wiebers DO, et al. Has there been a decline in subarachnoid hemorrhage mortality? Stroke 1989;20:718–724

24. Linn FH, Rinkel GJ, Algra A, et al. Incidence of subarachnoid hemorrhage: role of region, year, and rate of computed tomography: a meta-analysis. Stroke 1996;27:625–629

25. Ljunggren B, Brandt L, Kagstrom E, et al. Results of early operations for ruptured aneurysms. J Neurosurg 1981;54:473–470

26. Ljunggren B, Saveland H, Brandt L. Aneurysmal subarachnoid hemorrhage–historical background from a Scandinavian horizon. Surg Neurol 1984;22:605–616

27. Ljunggren B, Saveland H, Brandt L, et al. Aneurysmal subarachnoid hemorrhage. Total annual outcome in a 1.46 million population. Surg Neurol 1984;22:435–438

28. Mayberg MR, Batjer HH, Dacey R, et al. Guidelines for the management of aneurysmal subarachnoid hemorrhage. A statement for healthcare professionals from a special writing group of the Stroke Council, American Heart Association. Stroke 1994;25: 2315–2328

29. Ohno K, Suzuki R, Masaoka H, et al. A review of 102 consecutive patients with intracranial aneurysms in a community hospital in Japan. Acta Neurochir (Wien) 1988;94:23–27

30. Sarti C, Tuomilehto J, Salomaa V, et al. Epidemiology of subarachnoid hemorrhage in Finland from 1983 to 1985. Stroke 1991;22:848–853

31. Kassell NF, Torner JC. Epidemiology of intracranial aneurysms. Int Anesthesiol Clin 1982;20:13–17

32. Kassell NF, Torner JC, Haley EC Jr, et al. The International Cooperative Study on the Timing of Aneurysm Surgery. Part 1: Overall management results. J Neurosurg 1990;73:18–36

33. Weir B. Intracranial aneurysms and subarachnoid hemorrhage: an overview. In: Wilkins RH, Rengachary SS, Eds. Neurosurgery. New York: McGraw-Hill; 1994: Vol 2, 1308–1329

34. Kassell NF, Torner JC. Aneurysmal rebleeding: a preliminary report from the Cooperative Aneurysm Study. Neurosurgery 1983; 13:479–481

35. Kassell NF, Torner JC. The International Cooperative Study on Timing of Aneurysm Surgery—an update. Stroke 1984;15:566–570

36. Locksley HB. Natural history of subarachnoid hemorrhage, intracranial aneurysms and arteriovenous malformations. J Neurosurg 1966;25:321–368

37. Jane JA, Kassell NF, Torner JC, et al. The natural history of aneurysms and arteriovenous malformations. J Neurosurg 1985; 62:321–323

38. Jane JA, Winn HR, Richardson AE. The natural history of intracranial aneurysms: rebleeding rates during the acute and long term period and implication for surgical management. Clin Neurosurg 1977;24:176–184

39. Kassell NF, Drake CG. Timing of aneurysm surgery. Neurosurgery 1982;10:514–519

40. Martland H. Spontaneous subarachnoid hemorrhage and congenital "berry aneurysms" of the circle of Willis. Am J Surg 1939;43: 10–19

41. Okawara SH. Warning signs prior to rupture of an intracranial aneurysm. J Neurosurg 1973;38:575–580

42. Symonds CP. Spontaneous subarachnoid hemorrhage. Q J Med 1924;18:93

43. Verweij RD, Wijdicks EF, van Gijn J. Warning headache in aneurysmal subarachnoid hemorrhage. A case-control study. Arch Neurol 1988;45:1019–1020

44. Leblanc R. The minor leak preceding subarachnoid hemorrhage. J Neurosurg 1987;66:35–39

45. Fisher CM, Kistler JP, Davis JM. Relation of cerebral vasospasm to subarachnoid hemorrhage visualized by computerized tomographic scanning. Neurosurgery 1980;6:1–9

46. Hunt WE, Hess RM. Surgical risk as related to time of intervention in the repair of intracranial aneurysms. J Neurosurg 1968;28:14–20

47. Teasdale GM, Drake CG, Hunt W, et al. A universal subarachnoid hemorrhage scale: report of a committee of the World Federation of Neurosurgical Societies. J Neurol Neurosurg Psychiatry 1988; 51:1457

48. Bailes JE, Spetzler RF, Hadley MN, et al. Management morbidity and mortality of poor-grade aneurysm patients. J Neurosurg 1990;72:559–566

49. Kassell NF, Torner JC. The International Cooperative study on timing of aneurysm surgery. Acta Neurochir (Wien) 1982;63:119–123

50. Haley EC Jr, Kassell NF, Torner JC. A randomized controlled trial of high-dose intravenous nicardipine in aneurysmal subarachnoid hemorrhage. A report of the Cooperative Aneurysm Study. J Neurosurg 1993;78:537–547

51. Ljunggren B, Saveland H, Brandt L, et al. Early operation and overall outcome in aneurysmal subarachnoid hemorrhage. J Neurosurg 1985;62:547–551

52. Ljunggren BC, Brandt JL, Saveland HG. Outcome in patients subjected to early aneurysm operation and intravenous nimodipine. Minerva Med 1986;77:1087–1092

53. Saveland H, Brandt L. Which are the major determinants for outcome in aneurysmal subarachnoid hemorrhage? A prospective total management study from a strictly unselected series. Acta Neurol Scand 1994;90:245–250

54. Le Roux PD, Elliott JP, Newell DW, et al. Predicting outcome in poor-grade patients with subarachnoid hemorrhage: a retrospective review of 159 aggressively managed cases. J Neurosurg 1996;85: 39–49

55. Le Roux PD, Winn HR. Management of the ruptured aneurysm. Neurosurg Clin N Am 1998;9:525–540

56. Le Roux PD, Elliot JP, Newell DW, et al. The incidence of surgical complications is similar in good and poor grade patients undergoing repair of ruptured anterior circulation aneurysms: a retrospective review of 355 patients. Neurosurgery 1996;38:887–893, 893–885

57. Adams HP Jr, Kassell NF, Torner JC, et al. CT and clinical correlations in recent aneurysmal subarachnoid hemorrhage: a preliminary report of the Cooperative Aneurysm Study. Neurology 1983;33:981–988

58. Masson RL Jr, Day AL. Aneurysmal intracerebral hemorrhage. Neurosurg Clin N Am 1992;3:539–550

59. Le Roux PD, Dailey AT, Newell DW, et al. Emergent aneurysm clipping without angiography in the moribund patient with intracerebral hemorrhage: the use of infusion computed tomography scans. Neurosurgery 1993;33:189–197

60. Batjer HH, Kopitnik TA, Giller CA, et al. Surgery for paraclinoidal carotid artery aneurysms. J Neurosurg 1994;80:650–658

61. Cawley CM, Zipfel GJ, Day AL. Surgical treatment of paraclinoid and ophthalmic aneurysms. Neurosurg Clin N Am 1998;9:765–783

62. Day AL. Aneurysms of the ophthalmic segment. A clinical and anatomical analysis. J Neurosurg 1990;72:677–691

63. Day AL. Clinicoanatomic features of supraclinoid aneurysms. Clin Neurosurg 1990;36:256–274

64. Zipfel GJ, Day AL. Surgical treatment of clinoidal and ophthalmic segment internal carotid artery aneurysms. In Le Roux PD, Winn HR, Newell DW, Eds. Management of Cerebral Aneurysms. Philadelphia: Saunders; 2004, 731–745

65. Nagasawa S, Deguchi J, Arai M, et al. Topographic anatomy of paraclinoid carotid artery aneurysms: usefulness of MR angiographic source images. Neuroradiology 1997;39:341–343

66. White JA, Horowitz MB, Samson D. Dural waisting as a sign of subarachnoid extension of cavernous carotid aneurysms: a follow-up case report. Surg Neurol 1999;52:607–609, 609–610

67. Yasargil MG. Microneurosurgery. New York: Thieme-Stratton; 1987, Vol 1 & 2

68. Iwanaga H, Wakai S, Ochiai C, et al. Ruptured cerebral aneurysms missed by initial angiographic study. Neurosurgery 1990;27:45–51

69. Perlmutter D, Rhoton AL Jr. Microsurgical anatomy of the distal anterior cerebral artery. J Neurosurg 1978;49:204–228

70. Yasargil MG, Carter LP. Saccular aneurysms of the distal anterior cerebral artery. J Neurosurg 1974;40:218–223

71. Connolly ES Jr, Solomon RA. Management of symptomatic and asymptomatic unruptured aneurysms. Neurosurg Clin N Am 1998;9:509–524

72. Solomon RA, Fink ME, Pile-Spellman J. Surgical management of unruptured intracranial aneurysms. J Neurosurg 1994;80: 440–446

73. Wirth FP. Surgical treatment of incidental intracranial aneurysms. Clin Neurosurg 1986;33:125–135

74. Khanna RK, Malik GM, Qureshi N. Predicting outcome following surgical treatment of unruptured intracranial aneurysms: a proposed grading system. J Neurosurg 1996;84:49–54

75. Raaymakers TW, Rinkel GJ, Limburg M, et al. Mortality and morbidity of surgery for unruptured intracranial aneurysms: a meta-analysis. Stroke 1998;29:1531–1538

76. Acevedo JC, Turjman F, Sindou M. Postoperative arteriography in surgery for intracranial aneurysm. Prospective study in a consecutive series of 267 operated aneurysms Neurochirurgie 1997;43: 275–284. French

77. David CA, Vishteh AG, Spetzler RF, et al. Late angiographic follow-up review of surgically treated aneurysms. J Neurosurg 1999; 91:396–401

78. Le Roux PD, Elliott JP, Eskridge JM, et al. Risks and benefits of diagnostic angiography after aneurysm surgery: a retrospective analysis of 597 studies. Neurosurgery 1998;42:1248–1254, 1254–1245

79. Le Roux PD, Winn HR. Intracranial aneurysms and subarachnoid hemorrhage management of the poor grade patient. Acta Neurochir Suppl 1999;72:7–26

80. Batjer H, Samson D. Intraoperative aneurysmal rupture: incidence, outcome, and suggestions for surgical management. Neurosurgery 1986;18:701–707

81. Molyneux A, Kerr R, Stratton I, et al. International Subarachnoid Aneurysm Trial (ISAT) of neurosurgical clipping versus endovascular coiling in 2143 patients with ruptured intracranial aneurysms: a randomised trial. Lancet 2002;360:1267–1274

82. Drake CG, Allcock JM. Postoperative angiography and the "slipped" clip. J Neurosurg 1973;39:683–689

83. Drake CG, Friedman AH, Peerless SJ. Failed aneurysm surgery. Reoperation in 115 cases. J Neurosurg 1984;61:848–856

84. Macdonald RL, Wallace MC, Kestle JR. Role of angiography following aneurysm surgery. J Neurosurg 1993;79:826–832

85. Klopfenstein JD, Spetzler RF, Kim LJ, et al. Comparison of routine and selective use of intraoperative angiography during aneurysm surgery: a prospective assessment. J Neurosurg 2004;100:230–235

86. Sahs AL, Perret G, Locksley HB. Intracranial Aneurysms and Subarachnoid Hemorrhage: A Cooperative Study. Philadelphia: JB Lippincott; 1969

87. Salazar JL. Surgical treatment of asymptomatic and incidental intracranial aneurysms. J Neurosurg 1980;53:20–21

88. Eskesen V, Rosenorn J, Schmidt K, et al. Clinical features and outcome in 48 patients with unruptured intracranial saccular aneurysms: a prospective consecutive study. Br J Neurosurg 1987; 1:47–52

89. Inagawa T, Hada H, Katoh Y. Unruptured intracranial aneurysms in elderly patients. Surg Neurol 1992;38:364–370

90. Nakagawa T, Hashi K. The incidence and treatment of asymptomatic, unruptured cerebral aneurysms. J Neurosurg 1994;80: 217–223

91. Yoshimoto T, Uchida K, Kaneko U, et al. An analysis of follow-up results of 1000 intracranial saccular aneurysms with definitive surgical treatment. J Neurosurg 1979;50:152–157

92. Sundt TM Jr, Kobayashi S, Fode NC, et al. Results and complications of surgical management of 809 intracranial aneurysms in 722 cases. Related and unrelated to grade of patient, type of aneurysm, and timing of surgery. J Neurosurg 1982;56:753–765

93. Ropper AH, Zervas NT. Outcome 1 year after SAH from cerebral aneurysm. Management morbidity, mortality, and functional status in 112 consecutive good-risk patients. J Neurosurg 1984;60: 909–915

94. Rosenorn J, Eskesen V, Schmidt K, et al. Clinical features and outcome in 1076 patients with ruptured intracranial saccular aneurysms: a prospective consecutive study. Br J Neurosurg 1987; 1:33–45

95. Disney L, Weir B, Petruk K. Effect on management mortality of a deliberate policy of early operation on supratentorial aneurysms. Neurosurgery 1987;20:695–701

96. Chyatte D, Fode NC, Sundt TM Jr. Early versus late intracranial aneurysm surgery in subarachnoid hemorrhage. J Neurosurg 1988;69:326–331

97. Ohman J, Heiskanen O. Timing of operation for ruptured supratentorial aneurysms: a prospective randomized study. J Neurosurg 1989;70:55–60

98. Lee KC. Surgery of intracranial aneurysms at Yonsei University: 780 cases. Keio J Med 1991;40:1–5

99. Saveland H, Hillman J, Brandt L, et al. Overall outcome in aneurysmal subarachnoid hemorrhage. A prospective study from neurosurgical units in Sweden during a 1-year period. J Neurosurg 1992;76:729–734

100. Krupp W, Heienbrok W, Muke R. Management results attained by predominantly late surgery for intracranial aneurysms. Neurosurgery 1994;34:227–233, 233–224

9

Endovascular Treatment of Anterior Circulation Aneurysms

REZA JAHAN, GARY DUCKWILER, AND FERNANDO VINUELA

Objectives: Upon completion of this chapter, the reader should be able to describe the endovascular techniques utilized in the treatment of anterior circulation aneurysms, including parent artery occlusion, endosaccular coiling, and stent-assisted techniques. The reader will also review the results that can be expected with these techniques.

Accreditation: The AANS* is accredited by the Accreditation Council for Continuing Medical Education (ACCME) to sponsor continuing medical education for physicians.

Credit: The AANS designates this educational activity for a maximum of 15 credits in Category 1 credit toward the AMA Physician's Recognition Award. Each physician should claim only those hours of credit that he/she spent in the educational activity.

The Home Study Examination is online on the AANS Web site at: http://www.aans.org/education/books/controversy.asp

* The acronym AANS refers to both the American Association of Neurological Surgeons and the American Association of Neurosurgeons.

The prevalence of intracranial aneurysms in the general population is not well known. Most autopsy studies estimate the prevalence to be ~2 to 5% .[1-3] The largest study published thus far found intracranial aneurysms in 1.6% of 87,772 autopsies.[4] Intracranial aneurysms are a major cause of nontraumatic subarachnoid bleeding, with morbidity and mortality exceeding 50%.[5-8] Neurosurgical clipping has been established as the "gold standard" for treatment of intracranial aneurysms.[9] Due to the high surgical morbidity and mortality in selected patients, much interest has developed in endovascular treatment of intracranial aneurysms. This technique allowed treatment of aneurysms in high-risk patients. The current technique of endovascular coiling of aneurysms was first performed in 1990 and reported by Guglielmi et al[10,11] Since then, endovascular coiling has been shown to have a major role in management of intracranial aneurysms. Recently, it has been shown to be a safer procedure compared with surgical clipping in selected patients with ruptured intracranial aneurysms.[12]

Despite attempts at understanding the natural history of aneurysms, the fate of an aneurysm is still unpredictable in an individual patient. In general, treatment is undertaken when the risk of treatment does not exceed the predicted morbidity of the aneurysm. In this chapter, endovascular treatment of aneurysms in the anterior circulation will be discussed.

■ Endovascular Treatment Background

Approximately 90% of intracranial aneurysms occur in the anterior circulation with the majority in the anterior communicating and posterior communicating location.[13] Generally, endovascular treatment of aneurysms in the anterior circulation consists of occlusion of the aneurysm and the parent artery or obliteration of the aneurysm sac with preservation of the parent artery.

Parent Vessel Occlusion

The first reports of endovascular occlusion of a parent artery were described in the 1970s.[14–17] Since then, various authors have substantiated the utility of the technique in the treatment of selected intracranial aneurysms.[18–20] In the anterior circulation, for aneurysms below the circle of Willis off of the internal carotid artery (ICA), the procedure involves temporary balloon occlusion (TBO) of the ICA to assess collateral flow through the circle of Willis. This procedure is performed with the patient fully awake. This allows the operator to perform neurological assessment of the patient while the ICA is temporarily occluded. Abrupt occlusion of the ICA is not performed as it results in a 26% stroke rate and 12% mortality.[21] Several techniques have been developed to increase the sensitivity of the test and ensure that few patients suffer delayed ischemic symptoms from occlusion of the ICA. These include neurological testing for 15 or 30 minutes, electroencephalographic monitoring, and induced systemic hypotension during balloon occlusion.[18–20,22–25] Physiological studies to assess cerebral blood flow and cerebrovascular reserve during balloon occlusion have also been performed. These include utilization of transcranial doppler, Tc HMPAO SPECT, and Xenon-enhanced CT.[24,26–28] Based on these physiological studies it has been proposed to separate patients undergoing TBO into low-, moderate-, and high-risk patients.[24,29] The high-risk group would be those that do not tolerate the TBO with neurological deterioration during the test. The moderate-risk group would be those that neurologically tolerate the TBO but who on blood flow studies show a significant and asymmetric decrease in cerebral blood flow to less than 30 ml/100 g of tissue per minute. The low-risk group would tolerate the TBO but show a mild asymmetric decrease in cerebral blood flow (>30 ml/100 g of tissue per minute). In light of this classification into low-, moderate-, and high-risk patients, two approaches have emerged in the management of patients undergoing TBO; a selective approach and a universal approach. In a selective approach those with moderate or high risk would undergo external carotid to internal carotid artery bypass (EC/IC bypass) prior to ICA occlusion.[25,30] This is justified by studies showing a low risk of ischemic complications in patients undergoing TBO and parent vessel occlusion.[30–32] In addition, long-term follow-up hemodynamic studies of patients who are undergoing elective occlusion of the ICA have shown no diminishment in cerebrovascular reserve.[33]

In contrast to the selective approach, in the universal approach, all patients undergoing parent vessel occlusion would undergo EC/IC bypass.[34] The universal approach is justified by studies that show that even the low-risk patients as identified by TBO incur a significant risk of long-term ischemic complications following parent vessel occlusion without bypass.[34] In addition, there are theoretical advantages of EC/IC bypass in these patients. First, the bypass reduces flow and turbulence through the circle of Willis, increasing the potential for aneurysmal thrombosis and shrinkage. Furthermore, it reduces the risk of development of contralateral flow related aneurysms due to increased circulation through the circle of Willis.[25,34,35]

The techniques of TBO and parent vessel occlusion have been described extensively. Early reports involved the use of detachable balloons for testing, followed by occlusion of the vessel with the same balloon.[14–17,20] Alternatively, a separate double-lumen balloon can be used for test occlusion followed by a detachable balloon for occlusion.[20] However, permanent occlusion is achieved by utilization of detachable coils. This removes the technical and clinical complications related to premature detachment of the balloon or deflation and distal migration of detachable balloons. The balloons used for test occlusion are typically compliant balloons necessary to minimize damage to the ICA during inflation. Systemic heparinization is necessary to prevent thromboembolic complications during balloon occlusion. Following the procedure, the heparin can be reversed with protamine sulfate or digested.

In the anterior circulation, parent vessel occlusion is typically reserved for wide-neck symptomatic cavernous aneurysms or giant wide-neck aneurysms of the supraclinoid ICA. The objectives of treatment are twofold. The first objective is to prevent bleeding from the aneurysm, particularly with supraclinoid ICA aneurysms. Occlusion of the parent artery allows thrombosis of the aneurysm, and transmural stress due to flow in the aneurysm is removed. To accomplish this, one must ensure that substantial collateral flow to the aneurysm is absent. This may require, at times, occlusion above and below the aneurysm with trapping of the aneurysm to exclude it from the circulation. Furthermore, with giant ophthalmic aneurysms, continued flow to the aneurysm can be seen through the ophthalmic artery following occlusion of the ICA below the ophthalmic artery. In this instance, coils would be first placed into the aneurysm and then allowed to fall into the ICA for occlusion of the parent vessel.

The second objective of parent vessel occlusion is to shrink the aneurysm, thus removing its mass effect. This is particularly true with cavernous aneurysms. Cavernous aneurysms are not generally life threatening, as they rarely cause subarachnoid bleeding.[36] The treatment of cavernous aneurysms is aimed at alleviation of symptoms related to mass effect, carotid cavernous fistula, decreased visual acuity, or headaches not responding to medical therapy.[22,36] Most cavernous aneurysms are large or giant at the time of diagnosis and thus require parent vessel occlusion. Small asymptomatic cavernous aneurysms do not pose an immediate risk to the patient and thus can be observed conservatively and only treated if showing evidence of growth or becoming symptomatic.[37] Aneurysms treated by carotid occlusion have been shown to involute with reduction of mass effect.[27,37,38]

In conclusion, the utilization of parent vessel occlusion in the management of anterior circulation aneurysms must be individualized for each patient to allow maximum protection of the patient from acute and chronic ischemic complications and to minimize technical complications from the TBO, parent vessel occlusion, and EC/IC bypass surgery.

Endovascular Occlusion of the Aneurysm Sac

General Considerations

Over the past decade, endovascular occlusion of aneurysms with microcoils has become an acceptable alternative to surgical clipping. Guglielmi et al first reported utilization of detachable coils in 1991.[10,11] The Food and Drug Administration approved the platinum coil in 1995 for treatment of intracranial aneurysms. Since then, there has been much controversy over the selection of patients for endovascular coiling versus clipping. The results of a major trial comparing endovascular coiling to surgical clipping showed that in a population of patients with subarachnoid bleeding with aneurysms suitable for coiling and clipping, endovascular occlusion was safer at 1 year follow-up.[12] It is most certain that coiling will continue to play a major role in the management of patients with aneurysms. This role will likely grow in the future as improvements in technology address the current limitations of the coiling procedure.

As the technology evolves, the selection criteria for patients undergoing coiling continue to be revised. With the introduction of Guglielmi detachable coils (GDC) in early 1990, patient selection was primarily based on the patient's medical condition and the location of the aneurysm. In short, this included patients that were not good surgical candidates. Initial success in a population of patients with complete occlusion of the aneurysm was reported in two large studies to be 50%[39] and 56%.[40] Based on early technical experience and angiographic outcomes, it was noted that aneurysm anatomy and morphology play a significant role in the determination of successful occlusion.[41] An aneurysm with neck width of 4 mm or greater is considered wide-necked with initial endovascular occlusion possible in a few of these aneurysms, with high rates of recanalization.[41] Zubillaga et al reported the success rate of initial endovascular occlusion in narrow- and wide-neck aneurysms[41] to be 85% and 15%, respectively. In our own center's experience of 11 years with 916 aneurysms treated in 818

patients, small aneurysms (less than 10 mm) with small necks (less than 4 mm) had an initial success rate with complete occlusion in 75.4% of cases.[39] Complete occlusion was achieved in only 11.2% of small aneurysms with wide necks. On follow-up, small-neck aneurysms had a recanalization rate of 5.1%, whereas wide-neck aneurysms had recanalization rates of 20%.

Neck width is not the only morphological determinant of successful occlusion. For instance, an aneurysm with a 3 mm neck and a 3 mm body diameter would have unfavorable morphology for coiling, although the neck diameter is less than 4 mm. Thus, the ratio of the aneurysm sac width to the width of the aneurysm neck should also be considered. Aneurysms with a sac-to-neck ratio less than 2:1 should be considered wide necked. Debrun et al reported their results of embolization of 339 aneurysms in 329 patients,[40] dividing the aneurysms into those with sac-to-neck ratio greater or less than 2:1. In a group of patients selected for treatment primarily based on aneurysm geometry, a complete occlusion rate of 80% was noted when the sac-to-neck ratio was at least 2, and 58% when the ratio was less than 2.

The reason for the low initial success rate and recanalization in wide-neck aneurysms is multifactorial. Wide-neck aneurysms do not allow dense packing of the aneurysm. Studies have shown that there is a direct correlation between aneurysm packing density and recanalization rates.[42,43] Even in narrow-neck aneurysms only ~20 to 30% of the aneurysm volume is filled with platinum coils, with the remaining 70 to 80% being filled with thrombus.[44] As the majority of the aneurysm is filled with thrombus, natural thrombolytic processes can act on this thrombus and recanalize the aneurysm. This is particularly true in large and giant aneurysms where the thrombus remains unorganized for a long period following embolization.[44–49] There have been mainly two approaches to address this limitation of platinum coil technology. The first is to hasten the conversion of the thrombus to collagen scar tissue, providing a stable firm scaffold that resists coil compaction and recanalization.[49] The second is filling the aneurysm cavity with complete or near-complete exclusion of thrombus.[50,51]

The first approach, enhancing the organization of thrombus, relies on surface modification of the platinum coil to accomplish this goal. Platinum coils are biologically inert and produce little or no inflammatory response. The utilization of biologically active material as an embolic agent to promote scar formation inside the aneurysm has been reported by Murayama et al[49] The Guglielmi platinum detachable coils were covered with a bioabsorbable polymer that enhances the intra-aneurysmal inflammatory response. Histologic studies in animals showed that this material enhanced clot maturation. The new coils, called Matrix detachable coils, are now being utilized for embolization of aneurysms. Definitive clinical data to show reduced recanalization rates with Matrix coils remain to be seen. There has not yet been a direct trial comparing the platinum coils to the new Matrix coils.

The second approach, enhanced filling of the aneurysm has been reported by Kallmes et al[50,51] As stated above, recanalization of aneurysms is in part related to the density of the packing with embolic material. As the majority of the aneurysm filled with platinum coils is thrombus, recanalization can occur as the clot is lysed. The hydrocoil embolic system (HES) was developed to address this.[51] The HES is a hybrid hydrogel–platinum coil device with the hydrogel expanding in blood to about three times its initial diameter. Thus, the majority of the aneurysm volume is filled with the hydrogel, with small amounts of thrombus within the aneurysm cavity. Initial clinical experience with the HES has been reported in 11 patients.[50] Volumetric packing was improved with the HES compared with standard platinum coils. Long-term follow-up studies to show reduced recanalization rates with the HES have not been reported.

Morphological factors other than neck size and sac-to-neck ratio have been reported to be important determinants of anatomical outcome after coiling. Gonzalez et al reported results of embolization of anterior communicating artery aneurysms.[52] Over a 12-year period of treating over 1000 intracranial aneurysms, 135 anterior communicating aneurysms were identified. These were divided into those pointing anteriorly versus those pointing posteriorly with respect to the axis of the pericallosal artery, as described by Proust et al[53] In addition, aneurysms were classified with respect to orientation of the neck. This included aneurysms with necks that were arising from the anterior communicating artery (pure anterior communicating artery aneurysms) and those with the neck pointing toward an A1 segment of the anterior cerebral artery (ie, arising from the junction of the A1 and A2 segments). Orientation of the dome and neck had a significant impact on anatomical success and recanalization. For instance, aneurysms with the neck oriented toward an A1 have significant less risk of recanalization, while pure anterior communicating artery aneurysms have a significant risk of recanalization. Anterior communicating aneurysms pointing anteriorly have significant better anatomic results with higher rates of complete occlusion. Posteriorly pointing anterior communicating aneurysms have a higher risk of incomplete occlusion and higher recanalization.

Other configurations unfavorable to successful coiling include the branching pattern near the neck of the aneurysm. This is particularly true of middle cerebral and posterior communicating aneurysms. The branching vessels can obscure visualization of the aneurysm neck, increasing the risk of coil protrusion into the parent artery or adjacent branch vessel. This is often the case with middle cerebral artery aneurysms. A branch arising near the neck of the aneurysm, which commonly occurs with

posterior communicating artery aneurysms, is an unfavorable configuration for coiling as well. These facts are well reflected in a reported series of aneurysm embolizations. Debrun et al reported their experience of coiling 339 aneurysms, and middle cerebral and posterior communicating artery aneurysms were underrepresented due to this anatomical limitation with branching at the neck region.[40] In the randomized International Subarachnoid Aneurysm Trial (ISAT),[12] middle cerebral aneurysms constituted only 14% of the aneurysms treated as the branching pattern at the middle cerebral artery trifurcation resulted in unfavorable configuration for coiling. The majority of patients with middle cerebral artery aneurysms were sent to surgery in the ISAT.

Treatment of Wide-Neck Aneurysms

As the above discussion indicates, the endovascular treatment of cerebral aneurysms with coils has significant challenges. This is particularly true with respect to the treatment of wide-neck aneurysms. Several technical advances have improved the successful treatment of wide-neck aneurysms. These include the introduction of three-dimensional coils, which, with their complex three-dimensional shape provided some additional flexibility with respect to the ability to treat patients with wide-neck aneurysms.[54] Moret et al[55] developed a balloon remodeling technique by which the parent vessel could be protected with the use of a nondetachable balloon catheter. Then, in 1994, the application of endovascular stents for the treatment of experimental carotid sidewall aneurysms in animals was first reported,[56–58] followed by a report by Higashida et al describing the first use of endovascular stents to treat wide-neck aneurysms in humans.[59] These technical advances have allowed for endovascular treatment of broad-neck aneurysms that otherwise would not have been amenable to safe treatment with coiling.

The application of an endovascular stent to support the coil embolization deserves further mention, as it has significantly broadened the range of aneurysms amenable to the coiling procedure. Stent-supported coiling of cerebral aneurysms provides several important theoretical and technical advantages. First, the stent provides for protection of the parent vessel during coiling, and this, in part, facilitates more complete aneurysm packing. Second, the stent can produce flow redirection with disruption of the aneurysm inflow and outflow zones contributing to stasis and thrombosis in the aneurysm. Third, the stent may provide a scaffold across the neck of the aneurysm for endothelial growth. Balloon remodeling can often facilitate adequate embolization of complex aneurysms; however, it does not provide the durable advantages achieved with the application of an endovascular stent.

Thus, stent-assisted coiling has been utilized to increase the success of acute aneurysm occlusion and reduce recanalization.[60,61] Initially, only balloon-expandable coronary stents were available for use. Although success in selected cases was reported, the inflexibility of these stents made navigation through the cerebrovasculature difficult. Recently, stents specifically designed for use in the cerebrovasculature have become available.[60,61] Initial experience with the first generation of these stents reported an overall complication rate of 10.7%.[61] Of 56 patients treated, there were three ischemic events and one death related to stent placement. Fiorella et al reported stent-assisted coiling in 19 patients with 22 aneurysms.[60] Two clinically significant events were reported, both of which were secondary to thrombo-embolic events related to stent placement. One of these patients died after thrombolysis was attempted, while the other made an excellent recovery.

The stent used in these reports was the Neuroform stent from Boston Scientific Corporation (Natick, MA). The flexibility of this stent greatly facilitates navigation of the tortuous cerebral vasculature not accessible with balloon-expandable stents. In addition, even the tortuous arterial segments themselves, such as the carotid siphon, can be stented. The challenge with this technology has been the actual stent deployment rather than navigation to the site of interest. However, a second-generation Neuroform stent is now available with an improved delivery catheter, which allows for better-controlled stent deployment. Long-term follow-up of patients has not been yet reported, and it remains to be seen whether stent-assisted coiling reduces recanalization rates of wide-neck aneurysms.

Clinical Outcomes of Embolization of Anterior Circulation Aneurysms

Published clinical data suggest that endovascular embolization of ruptured and unruptured cerebral aneurysms carries permanent procedural morbidities of 3 to 9%, mortality up to 8%, and rehemorrhage rates up to 4%.[62-75] Although these studies do not report results based on anatomic location of the aneurysm (i.e., anterior vs. posterior circulation), morbidity and mortality with respect to aneurysm location can be inferred from several reported studies. Murayama et al reported the experience at our institution over an 11-year period with 818 patients harboring 916 aneurysms.[39] Six hundred forty-eight aneurysms (71%) were anterior circulation aneurysms. In-hospital morbidity and mortality was reported as 91% of patients having no change or improved clinical condition after embolization. Six percent of patients had a new neurological deficit, and mortality was 3%. Dividing this group into those with acute subarachnoid hemorrhage (SAH) and those with

incidental aneurysms, in-hospital morbidity and mortality in those with acute SAH were 7.2% and 6.4% and, in those with incidental aneurysms, 4.5% and 0.8%, respectively. Long-term clinical follow-up was obtained in 768 of the 818 patients from 3 months to 8 years post-embolization. Compared with postdischarge from the hospital, of 768 patients, 131 (17.1%) had clinical improvement, 531 (69.1%) were unchanged, and 37 (4.8%) had neurological deficits. Mortality was 5.7%, and the incidence of delayed rupture was 1.6% (12 patients). Ten of the 12 delayed ruptures were large and giant aneurysms. The introduction of the balloon-assisted technique was assessed in this series. Since 1996, this technique has improved results of aneurysm embolization, with the greatest benefit noted in small aneurysms with wide necks. In this group of aneurysms, a 60% rate of complete occlusion was noted, compared with 41.2% prior to the introduction of the balloon-assisted technique. Most notable in this series is the rate of recanalization of giant aneurysms, which was noted to be higher than 50%. This is an unacceptable rate of recurrence, particularly because the majority of late ruptures in this series were large and giant aneurysms. Parent artery occlusion or direct clipping may be the best treatment currently for the cure of giant anterior circulation aneurysms.

Our center has evaluated coil embolization morbidity and mortality with respect to aneurysm location.[76] Comparing 585 aneurysms in the anterior circulation to 239 aneurysms in the posterior circulation, morbidity was 5.6% (anterior circulation) versus 7.1% (posterior circulation). Mortality was 1.4% in the anterior circulation versus 3.3% in the posterior circulation. Thus, there was no significant difference in morbidity and mortality as a function of aneurysm location. This is in sharp contrast to surgical experience, where aneurysm location plays a major role in outcome. With current catheter technology, catheterization of intracranial vessels, whether in the anterior or posterior circulation, can be safely performed. Morphological characteristics of the aneurysm are the most important factor determining success in anatomic occlusion and morbidity and mortality rates, as discussed in the previous sections.

Questions regarding morbidity and mortality in relation to any medical procedure are best addressed in a randomized clinical trial. The International Subarachnoid Aneurysm Trial evaluated neurosurgical clipping versus coiling in 2143 patients with ruptured intracranial aneurysms.[12] These were patients who had ruptured aneurysms that were suitable for neurosurgical clipping and endovascular coiling. The majority of patients randomized in the study had anterior circulation aneurysms. Of the 2143 aneurysms randomized, 2.7% were of posterior circulation. The remainder was anterior circulation aneurysms with 50.5% anterior cerebral artery, 32.5% internal carotid artery, and 14.1% middle cerebral artery. The majority of the patients were of good clinical grade, and the median age in each arm of the study was 52 years. At 1 year, data were available on 1594 patients with poor outcome defined as Modified Rankin Scale 3 to 6 in 23.7% of endovascular patients and 30.6% of surgical patients. The relative and absolute risk reductions in dependency or death in favor of endovascular treatment were 22.6% and 6.9%, respectively. The risk of rebleeding after 1 year was 2 per 1276 and 0 per 1081 patient-years for patients allocated endovascular and neurosurgical treatment, respectively. It must be emphasized that this risk of rebleeding has been taken into account in the final analysis of outcome at 1 year, with endovascular treatment showing better clinical results. The ISAT study with over 4000 patient-year follow-ups now has assessed the risk of rebleeding in the endovascular versus surgical patients to be 0.15% and 0.07% per year, respectively. Thus, it is calculated that to lose the benefit gained by endovascular treatment due to rebleeding would require at least 70 years.

In summary, the study showed that in the population of patients with ruptured aneurysms suitable for both endovascular and surgical treatment, the outcome in terms of survival free of disability at 1 year is significantly better with endovascular coiling. It must be emphasized that the population of patients in this study were young and had ruptured aneurysms (mostly anterior circulation aneurysms) that were suitable for endovascular or surgical treatment, with good clinical grade.

Many aspects related to subarachnoid bleeding remain to be evaluated in a population of patients treated in the ISAT study. This includes the incidence of epilepsy, assessment of symptomatic cerebral vasospasm, and evaluation of outcomes in predefined groups of patients. Neuropsychological assessment of patients also remains to be evaluated to better understand differences in cognitive outcome related to surgical versus endovascular treatment.

There has yet been no study to compare endovascular and surgical treatment of unruptured aneurysms. In addition, there has been no randomized trial to compare endovascular and surgical treatment of aneurysms in poor-grade patients. As mentioned above, the majority of patients in the ISAT were of good clinical grade. There have been single-center studies that have addressed this issue. Groden et al[77] compared operative and endovascular treatment of anterior circulation aneurysms in poor-grade patients (Hunt and Hess grade IV and V). They reported on the treatment of 40 patients, 21 treated surgically and 19 treated by endovascular means. The incidence of cerebral vasospasm did not differ significantly between the two groups. There was one surgical- and three endovascular procedural-related complications with clinical consequences. Clinical outcome

was assessed at 6 months. Good outcome was obtained in six (29%) of the surgically treated patients and six (30%) of the endovascularly treated patients. Outcome was similar after surgical and endovascular approaches. In this population, surgery was the treatment of choice in patients with intracerebral bleeding with mass effect for whom hematoma evacuation may be necessary. Alternatively, endovascular treatment is considered in certain poor-grade patients within the first 72 hours of hemorrhage where an edematous brain is a major argument against early surgery. The risks of surgery in the elderly would also indicate a endovascular approach in this population, as would the presence of severe vasospasm requiring an angioplasty, which can be performed in the same session that the embolization is done.

■ Conclusion

Endovascular treatment of aneurysms was initially introduced to provide a viable option for patients considered a high risk for surgical treatment. The technology has advanced rapidly to where endovascular therapy is now playing a major role in the management of patients with cerebral aneurysms. The selection of patients for endovascular therapy is continuing to be defined. Techniques of balloon-supported and stent-assisted coiling have improved anatomical outcomes following embolization. In addition, coil modifications such as the polymer-coated coils are now introduced to further improve immediate and long-term anatomical results of coiling procedure. To become the first line of treatment for cerebral aneurysms, endovascular embolization must provide a permanent occlusion of the treated aneurysm. A single endovascular tool is not likely to accomplish this but, rather, a combination of techniques such as stents and polymer-coated coils. A randomized trial in a population of patients with ruptured aneurysms has shown improved clinical outcome at 1 year in the endovascularly treated group compared with the surgically treated group. Randomized trials to compare the endovascular and surgical treatment of unruptured aneurysms are in the planning stages.

■ References

1. Chason JL, Hindman WM. Berry aneurysms of the Circle of Willis. Neurology 1958;8:41–44
2. de la Monte SM, Moore GW, Mong MA, Hutchins GM. Risk factors for the development and rupture of intracranial berry aneurysms. Am J Med 1985;78:957–964
3. Di Bonito L, Giarelli L. Pathogenesis of cerebral hemorrhage considered in the light of objective lesions in the arteries of the brain (in 226 cases studied by autopsy). Minerva Med 1975;66: 4391–4398. Italian

4. Jellinger K. Pathology and aetiology of intracranial aneurysms. In: Pia HW, Langmaid C, Zierski J, eds. Cerebral Aneurysms: Advances in Diagnosis and Therapy. New York, NY: Springer; 1979:5–19

5. Kassell NF, Torner JC. Aneurysmal rebleeding: a preliminary report from the cooperative aneurysm study. Neurosurgery 1983;13:479–481

6. Sahs A. Intracranial Aneurysms and Subarachnoid Hemorrhage: A Cooperative Study. Philadelphia: JB Lippincott Co; 1969

7. Nishioka H, Torner JC, Graf CJ, Kassell NF, Sahs AL, Goettler LC. Cooperative study of intracranial aneurysms and subarachnoid hemorrhage: a long-term prognostic study. II. Ruptured intracranial aneurysms managed conservatively. Arch Neurol 1984;41:1142–1146

8. Ropper AH, Zervas NT. Outcome 1 year after SAH from cerebral aneurysm. Management morbidity, mortality, and functional status in 112 consecutive good-risk patients. J Neurosurg 1984;60: 909–915

9. Zabramski JM, Spetzler RF. Intracranial aneurysms: surgical management. In: Barnett HJM, Mohr JP, Bennett MS, Yatsu FM, eds. Stroke, Pathophysiology, Diagnosis, and Management. Philadelphia: Churchill Livingstone; 1998:1263–1298

10. Guglielmi G, Vinuela F, Dion J, Duckwiler G. Electrothrombosis of saccular aneurysms via endovascular approach. Part 2: preliminary clinical experience. J Neurosurg 1991;75:8–14

11. Guglielmi G, Vinuela F, Sepetka I, Macellari V. Electrothrombosis of saccular aneurysms via endovascular approach. Part 1: electrochemical basis, technique, and experimental results. J Neurosurg 1991;75:1–7

12. Molyneux A, Kerr R, Stratton I, et al. International Subarachnoid Aneurysm Trial (ISAT) of neurosurgical clipping versus endovascular coiling in 2143 patients with ruptured intracranial aneurysms: a randomised trial. Lancet 2002;360:1267–1274

13. Weir BK. Intracranial aneurysms and subarachnoid hemorrhage. In: Wilkins W, Rengachary SS, eds. Neurosurgery. New York, NY: McGraw-Hill; 1985:1308–1329

14. Debrun G, Lacour P, Caron JP, Hurth M, Comoy J, Keravel Y. Inflatable and released balloon technique experimentation in dog—application in man. Neuroradiology 1975;9:267–271

15. Debrun G, Lacour P, Caron JP, Hurth M, Comoy J, Keravel Y. Detachable balloon and calibrated-leak balloon techniques in the treatment of cerebral vascular lesions. J Neurosurg 1978;49: 635–649

16. Debrun G, Fox A, Drake C, Peerless S, Girvin J, Ferguson G. Giant unclippable aneurysms: treatment with detachable balloons. AJNR Am J Neuroradiol 1981;2:167–173

17. Serbinenko FA. Balloon catheterization and occlusion of major cerebral vessels. J Neurosurg 1974;41:125–145

18. Higashida RT, Halbach VV, Dowd C, et al. Endovascular detachable balloon embolization therapy of cavernous carotid artery aneurysms: results in 87 cases. J Neurosurg 1990;72:857–863

19. Berenstein A, Ransohoff J, Kupersmith M, Flamm E, Graeb D. Transvascular treatment of giant aneurysms of the cavernous carotid and vertebral arteries. Functional investigation and embolization. Surg Neurol 1984;21:3–12

20. Fox AJ, Vinuela F, Pelz DM, et al. Use of detachable balloons for proximal artery occlusion in the treatment of unclippable cerebral aneurysms. J Neurosurg 1987;66:40–46

21. Linskey ME, Jungreis CA, Yonas H, et al. Stroke risk after abrupt internal carotid artery sacrifice: accuracy of preoperative assessment with balloon test occlusion and stable xenon-enhanced CT. AJNR Am J Neuroradiol 1994;15:829–843

22. Vazquez Anon V, Aymard A, Gobin YP, et al. Balloon occlusion of the internal carotid artery in 40 cases of giant intracavernous aneurysm: technical aspects, cerebral monitoring, and results. Neuroradiology 1992;34:245–251

23. Higashida RT, Halbach VV, Barnwell SL, et al. Treatment of intracranial aneurysms with preservation of the parent vessel:

results of percutaneous balloon embolization in 84 patients. AJNR Am J Neuroradiol 1990;11:633–640

24. Mathis JM, Barr JD, Jungreis CA, et al. Temporary balloon test occlusion of the internal carotid artery: experience in 500 cases. AJNR Am J Neuroradiol 1995;16:749–754

25. Barnett DW, Barrow DL, Joseph GJ. Combined extracranial-intracranial bypass and intraoperative balloon occlusion for the treatment of intracavernous and proximal carotid artery aneurysms. Neurosurgery 1994;35:92–97

26. Giller CA, Steig P, Batjer HH, Samson D, Purdy P. Transcranial Doppler ultrasound as a guide to graded therapeutic occlusion of the carotid artery. Neurosurgery 1990;26:307–311

27. Larson JJ, Tew JM Jr, Tomsick TA, van Loveren HR. Treatment of aneurysms of the internal carotid artery by intravascular balloon occlusion: long-term follow-up of 58 patients. Neurosurgery 1995; 36:26–30

28. Erba SM, Horton JA, Latchaw RE, et al. Balloon test occlusion of the internal carotid artery with stable xenon/CT cerebral blood flow imaging. AJNR Am J Neuroradiol 1988;9:533–538

29. Horton JA, Jungreis CA, Pistoia F. Balloon test occlusion. In: Sekhar LN, Janecka IP, eds. Surgery of Cranial Based Tumors. New York, NY: Raven Press; 1993:33–36

30. Drake CG, Peerless SJ, Ferguson GG. Hunterian proximal arterial occlusion for giant aneurysms of the carotid circulation. J Neurosurg 1994;81:656–665

31. Oldershaw JB, Voris HC. Internal carotid artery ligation: a follow-up study. Neurology 1966;16:937–938

32. Roski RA, Spetzler RF, Nulsen FE. Late complications of carotid ligation in the treatment of intracranial aneurysms. J Neurosurg 1981;54:583–587

33. Bavinzski G, Killer M, Ferraz-Leite H, Gruber A, Gross CE, Richling B. Endovascular therapy of idiopathic cavernous aneurysms over 11 years. AJNR Am J Neuroradiol 1998;19:559–565

34. Lawton MT, Hamilton MG, Morcos JJ, Spetzler RF. Revascularization and aneurysm surgery: current techniques, indications, and outcome. Neurosurgery 1996;38:83–92

35. Spetzler RF, Schuster H, Roski RA. Elective extracranial-intracranial arterial bypass in the treatment of inoperable giant aneurysms of the internal carotid artery. J Neurosurg 1980;53:22–27

36. Kupersmith MJ, Hurst R, Berenstein A, Choi IS, Jafar J, Ransohoff J. The benign course of cavernous carotid artery aneurysms. J Neurosurg 1992;77:690–693

37. Vargas ME, Kupersmith MJ, Setton A, Nelson K, Berenstein A. Endovascular treatment of giant aneurysms which cause visual loss. Ophthalmology 1994;101:1091–1098

38. van Rooij WJ, Sluzewski M, Metz NH, et al. Carotid balloon occlusion for large and giant aneurysms: evaluation of a new test occlusion protocol. Neurosurgery 2000;47:116–121

39. Murayama Y, Nien YL, Duckwiler G, et al. Guglielmi detachable coil embolization of cerebral aneurysms: 11 years' experience. J Neurosurg 2003;98:959–966

40. Debrun GM, Aletich VA, Kehrli P, Misra M, Ausman JI, Charbel F. Selection of cerebral aneurysms for treatment using Guglielmi detachable coils: the preliminary University of Illinois at Chicago experience. Neurosurgery 1998;43:1281–1295

41. Fernandez Zubillaga A, Guglielmi G, Vinuela F, Duckwiler GR. Endovascular occlusion of intracranial aneurysms with electrically detachable coils: correlation of aneurysm neck size and treatment results. AJNR Am J Neuroradiol 1994;15:815–820

42. Tamatani S, Ito Y, Abe H, Koike T, Takeuchi S, Tanaka R. Evaluation of the stability of aneurysms after embolization using detachable coils: correlation between stability of aneurysms and embolized volume of aneurysms. AJNR Am J Neuroradiol 2002; 23:762–767

43. Kawanabe Y, Sadato A, Taki W, Hashimoto N. Endovascular occlusion of intracranial aneurysms with Guglielmi detachable

coils: correlation between coil packing density and coil compaction. Acta Neurochir (Wien) 2001;143:451–455

44. Bavinzski G, Talazoglu V, Killer M, et al. Gross and microscopic histopathological findings in aneurysms of the human brain treated with Guglielmi detachable coils. J Neurosurg 1999;91: 284–293

45. Tenjin H, Fushiki S, Nakahara Y, et al. Effect of Guglielmi detachable coils on experimental carotid artery aneurysms in primates. Stroke 1995;26:2075–2080

46. Molyneux AJ, Ellison DW, Morris J, Byrne JV. Histological findings in giant aneurysms treated with Guglielmi detachable coils. Report of two cases with autopsy correlation. J Neurosurg 1995;83:129–132

47. Mawad ME, Mawad JK, Cartwright J Jr, Gokaslan Z. Long-term histopathologic changes in canine aneurysms embolized with Guglielmi detachable coils. AJNR Am J Neuroradiol 1995;16:7–13

48. Castro E, Fortea F, Villoria F, Lacruz C, Ferreras B, Carrillo R. Long-term histopathologic findings in two cerebral aneurysms embolized with Guglielmi detachable coils. AJNR Am J Neuroradiol 1999;20:549–552

49. Murayama Y, Tateshima S, Gonzalez NR, Vinuela F. Matrix and bioabsorbable polymeric coils accelerate healing of intracranial aneurysms: long-term experimental study. Stroke 2003;34:2031–2037

50. Cloft HJ, Kallmes DF. Aneurysm packing with HydroCoil Embolic System versus platinum coils: initial clinical experience. AJNR Am J Neuroradiol 2004;25:60–62

51. Kallmes DF, Fujiwara NH. New expandable hydrogel-platinum coil hybrid device for aneurysm embolization. AJNR Am J Neuroradiol 2002;23:1580–1588

52. Gonzalez NR, Martin N, Duckwiler G, et al. Treatment of anterior communicating artery aneurysms with coil embolization: Experience in 135 cases. Paper presented at: Annual Meeting of the American Society of Interventional and Therapeutic Neuroradiology; February 1–4, 2004; San Diego, CA.

53. Proust F, Debono B, Hannequin D, et al. Treatment of anterior communicating artery aneurysms: complementary aspects of microsurgical and endovascular procedures. J Neurosurg 2003;99:3–14

54. Malek AM, Higashida RT, Phatouros CC, Dowd CF, Halbach VV. Treatment of an intracranial aneurysm using a new three-dimensional-shape Guglielmi detachable coil. Neurosurgery 1999;44:1142–1145

55. Moret J, Cognard C, Weill A, Castaings L, Rey A. Reconstruction technic in the treatment of wide-neck intracranial aneurysms. J Neuroradiol 1997;24:30–44

56. Wakhloo AK, Schellhammer F, de Vries J, Haberstroh J, Schumacher M. Self-expanding and balloon-expandable stents in the treatment of carotid aneurysms. AJNR Am J Neuroradiol 1994;15:493–502

57. Szikora I, Guterman LR, Wells KM, Hopkins LN. Combined use of stents and coils to treat experimental wide-necked carotid aneurysms. AJNR Am J Neuroradiol 1994;15:1091–1102

58. Turjman F, Massoud TF, Ji C, Guglielmi G, Viñuela F, Robert J. Combined stent implantation and endosaccular coil placement for treatment of experimental wide-necked aneurysms. AJNR Am J Neuroradiol 1994;15:1087–1090

59. Higashida RT, Smith W, Gress D, et al. Intravascular stent and endovascular coil placement for a ruptured fusiform aneurysm of the basilar artery. J Neurosurg 1997;87:944–949

60. Fiorella D, Albuquerque FC, Han P, McDougall CG. Preliminary experience using the Neuroform stent for the treatment of cerebral aneurysms. Neurosurgery 2004;54:6–16

61. Benitez RP, Silva MT, Klem J, Veznedaroglu E, Rosenwasser RH. Endovascular occlusion of wide-necked aneurysms with a new intracranial microstent (Neuroform) and detachable coils. Neurosurgery 2004;54:1359–1367

62. Bavinzski G, Killer M, Gruber A, Reinprecht A, Gross CE, Richling B. Treatment of basilar artery bifurcation aneurysms by using Guglielmi detachable coils: a 6-year experience. J Neurosurg 1999;90:843–852

63. Guglielmi G, Vinuela F, Duckwiler G, et al. Endovascular treatment of posterior circulation aneurysms by electrothrombosis using electrically detachable coils. J Neurosurg 1992;77:515–524

64. Byrne JV, Adams CB, Kerr RS, Molyneux AJ. Endosaccular treatment of inoperable intracranial aneurysms with platinum coils. Br J Neurosurg 1995;9:585–592

65. Byrne JV, Molyneux AJ, Brennan RP, Renowden SA. Embolisation of recently ruptured intracranial aneurysms. J Neurol Neurosurg Psychiatry 1995;59:616–620

66. Graves VB, Strother CM, Duff TA, Perl J II. Early treatment of ruptured aneurysms with Guglielmi detachable coils: effect on subsequent bleeding. Neurosurgery 1995;37:640–647

67. Martin D, Rodesch G, Alvarez H, Lasjaunias P. Preliminary results of embolisation of nonsurgical intracranial aneurysms with GD coils: the 1st year of their use. Neuroradiology 1996;38(Suppl 1): S142–S150

68. McDougall CG, Halbach VV, Dowd CF, Higashida RT, Larsen DW, Hieshima GB. Endovascular treatment of basilar tip aneurysms using electrolytically detachable coils. J Neurosurg 1996;84:393–399

69. Pierot L, Boulin A, Castaings L, Rey A, Moret J. Selective occlusion of basilar artery aneurysms using controlled detachable coils: report of 35 cases. Neurosurgery 1996;38:948–953

70. Malisch TW, Guglielmi G, Vinuela F, et al. Intracranial aneurysms treated with the Guglielmi detachable coil: midterm clinical results in a consecutive series of 100 patients. J Neurosurg 1997;87:176–183

71. Nichols DA, Brown RD Jr, Thielen KR, Meyer FB, Atkinson JL, Piepgras DG. Endovascular treatment of ruptured posterior circulation aneurysms using electrolytically detachable coils. J Neurosurg 1997;87:374–380

72. Raymond J, Roy D, Bojanowski M, Moumdjian R, L'Esperance G. Endovascular treatment of acutely ruptured and unruptured aneurysms of the basilar bifurcation. J Neurosurg 1997;86:211–219

73. Raymond J, Roy D. Safety and efficacy of endovascular treatment of acutely ruptured aneurysms. Neurosurgery 1997;41:1235–1245

74. Vinuela F, Duckwiler G, Mawad M. Guglielmi detachable coil embolization of acute intracranial aneurysm: perioperative anatomical and clinical outcome in 403 patients. J Neurosurg 1997;86:475–482

75. Eskridge JM, Song JK. Endovascular embolization of 150 basilar tip aneurysms with Guglielmi detachable coils: results of the Food and Drug Administration multicenter clinical trial. J Neurosurg 1998;89:81–86

76. Murayama Y, Vinuela F. Intraaneurysmal endovascular therapy. In: Marks MP, Do HM, eds. Endovascular and Percutaneous Therapy of the Brain and Spine. Philadelphia: Lippincott Williams & Wilkins; 2002:141–162

77. Groden C, Kremer C, Regelsberger J, Hansen HC, Zeumer H. Comparison of operative and endovascular treatment of anterior circulation aneurysms in patients in poor grades. Neuroradiology 2001;43:778–783

10

Surgical Treatment of Posterior Circulation Aneurysms

HOWARD A. RIINA AND ROBERT F. SPETZLER

Objectives: Upon completion of this chapter, the reader should be able to distinguish the surgical approaches used to expose aneurysms in the posterior circulation.

Accreditation: The AANS* is accredited by the Accreditation Council for Continuing Medical Education (ACCME) to sponsor continuing medical education for physicians.

Credit: The AANS designates this educational activity for a maximum of 15 credits in Category 1 credit toward the AMA Physician's Recognition Award. Each physician should claim only those hours of credit that he/she spent in the educational activity.

The Home Study Examination is online on the AANS Web site at: http://www.aans.org/education/books/controversy.asp

* The acronym AANS refers to both the American Association of Neurological Surgeons and the American Association of Neurosurgeons.

Aneurysms of the posterior circulation are among the most difficult lesions encountered by cerebrovascular surgeons. Their treatment requires in-depth preoperative and intraoperative planning, and their successful obliteration requires adherence to the basic tenets of aneurysm surgery. As with the treatment of all intracranial aneurysms, these basic tenets include but are not limited to vascular control, sharp dissection, and meticulous preservation of perforating vessels, selective intraoperative angiography, and intraoperative monitoring. When possible, we prefer to clip lesions involving the posterior circulation directly. However, giant aneurysms in this location may require trapping, excision, aneurysmorrhaphy, or vessel occlusion.

■ Preoperative Considerations

Treatment of aneurysms involving the posterior circulation involves a thorough review of all imaging studies before surgery. In the current health care market, most patients present with computed tomography (CT) of the brain as well as magnetic resonance (MR) images.[1] Traditionally, patients subsequently undergo digital subtraction angiography to help delineate their vascular lesion. Recently, however, patients have undergone surgery based solely on MR angiography or CT angiography. Recent advances in the imaging quality of CT angiograms have made this study particularly useful in treating lesions of the posterior circulation.[2] In addition to providing the standard information about aneurysm size and morphology as well as location of branching vessels, CT angiography also provides information about surrounding bony structures that is crucial in preoperative planning and in understanding the anatomy of the lesion. In the treatment of aneurysms involving the posterior circulation, a thorough understanding of the anatomy is imperative for determining the appropriate operative approach.

■ Cerebral Protection

At our institution, all aneurysm patients receive intravenous barbiturates (thiopental) titrated to electroencephalographic burst suppression. Barbiturates are known to reduce cerebral injury from prolonged ischemia.[3] Therefore, they are most effective when administered before periods of temporary ischemia, as in the case of temporary vessel occlusion.[4] In addition, we favor slight hypertension during periods of temporary vessel occlusion, as this serves to enhance cerebral protection as well.

A ventriculostomy is placed in patients presenting with significant subarachnoid hemorrhage when they enter the institute. Spinal fluid drainage facilitates brain relaxation and helps minimize brain retraction.

■ Surgical Approaches to Posterior Circulation Aneurysms

We employ one of four surgical approaches when treating aneurysms of the posterior circulation: the extended orbitozygomatic approach, transpetrosal approaches, retrosigmoid approach, and extended far-lateral approach. We choose an approach based on the relation of the lesion to the basilar artery and clivus. Lesions of the posterior circulation can be placed into one of three distinct conceptual zones based on the basilar artery (**Fig. 10–1**).

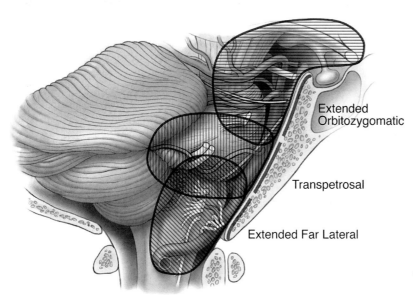

FIGURE 10–1 Three conceptual zones of the basilar artery and approaches to lesions in these zones (with permission from Barrow Neurological Institute).

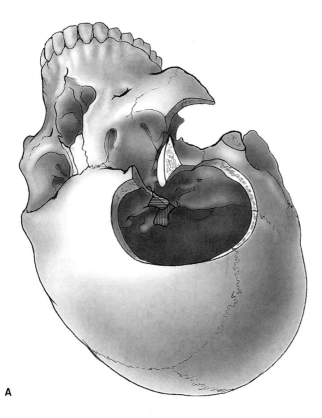

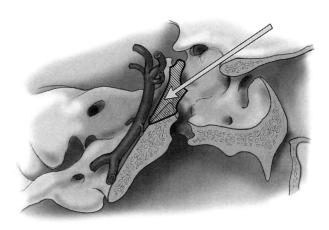

FIGURE 10–2 (A) The extended orbitozygomatic approach. **(B)** The approach includes removal of both the anterior and posterior clinoid as well as a portion of the dorsum sella (with permission from Barrow Neurological Institute).

The upper basilar zone comprises the upper two-fifths of the basilar artery. The midbasilar zone represents the middle fifth of the basilar artery. Finally, the vertebrobasilar zone represents the lower two-fifths of the basilar artery and includes all lesions involving the intradural segment of the vertebral artery.

Aneurysms of the upper basilar zone are approached through an extended orbitozygomatic approach (**Fig. 10–2**). The extended orbitozygomatic approach is modified to include removal of both the anterior and posterior clinoid processes as well as the portion of the dorsum sella.[5]

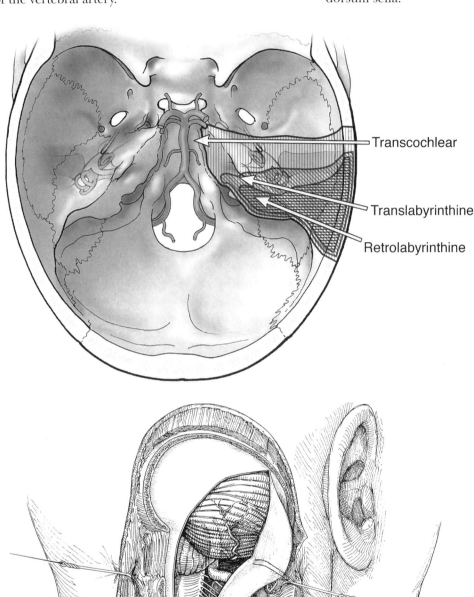

Transcochlear

Translabyrinthine

Retrolabyrinthine

FIGURE 10–3 The three transpetrosal approaches to lesions of the midbasilar zone: (1) transcochlear, (2) translabyrinthine, and (3) retrolabyrinthine (with permission from Barrow Neurological Institute).

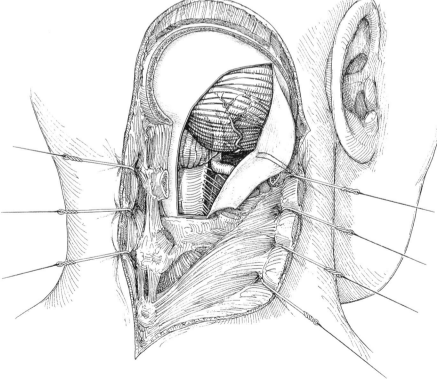

FIGURE 10–4 The far-lateral approach to lesions of the vertebrobasilar zone (with permission from Barrow Neurological Institute).

Retrosigmoid approach is used routinely for AICA aneurysms. Transpetrosal-type approaches are used to approach giant lesions that involve the midbasilar zone. We employ one of three transpetrosal approaches (**Fig. 10–3**): (1) the retrolabyrinthine approach, (2) the translabyrinthine approach,[6] and (3) the transcochlear approach.[7,8] A retrolabyrinthine-type approach provides exposure to the neck of the midbasilar aneurysm and spares the semicircular canals and cochlea. The translabyrinthine approach removes the semicircular canals and requires the sacrifice of hearing. The transcochlear approach requires removal of much of the petrous bone and, in so doing, provides maximum exposure of the brain stem and clivus. This approach,

however, requires removal of the cochlea and significant manipulation of the seventh nerve.

To approach lesions in the anterolateral brain stem or part of the vertebrobasilar zone, we use the far-lateral approach (**Fig. 10–4**).[9,10] The far-lateral approach requires removal of the posterior one-half to two-thirds of the occipital condyle and resection of the foramen magnum laterally toward the occipital condyle. In addition, the arch of C1 is removed laterally to the sulcus arteriosus of the vertebral artery.

The previously described three approaches are all primary techniques in approaching lesions of the posterior circulation. When a giant complex lesion lies between zones, a combined approach may rarely be required.[8,11]

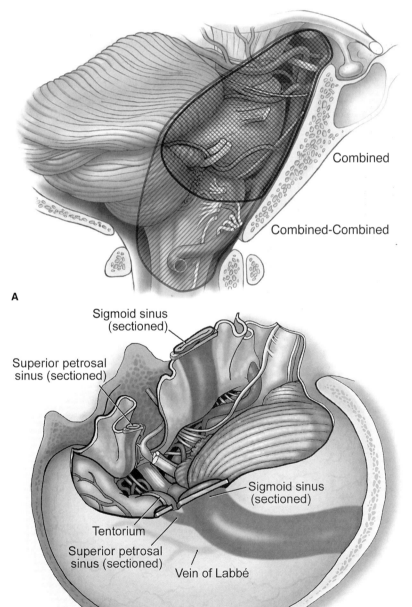

A

Combined

Combined-Combined

Sigmoid sinus
(sectioned)

Superior petrosal
sinus (sectioned)

Sigmoid sinus
(sectioned)

Tentorium

Superior petrosal
sinus (sectioned)

Vein of Labbé

B

FIGURE 10–5 (A) The combined and combined–combined approaches to posterior circulation lesions. **(B)** Combined far-lateral approach after bone removal and sectioning of both the tentorium and sigmoid sinus[10A] (with permission from the *Journal of Neurosurgery*).

A combined approach offers both supra- and infratentorial exposure by combining one of the transpetrosal approaches with a supratentorial craniotomy. The tentorium can then be divided to connect the two compartments. Lesions affecting the vertebrobasilar junction can be approached by a combined far-lateral approach with a supra- and infratentorial approach (**Fig. 10–5**).

■ References

1. Brugieres P, Blustajn J, Le Guerinel C, et al. Magnetic resonance angiography of giant intracranial aneurysms. Neuroradiology 1998;40:96–102

2. Villablanca JP, Martin N, Jahan R, et al. Volume-rendered helical computerized tomography angiography in the detection and characterization of intracranial aneurysms. J Neurosurg 2000;93:254–264

3. Selman WR, Spetzler RF, Roski RA, et al. Barbiturate coma in focal cerebral ischemia. Relationship of protection to timing of therapy. J Neurosurg 1982;56:685–690

4. Spetzler RF, Hadley MN. Protection against cerebral ischemia: the role of barbiturates. Cerebrovasc Brain Metab Rev 1989;1:212–229

5. Zabramski JM, Kiris T, Sankhla SK, et al. Orbitozygomatic craniotomy. Technical note. J Neurosurg 1998;89:336–341

6. House WF. Translabyrinthine approach. In: House WF, Luetje CM, eds. Acoustic Tumors. Baltimore: University Park; 1979:43–87

7. House WF, Hitselberger WE. The transcochlear approach to the skull base. Arch Otolaryngol 1976;102:334–342

8. Lawton MT, Daspit CP, Spetzler RF. Transpetrosal and combination approaches to skull base lesions. Clin Neurosurg 1996;43:91–112

9. Heros RC. Lateral suboccipital approach for vertebral and vertebrobasilar artery lesions. J Neurosurg 1986;64:559–562

10. Spetzler RF, Grahm TW. The far-lateral approach to the inferior clivus and upper cervical region: Technical note. BNI Q 1990;6(4):35–38

10A. Baldwin HZ, et al. The far lateral/combined supra- and infratentorial approach: a human cadaveric prosection model for routes of access to the petroclival region and ventral brain stem. J Neurosurg 1994;81:60–68

11. Hitselberger WE, House WF. A combined approach to the cerebellopontine angle. A suboccipital-petrosal approach. Arch Otolaryngol 1966;84(3):267–285

11

Endovascular Treatment of Posterior Circulation Aneurysms

ITALO LINFANTE, COLE B. GRAHAM III, AND AJAY K. WAKHLOO

Objectives: Upon completion of this chapter, the reader should be able to explain the indications for and results with endovascular coiling of posterior circulation aneurysms, including ruptured, unruptured, and dissecting aneurysms.

Accreditation: The AANS* is accredited by the Accreditation Council for Continuing Medical Education (ACCME) to sponsor continuing medical education for physicians.

Credit: The AANS designates this educational activity for a maximum of 15 credits in Category 1 credit toward the AMA Physician's Recognition Award. Each physician should claim only those hours of credit that he/she spent in the educational activity.

The Home Study Examination is online on the AANS Web site at: http://www.aans.org/education/books/controversy.asp

* The acronym AANS refers to both the American Association of Neurological Surgeons and the American Association of Neurosurgeons.

In this chapter, we briefly review the natural history of both ruptured and unruptured posterior circulation aneurysms. We then present the latest data supporting endovascular treatment for both types of aneurysms.

■ Intracranial Aneurysms: Epidemiological Data

Crude annual incidence rates of aneurysmal subarachnoid hemorrhage (SAH) have been estimated at between 10 to 15 cases per 100,000, with gender, ethnic, and geographical variations.[1] Approximately 15,000,000 Americans have an intracranial aneurysm; the exact number, however, is probably underestimated.[2] Aneurysms of the posterior circulation range between 8 and 15% of all intracranial aneurysms, according to several authors.[3–5] The majority of these aneurysms are located in the basilar apex, followed by the superior cerebellar arteries, the posterior inferior cerebellar arteries, the vertebrobasilar junction, the vertebral arteries, and the posterior cerebral arteries.

■ Ruptured Aneurysms

Prognosis in Ruptured Posterior Circulation Aneurysms

In the United States, every year ~50% of the 28,000 patients with SAH secondary to ruptured intracranial aneurysms die or are severely disabled. It is well established that the outcome of all ruptured intracerebral aneurysms depends on several factors, such as (1) age, (2) accessibility to a care facility, (3) the patient's clinical status (according to the Hunt and Hess grading system),[6] (4) the amount of intracerebral hemorrhage (according to the Fisher's grading scale), (5) aneurysmal location, and (6) the presence of vasospasm.

Access to a care facility is still a primary problem. Approximately 12% of patients die before reaching a hospital, 40% of patients expire within 30 days from the rupture, and ~30% of the survivors are left with major neurological deficits.[7] In addition, between 5 and 15% of all patients presenting with the clinical symptoms of stroke are found to have SAH due to a ruptured intracranial aneurysm. Early treatment within 24 to 72 hours has been advocated for these patients because of the high risk of repeat rupture within the first 2 weeks of SAH.[8]

For ruptured posterior circulation aneurysms, the prognosis is even more dismal. According to Schievink et al, these patients can expect survival rates of 32% within the first 48 hours of hemorrhage, 11% within the first 30 days, and have mortality rates three times that of ruptured anterior circulation aneurysms.[9] The close proximity of the brainstem and the propensity for hemorrhage into and expansion of the fourth ventricle is one of the factors explaining their poor outcomes. In addition, the decreased level of consciousness that often follows the rupture of posterior circulation aneurysms prevents the patient from seeking care urgently.

Treatment of Ruptured Posterior Circulation Aneurysms

The surgical approach to these lesions with traditional microsurgical techniques is technically challenging and anatomically unfavorable. In particular, approach to posterior circulation aneurysms requires a considerable amount of brain retraction and frequent protracted arterial occlusion, thus resulting in significant morbidity and mortality even in the best surgical hands. Consequently, the poor surgical results for ruptured posterior circulation aneurysms led to early studies using endovascular embolization to provide at least some protection from early rebleeding.[10]

The endovascular approach to intracranial aneurysms was originally reserved for the treatment of large, nonsurgical, giant aneurysms and used the method of endovascular "Hunterian" occlusion of the parent artery with detachable balloons.[11,12] However, in 1991 Guido Guglielmi revolutionized the field of endovascular embolization of intracranial aneurysms with the development of detachable platinum coils.[13,14] The first studies evaluating the endovascular treatment of aneurysms were largely descriptive and included patients with aneurysms that were considered too difficult to clip, had poor neurological status, had advancing age, or were otherwise predisposed to a poor overall prognosis.[15] As a result, in the early experience with Guglielmi detachable coils (GDC) reported by Viñuela et al,[16] 57% of the 403 patients treated in eight centers in the United States had aneurysms of the posterior circulation, a percentage that far exceeds the expected range of 8 to 15%.[3,4,15]

In a study evaluating the treatment of acutely ruptured and unruptured aneurysms of the basilar tip, Raymond et al treated 23 patients with acutely ruptured aneurysms using GDC and prevented rebleeding in all patients (mean follow-up: 15.5 months).[17] The mortality and poor outcome rates were 8.7% each, respectively, and

were attributed to intracranial hypertension related to the initial SAH and vasospasm. One death and one minor permanent deficit, but with good outcome, were attributed directly to endovascular treatment. These results compared favorably to the largest series of surgically treated basilar tip aneurysms compiled by Peerless et al[18] In this study of 1767 vertebrobasilar aneurysms, 113 were treated surgically within 1 week of SAH. The mortality (8%) and morbidity (9.7%) rates were related to the initial or recurrent SAH, vasospasm, or technical complications.

The rate of complete aneurysm obliteration by open neurosurgery for all aneurysms has been reported to be as high as 96%.[19,20] The resulting surgical remnant with "failed" aneurysm surgery may result in a significant rate of repeat hemorrhage,[20,21] estimated to be 0.8% per year.[22] Complete obliteration rates higher than 70% using endovascular coiling were once difficult to achieve even in a series consisting of small aneurysms (<10 mm) bearing small necks (<4 mm).[16] When aneurysms are large (10–25 mm) and giant (>25 mm), obliteration rates drop to 57% and 50%, respectively. However, it has been reported repeatedly that long-lasting, complete obliteration of the aneurysm after coil embolization is likely related to packing density. With experience, operators have recorded a decreased frequency of aneurysm neck remnants and increased the degree of coil packing. These factors have shown to play a major role in decreasing the likelihood of recanalization. Another critical factor in determining the frequency of recanalization is a neck size greater than 4 mm.[16] The literature suggests the rate of endovascular remnant rebleeding to be 0%, 4%, and 33% for patients with treated small, large, and giant aneurysms, respectively (average 3.5-year follow-up).[23] However, the advent of bioactive coils as well as of balloon- and stent-assisted coiling techniques continues to reduce these remnant rates (**Fig. 11–1A–C, Fig. 11–2A–F**). In addition, the high rates of aneurysm recurrence with endovascular therapy ought to be considered in light of (1) lower morbidity and mortality associated with endovascular therapy, (2) a rapidly advancing coil technology that is allowing safer and higher packing density, and (3) the ability to safely retreat these remnants at follow-up evaluation (**Fig. 11–3A–M**).

Cerebral vasospasm is the most common cause of morbidity and mortality in patients admitted to the hospital after developing SAH. The early surgical removal of subarachnoid clots and irrigation of the basal cisterns have been reported to reduce the incidence of vasospasm. In contrast to surgery, endovascular treatment of aneurysms does not allow removal of subarachnoid clots; therefore, it was considered less beneficial. However, Murajama et al measured the incidence of symptomatic vasospasm after early endovascular treatment of acutely ruptured aneurysms with GDCs.[24] Sixty-nine patients

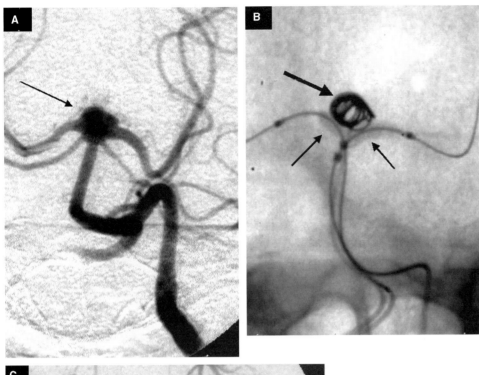

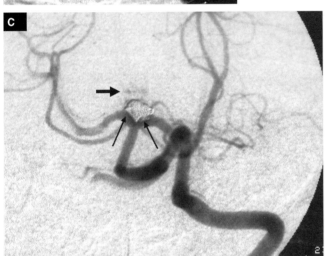

FIGURE 11–1 A 60-year-old woman with an unruptured basilar tip aneurysm. **(A)** Left vertebral artery (VA) injection shows a broad-base basilar tip aneurysm (arrow). **(B)** Placement of two non-detachable balloons from both VAs (small arrows) and coiling (large arrow) of the aneurysm via a microcatheter placed into the right VA. **(C)** Left VA injection shows complete aneurysmal obliteration with preservation of the perforating arteries (large arrow). In addition, the angiogram shows balloon-induced coil mass remodeling. There is a new coil interface with the aneurysmal base and the left P1 segment of the posterior cerebral artery (long arrows).

classified as Hunt and Hess Grades 1 to 3 underwent occlusion of intracranial aneurysms via GDCs within 72 hours of rupture. The amount of blood on the initial computerized tomography (CT) scan was classified by means of the Fisher's scale. Symptomatic vasospasm was defined as the onset of neurological deterioration verified with angiographic or transcranial Doppler studies. At 6-month clinical follow-up examination, 12 of these 16 patients experienced a good recovery, 2 were moderately disabled, and 2 had died of vasospasm. The authors concluded that the 23% incidence of symptomatic vasospasm in this series compares favorably to that found in conventional surgical series of patients with acute aneurysmal SAH.

Comparison of Open Surgery with Endovascular Treatment: Evidence from Randomized Trials

The first randomized clinical trial to compare open surgery with the endovascular treatment of acutely ruptured aneurysms was published in 1999.[25] The prospective randomized study consisted of 109 patients with SAH, an identified aneurysm, and potential for treatment using either modality. After treatment, the patients were followed clinically (3 months post SAH), angiographically (3, 12, and 36 months), and with neuropsychological testing (3 and 12 months). The technical mortality rate was 4% in the surgical group and 2% in the endovascular group. Significantly better initial angiographic results

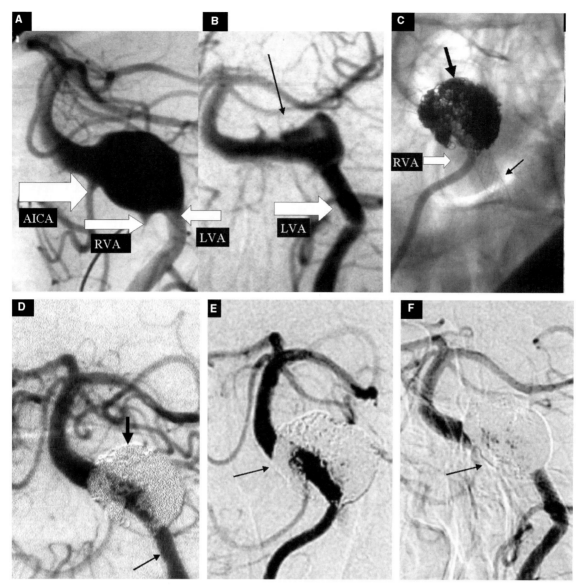

FIGURE 11–2 A 78-year-old man with a giant fusiform aneurysm of the vertebrobasilar junction, giving rise to headaches—a VI cranial nerve palsy. **(A)** Oblique view of the angiogram obtained with a left vertebral artery (VA) injection. The anterior inferior cerebellar artery (AICA) and the right and left VAs are indicated by the white arrows. The patient was initially treated with three low-porous stents (Magic Wallstent, Boston Scientific BSC, Natick, Massachusetts) deployed under the fusiform aneurysm via the left VA **(B)** Four-week follow-up angiogram obtained with a left VA injection shows partial thrombosis of the lesion (black arrow). The angiogram also shows straightening of the distal segment of the left VA and proximal segment of the basilar artery secondary to placement of the three stents. **(C)** Unsubtracted oblique view of a right VA injection shows coil embolization (large arrow) through the stent struts and the stents (small arrows). **(D)** Final oblique view of the left VA injection after coil embolization. **(E, F)** Sixteen-month follow-up angiogram with similar oblique view obtained with right **(E)** and left **(F)** VA injection that shows arterial remodeling and aneurysm obliteration (small arrows) with preservation of the parent vessel.

were achieved after endovascular treatment of patients with posterior circulation aneurysms ($N = 11$; $p = 0.045$).

Recently, the International Subarachnoid Aneurysm Trial (ISAT) provided level I evidence on the benefits of endovascular versus surgical treatment of ruptured intracranial aneurysms.[26] The study was a randomized, controlled trial of surgical clipping versus endovascular coiling for ruptured intracranial aneurysms. The multicenter study enrolled 2143 patients with aneurysms that were deemed suitable for either treatment modality. Random assignment included 1070 patients for clipping and 1073 patients for coiling. More than 50% of the aneurysms were less than 6 mm, and over 90% were less than 10 mm in diameter. Interestingly, the majority of aneurysms enrolled in the study involved the anterior cerebral artery (50.5%), followed by the internal carotid artery

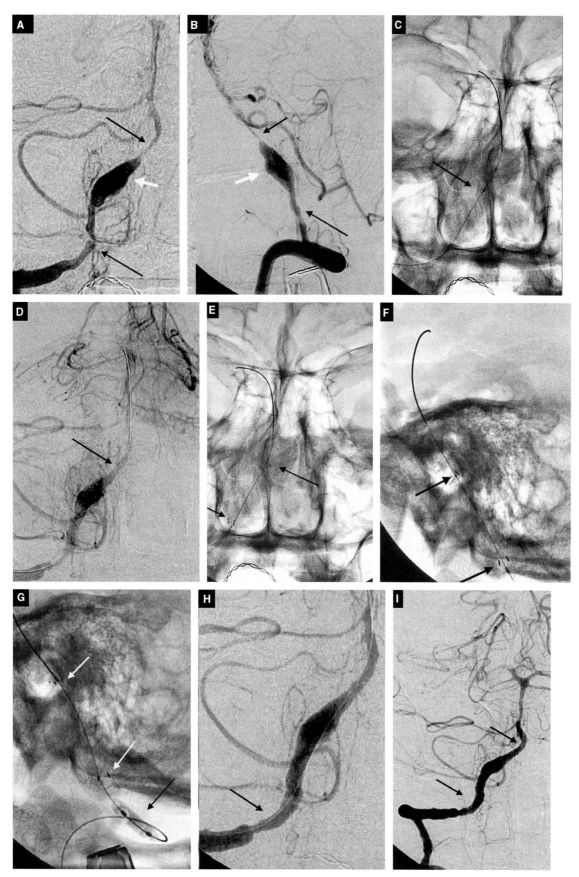

FIGURE 11–3 A 39-year-old woman with the second episode of subarachnoid hemorrhage secondary to a ruptured dissecting vertebral artery (VA) aneurysm. Clinically, the patient had altered mental status (Hunt and Hess grade 3). **(A, B)** Antero-posterior **(A)** and lateral **(B)** view of the right VA angiogram showing the right VA dissecting aneurysm (white arrow). In addition, the angiogram shows vasospasm of the VA and of the vertebrobasilar (VB) junction (black arrow). **(C, D)** Balloon angioplasty of the vasospasm of the VB junction (Maveric 2.5 × 9 mm; BSC, Natick, MA). **(E, F)** Deployment of the stent in the right VA (Neuroform 2; 2.5 × 20 mm). The arrows point to the proximal and distal margins of the stent. **(G, H)** Balloon angioplasty of the proximal segment of the VA (Maveric 2.5 × 9 mm).

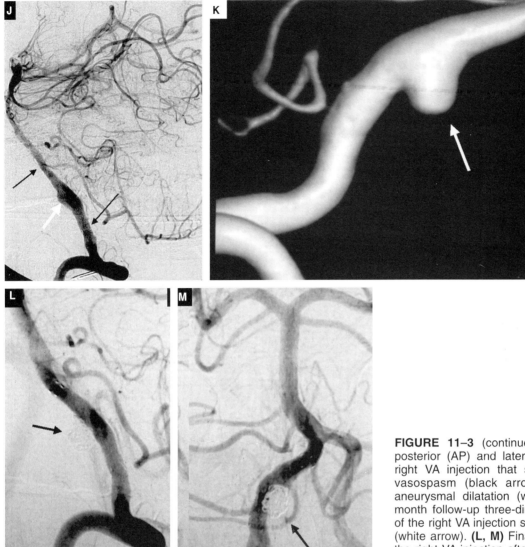

FIGURE 11–3 (continued) **(I, J)** Final antero-posterior (AP) and lateral (L) projections of the right VA injection that shows resolution of the vasospasm (black arrows) and mild residual aneurysmal dilatation (white arrow). **(K)** Three-month follow-up three-dimensional reconstruction of the right VA injection shows aneurysmal growth (white arrow). **(L, M)** Final AP and L projection of the right VA injection after coil embolization of the aneurysm through the stent struts.

(including posterior communicating artery aneurysms). Only a small number of aneurysms were located in the posterior circulation (2.7%). The fivefold reduction in the number of posterior circulation aneurysms (8 to 15% expected) reflects a selection bias. This is because the ISAT adjudicating committee considered it unethical to randomize posterior circulation aneurysms. Both neuroradiologists and neurosurgeons agreed that the majority of these aneurysms should be treated by coil embolization.

Most of the patients enrolled in ISAT were in excellent medical condition prior to the intervention. Clinical outcomes were assessed based on modified Rankin scale (mRS) at 2 months and 1 year. Recruitment into the trial was stopped after a planned interim analysis revealed significantly better death and disability rates in the endovascular group. Two hundred and forty-three of

793 (30.6%) patients treated with microvascular clipping were dependent or dead at 1-year follow-up, compared with 190 of 801 (23.7%) patients treated with coil embolization ($p = 0.0019$). The data yielded to a relative risk reduction for death or dependency of 22.6% and an absolute risk reduction of 6.9%. Although the randomization was halted, the follow-up continued. As more patients are being evaluated and more long-term follow-up data are available, the absolute risk reduction in endovascular treatment is even more evident.

■ Unruptured Aneurysms

Patients with unruptured intracranial aneurysms far outnumber those with ruptured aneurysms. There has been much debate over the management of unruptured aneurysms in the recent literature. The main discussion has focused on the variables that can predict when an unruptured aneurysm will rupture. The strongest predictors seem to be aneurysm size and location, as well as a patient's gender and history of previously ruptured intracranial aneurysms.

The International Study of Unruptured Intracranial Aneurysm (ISUIA) investigators provided the most comprehensive study on the natural history of unruptured aneurysms.[27] In a retrospective study of 1449 patients with 1937 aneurysms, two groups were followed: Group 1, without a history of SAH ($n = 727$), and Group 2, with a history of SAH from a different aneurysm ($n = 722$). Patients in Group 1 had a cumulative rupture rate of 0.05% per year for aneurysms that were less than 10 mm in diameter at the time of diagnosis. The rupture rate was 20 times higher for aneurysms greater than 10 mm in diameter (nearly 1% per year); patients with giant aneurysms (>25 mm) experienced a 6% rupture rate during the first year. Both size and location were predictive factors of future rupture in Group 1 patients. Aneurysms greater than 10 mm in diameter were more likely to rupture. Also, posterior circulation aneurysms were more likely to rupture independent of size.

Patients in Group 2 had a history of SAH, a properly treated aneurysm, and another unruptured aneurysm. The rupture rate for the untreated aneurysm was 11-fold higher (0.5% per year) for aneurysms less than 10 mm in diameter. Similar to the patients in Group 1, the rupture rate was less than 1% per year for aneurysms greater than 10 mm in diameter. Surprisingly, size was not an independent risk factor for Group 2 aneurysms. Location and patient age were independent risk factors for rupture; specifically, basilar tip aneurysms provided a 5.1 relative risk, and older age was a 1.31 relative risk for rupture.

Another study that evaluated aneurysm rupture risk regardless of size was published by Juvela et al, who followed the natural history of intracranial aneurysms for an average of nearly 20 years in 142 patients with 181 unruptured aneurysms.[28] The average annual incidence rate of rupture was 1.3%, and the relative risk of rupture increased with the size of aneurysms. Smoking, size of aneurysm, and patient age were concluded to be the most important risk factors for rupture.

Because of the discrepancy between the original ISUIA data on the frequency of rupture of small aneurysm and the data from the clinical practice,[27] the ISUIA investigators prospectively studied a larger cohort recently.[29] The data suggested the critical size for aneurysm ruptures to be ~7 mm. On the other hand, we need to consider that the error in size measurement of ~10% and the averaging of aneurysm size during the pulse cycle (increase in diameter during systole, and decrease during diastole) can effect a 10 to 15% change in diameter.[30] Obviously, another major factor confirmed by Wiebers et al is the higher risk of rupture, in general, for posterior circulation aneurysms relative to the anterior circulation. Based, most likely, on the initial angiogram and aneurysm architecture, surgeons decided to enroll some patients in the ISUIA long-term study and subjected other cases to surgery. The low annual risk of rupture reflects the excellent judgment of the involved physicians.

■ Posterior Circulation Aneurysms: Importance of Location

One major factor to consider when assessing endovascular techniques for treating posterior circulation aneurysms is the exact location of the aneurysm. In a comprehensive, systematic literature review of posterior circulation aneurysms by Lozier et al, the most commonly cited location for posterior circulation aneurysms was the basilar apex.[5] Other locations included the superior cerebellar, midbasilar (basilar trunk, including the anterior inferior cerebellar artery [AICA]) vertebrobasilar junction, posterior inferior cerebellar, and the vertebral artery.

Basilar apex aneurysms account for 5 to 8% of all intracranial aneurysms and are the most common type of aneurysm of the posterior circulation (51%).[9,31,32] These lesions are often nestled between critical thalamoperforator and thalamogeniculate arteries of the distal basilar trunk and P1 posterior cerebral segments. If left untreated, the overwhelming majority of patients with ruptured basilar apex aneurysms die or become severely disabled within 3 to 6 years.[33] According to Le Roux and Winn, the major cause of death in these patients was rebleeding, with risk factors for rebleeding to include poor clinical grade, large aneurysm size, and mass effect upon the third ventricle.[33] As a result, the early multicenter trials describing the endovascular occlusion of intracranial aneurysms were largely composed of basilar apex aneurysms.

Open neurosurgical morbidity and mortality rates for the treatment of ruptured basilar tip aneurysms have been notoriously poor. Kassell et al studied the open neurosurgical treatment of 266 vertebrobasilar aneurysms and described a 47.4% morbidity and mortality rate with no difference in rebleeding rate with respect to the timing of surgery.[4,34] Basilar aneurysms were predictors of mortality in the study. Therefore, the indications for treatment of unruptured basilar tip aneurysms is based on the fact that basilar tip aneurysms had a greater propensity to rupture in both the non-SAH and unrelated SAH groups described in the ISUIA study.

To evaluate the state of the art in the endovascular treatment of posterior circulation aneurysms as a whole, Lozier et al performed a MEDLINE literature search and reviewed the pooled data.[5] Twelve reports out of 18 were specific to the posterior circulation and described 495 aneurysms in 489 patients. The 18 reports included 12 single-center experiences limited to the posterior circulation[17,35-45]; six of these studies involved only the basilar apex, with 228 basilar apex aneurysms in 226 patients.[17,35-39] The indications for treatment in these six studies were variable and included anticipated surgical difficulty, poor neurological condition, failed clipping, poor medical condition, patient preference, and physician preference. The vast majority of the studies reviewed by Lozier cited anticipated surgical difficulty followed by failed clipping and physician preference as the main reasons for endovascular therapy.[5] In all studies, the aneurysms were characterized based on size. Lozier describes 57.5% of the basilar apex aneurysms in his review as small (<10 mm), 34.6% as large (11 to 25 mm), and 7.0% as giant (>25 mm); 60.1% harbored wide necks (>4 mm, regardless of aneurysm size). The Hunt and Hess grades were 33.2%, 31.4%, 22.1%, 8%, and 4.4% for grades 0, 1 or 2, 3, 4, and 5, respectively. Of the 220 embolized with GDC coils, 32 (14%) had complications directly related to the procedure, such as coil protrusion (9; 3.9%) and parent artery thrombosis (9; 3.9%). Intraprocedural aneurysm rupture occurred in seven (3.1%) cases, with two patients having a poor neurological outcome and two fatalities. Immediate postprocedure angiography revealed 100% occlusion in 43.2%, 90 to 99% occlusion in 44.6%, and less than 90% occlusion in 12.3%. The 6-month follow-up of 96 patients showed 36.5%, 36.5% and 27.1% for 100%, 90 to 99%, and over 90% occlusion, respectively. Thirty-two of the 34 (94.1%) recanalized aneurysms had a large neck, defined as >4 mm. The recurrence rate for narrow-neck aneurysms was estimated at between 7.7% and 2.5%. Using the Glasgow Outcome Scale,[46] five of the studies cited by Lozier followed clinical outcome for a mean of 26.1 months on 198 patients.[17,35-39] There was an overall 0.7% annual risk of SAH postembolization. For patients with treated ruptured aneurysms, 101 (80.2%) were independent, 11 (8.7%) were dependent, and 14 (11.1%) had expired on latest follow-up. For patients with unruptured aneurysms, that latest clinical follow-up revealed that 58 (90.6%) were independent, 2 (3.1%) were dependent, and 4 (6.3%) had expired.

In 1997 Eskridge et al, under an Investigational Device Exemption approved by the Food and Drug Administration (FDA), conducted a multicenter study that analyzed 150 basilar tip aneurysms treated with GDC.[47] Of the 67 unruptured aneurysms, 49 were symptomatic and less than 2.5 cm; 9 were symptomatic and giant (>2.5 cm). There was greater than 90% initial angiographic occlusion in 81% of the unruptured aneurysms. However, the mortality rate was 12% (6 of 49) in the symptomatic unruptured group; of the 9 patients with symptomatic unruptured giant aneurysms, 3 patients did not survive. It should be noted that these data reflect the early experience with GDC aneurysm treatment without the benefit of improved catheter and coil technology as well as balloon-assisted techniques.

In early 2003, Vallee et al described 55 basilar tip aneurysms in 53 patients treated by GDC occlusion with or without balloon assistance for the previous 6 years.[32] Forty-one (75%) of the aneurysms were ruptured (25%) and 14 unruptured. Of the 41 ruptured aneurysms, 32 (78.1%) were Hunt and Hess grade 2 or better. Fifty-two (95%) of the 55 aneurysms were treated with GDC; complete initial angiographic occlusion was achieved in 34 (77%) and near complete occlusion in 4 of the treated aneurysms (9%). On 6- to 12-month follow-up, 26 (79%) remained completely occluded. Multivariate analysis showed that neck size (large; >4 mm) was the only independent predictor of the initial occlusion rate and revascularization. Forty-eight (94%) of 51 patients treated remained asymptomatic or returned to their previous neurological status. Of the patients with ruptured aneurysms, 3 of 39 (8%) expired and 1 experienced significant morbidity. Mortality was strongly correlated with Hunt and Hess grade 4.

Posterior Circulation Aneurysms: Other Locations

In the comprehensive review by Lozier et al,[5] other locations other than the basilar apex include the superior cerebellar artery (50.6%), posterior inferior cerebellar artery (PICA) (6.4%), midbasilar (basilar trunk) (13.1%), vertebrobasilar junction (7.1%), vertebral artery (5.2%), posterior cerebral artery (3.4%), and others (0.7%). Because of the rarity of posterior circulation aneurysms in locations other than the basilar apex, the data available for these lesions are limited to single-center reports of a few cases. Mukonoweshuro et al described the endovascular treatment with GDC of 23 patients with PICA aneurysms.[48] They observed a 28-day procedure-related neurological morbidity of 13% (3 of 23 patients). Although one patient suffered permanent neurological deficits, there were no procedure-related deaths and no rebleeding observed for any of the treated aneurysms.

Dissecting Aneurysms of the Vertebrobasilar System

Dissecting aneurysms of the posterior circulation are uncommon. Since the initial description of their radiographical and pathological appearance by Yonas,[49] these lesions have been detected and described with increasing frequency. Dissecting aneurysms of the vertebrobasilar system remain high-risk lesions because of their natural history. Approximately 30 to 70% of patients with rupture will have rebleeding. Clinical presentation includes SAH, thromboembolic events, and cranial neuropathy secondary to mass effect. Most cases of dissecting aneurysms are idiopathic, but several other etiologies have been reported, such as trauma, hypertension, syphilis, fibromuscular dysplasia, and polyarthritis nodosa. Several approaches to the treatment of these aneurysms of the vertebrobasilar system have been used.

A single-center case series was reported by Rabinov et al in which they analyzed the data relative to 35 patients with intradural vertebrobasilar dissecting aneurysms who presented to Massachusetts General Hospital between 1992 and 2002.[50] Twenty-six were treated by endovascular means and 2 with open surgery. In the endovascular group, 14 were in a supra-PICA location, and 3 of these extended to the vertebrobasilar junction on the initial angiogram. Ten were located in an infra-PICA location, or no antegrade flow was seen in the PICA or anterior spinal artery. Two were located at the PICA with antegrade flow preserved in the branch. Twelve lesions were treated with trapping; another 14 were initially treated with proximal occlusion techniques, 2 of which eventually required trapping procedures. Follow-up images were obtained within 1 year of initial treatment in 24 patients. Mean follow-up for these patients was 3.5 years. Initial treatments were technically successful and without complication in all 26 patients. Follow-up examinations showed complete cure in 19 out of 24 patients. One patient died of global ischemia after presenting as Hunt and Hess grade 5 with subarachnoid hemorrhage. Two recurrent hemorrhages occurred in patients in the proximal occlusion group; one died, and the other underwent a trapping procedure. One patient developed contralateral vertebral dissection 24 hours after occlusion of a dissecting aneurysm of the dominant vertebral artery and died of a brain stem infarct. Another died of probable vasospasm, and the last died of an unknown cause 1 month after treatment. Two patients had recanalization despite an initial trapping procedure; both underwent further treatment. Mortality rate was 20% in the treated group (including the two patients treated surgically), with four out of five deaths occurring during the initial hospital course. Mortality rate was 50% in the six patients in the untreated group who were available for follow-up.

■ Conclusion

Posterior circulation aneurysms represent 8 to 15% of all intracranial aneurysms and have significantly higher morbidity and mortality compared with anterior circulation aneurysms. The approach to posterior circulation aneurysms with traditional microsurgical techniques is technically challenging, anatomically unfavorable, and results in significant morbidity and mortality even in the best surgical hands.

Over the past 20 years, the use of endovascular embolization to treat intracranial aneurysms has steadily increased, particularly since the development of coils. It has been estimated that more than 125,000 aneurysms worldwide have been treated with GDC coils. Since the initial description by Guido Guglielmi,[13,14] a rapidly advancing endovascular technology now facilitates the use of this approach for the treatment of the most complex and dangerous aneurysms.

Although the published endovascular experience in posterior circulation aneurysms is limited, at times incomplete, and mostly on basilar apex aneurysms, coil embolization emerges as the safest and most effective treatment for these lesions. Concerning published data from clinical trials, the ISAT provided level I evidence on the benefits of endovascular versus surgical treatment of ruptured intracranial aneurysms. The small number of posterior circulation aneurysms randomized in ISAT reflects a selection bias. In fact, the ISAT adjudicating committee considered it unethical to randomize posterior circulation aneurysms, as the majority of these lesions should be treated by coil embolization.

Regarding the vast majority of unruptured aneurysms, the general consensus is that posterior circulation aneurysms are considered at high risk for rupture and therefore should be treated. The drawback of the endovascular approach for the treatment of intracranial aneurysms in general, and in particular for posterior circulation aneurysms, is the rate of aneurysm recurrence. However, these data ought to be considered in light of (1) lower morbidity and mortality associated with endovascular therapy; (2) a rapidly advancing endovascular embolization technology that is allowing safer and higher packing density, and therefore lower recanalization rates; and (3) the ability to safely retreat these remnants at follow-up evaluation. Future studies with standardized methods of data presentation are definitely needed as endovascular embolization technology continues to improve.

■ References

1. Weir B. Intracranial aneurysms and subarachnoid hemorrhage: an overview. In: Wilkins RH, Rengachary SS, eds. Neurosurgery, 1st ed. New York, NY: McGraw-Hill; 1985:1308–1329
2. Phillips LH. The unchanging pattern of subarachnoid hemorrhage in a community. Neurology 1980;30:1034–1040
3. Youmans JR. Neurological Surgery: A Comprehensive Reference Guide to the Diagnosis and Management of Neurosurgical Problems, 4th ed. Philadelphia: Saunders; 1996
4. Kassell NF, Torner JC, Jane JA, Haley EC Jr, Adams HP. The International Cooperative Study on the Timing of Aneurysm Surgery. Part 2: surgical results. J Neurosurg 1990;73(1):37–47
5. Lozier AP, Connolly ES Jr, Lavine SD, Solomon RA. Guglielmi detachable coil embolization of posterior circulation aneurysms: a systematic review of the literature. Stroke 2002;33(10):2509–2518
6. Hunt WE, Hess RM. Surgical risk as related to time of intervention in the repair of intracranial aneurysms. J Neurosurg 1968;28(1):14–20
7. Schievink WI. Intracranial aneurysms. N Engl J Med 1997; 336(1):28–40
8. Mayberg MR, Batjer HH, Dacey R, et al. Guidelines for the management of aneurysmal subarachnoid hemorrhage. A statement for healthcare professionals from a special writing group of the Stroke Council, American Heart Association. Stroke 1994; 25(11):2315–2328
9. Schievink WI, Wijdicks EF, Piepgras DG, Chu CP, O'Fallon WM, Whisnant JP. The poor prognosis of ruptured intracranial aneurysms of the posterior circulation. J Neurosurg 1995;82(5):791–795

10. Graves VB, Strother CM, Duff TA, Perl JII. Early treatment of ruptured aneurysms with Guglielmi detachable coils: effect on subsequent bleeding. Neurosurgery 1995;37:640–648

11. Fox AJ, Viñuela F, Pelz DM, et al. Use of detachable balloons for the proximal artery occlusion in the treatment of unclippable aneurysms. J Neurosurg 1987;66:40–46

12. Halbach VV, Hieshima GB, Higashida RT. Treatment of intracranial aneurysms by balloon embolization. Semin Intervent Radiol 1987;4:261–268

13. Guglielmi G, Viñuela F, Sepetka I, Macellari V. Electrothrombosis of saccular aneurysms via endovascular approach. Part 1: electrochemical basis, technique, and experimental results. J Neurosurg 1991;75(1):1–7

14. Guglielmi G, Viñuela F, Dion J, et al. Electrothrombosis of saccular aneurysms via endovascular approach. Part 2: preliminary clinical experience. J Neurosurg 1991;75:8–14

15. Latchaw RE. Acutely ruptured intracranial aneurysm: should we treat with endovascular coils or with surgical clipping? Radiology 1999;211(2):306–308

16. Viñuela F, Duckwiler G, Mawad M. Guglielmi detachable coil embolization of acute intracranial aneurysm: perioperative anatomical and clinical outcome in 403 patients. J Neurosurg 1997;86(3):475–482

17. Raymond J, Roy D, Bojanowski M, Moumdjian R, L'Esperance G. Endovascular treatment of acutely ruptured and unruptured aneurysms of the basilar bifurcation. J Neurosurg 1997;86(2):211–219

18. Peerless SJ, Hernesniemi JA, Gutman FB, Drake CG. Early surgery for ruptured vertebrobasilar aneurysms. J Neurosurg 1994;80(4):643–649

19. Drake CG, Allcock JM. Postoperative angiography and the "slipped" clip. J Neurosurg 1973;39(6):683–689

20. Drake CG, Friedman AH, Peerless SJ. Failed aneurysm surgery. Reoperation in 115 cases. J Neurosurg 1984;61(5):848–856

21. Giannotta SL, Litofsky NS. Reoperative management of intracranial aneurysms. J Neurosurg 1995;83(3):387–393

22. Feuerberg I, Lindquist C, Lindqvist M, Steiner L. Natural history of postoperative aneurysm rests. J Neurosurg 1987;66(1):30–34

23. Malisch TW, Guglielmi G, Viñuela F, et al. Intracranial aneurysms treated with the Guglielmi detachable coil: midterm clinical results in a consecutive series of 100 patients. J Neurosurg 1997;87(2):176–183

24. Murayama Y, Malisch T, Guglielmi G, et al. Incidence of cerebral vasospasm after endovascular treatment of acutely ruptured aneurysms: report on 69 cases. J Neurosurg 1997;87(6):830–835

25. Vanninen R, Koivisto T, Saari T, Hernesniemi J, Vapalahti M. Ruptured intracranial aneurysms: acute endovascular treatment with electrolytically detachable coils—a prospective randomized study. Radiology 1999;211(2):325–336

26. Molyneux A, Kerr R, Stratton I, et al. International Subarachnoid Aneurysm Trial Collaborative Group (ISAT). ISAT of neurosurgical clipping versus endovascular coiling in 2143 patients with ruptured intracranial aneurysms: a randomised trial. Lancet 2002;360(9342):1267–1274

27. International Study of Unruptured Intracranial Aneurysms Investigators. Unruptured intracranial aneurysms—risk of rupture and risks of surgical intervention. N Engl J Med 1998;339(24):1725–1733

28. Juvela S, Porras M, Poussa K. Natural history of unruptured intracranial aneurysms: probability of and risk factors for aneurysm rupture. J Neurosurg 2000;93(3):379–387

29. Wiebers DO, Whisnant JP, Huston J III, et al; International Study of Unruptured Intracranial Aneurysms Investigators. Unruptured intracranial aneurysms: natural history, clinical outcome, and risks of surgical and endovascular treatment. Lancet 2003;362(9378):103–110

30. McCormick WF, Acosta-Rua GJ. The size of intracranial saccular aneurysms. An autopsy study. J Neurosurg 1970;33(4):422–427

31. Schievink WI, Wijdicks EF, Parisi JE, Piepgras DG, Whisnant JP. Sudden death from aneurysmal subarachnoid hemorrhage. Neurology 1995;45(5):871–874

32. Vallee JN, Aymard A, Vicaut E, Reis M, Merland JJ. Endovascular treatment of basilar tip aneurysms with Guglielmi detachable coils: predictors of immediate and long-term results with multivariate analysis 6-year experience. Radiology 2003;226(3):867–879

33. Le Roux PD, Winn HR. Management of cerebral aneurysms. How can current management be improved? Neurosurg Clin N Am 1998;9(3):421–433

34. Kassell NF, Torner JC, Haley EC Jr, Jane JA, Adams HP, Kongable GL. The International Cooperative Study on the Timing of Aneurysm Surgery. Part 1: overall management results. J Neurosurg 1990;73(1):18–36

35. Tateshima S, Murayama Y, Gobin YP, Duckwiler GR, Guglielmi G, Viñuela F. Endovascular treatment of basilar tip aneurysms using Guglielmi detachable coils: anatomic and clinical outcomes in 73 patients from a single institution. Neurosurgery 2000;47(6):1332–1339 discussion 1339–1342

36. Gruber DP, Zimmerman GA, Tomsick TA, van Loveren HR, Link MJ, Tew JM Jr. A comparison between endovascular and surgical management of basilar artery apex aneurysms. J Neurosurg 1999;90(5):868–874

37. McDougall CG, Halbach VV, Dowd CF, Higashida RT, Larsen DW, Hieshima GB. Endovascular treatment of basilar tip aneurysms using electrolytically detachable coils. J Neurosurg 1996;84(3):393–399

38. Bavinzski G, Killer M, Gruber A, Reinprecht A, Gross CE, Richling B. Treatment of basilar artery bifurcation aneurysms by using Guglielmi detachable coils: a 6-year experience. J Neurosurg 1999;90(5):843–852

39. Klein GE, Szolar DH, Leber KA, Karaic R, Hausegger KA. Basilar tip aneurysm: endovascular treatment with Guglielmi detachable coils—midterm results. Radiology 1997;205(1):191–196

40. Steiger HJ, Medele R, Bruckmann H, Schroth G, Reulen HJ. Interdisciplinary management results in 100 patients with ruptured and unruptured posterior circulation aneurysms. Acta Neurochir (Wien) 1999;141(4):359–366 discussion 366–367

41. Uda K, Murayama Y, Gobin YP, Duckwiler GR, Viñuela F. Endovascular treatment of basilar artery trunk aneurysms with Guglielmi detachable coils: clinical experience with 41 aneurysms in 39 patients. J Neurosurg 2001;95(4):624–632

42. Lempert TE, Malek AM, Halbach VV, et al. Endovascular treatment of ruptured posterior circulation cerebral aneurysms. Clinical and angiographic outcomes. Stroke 2000;31(1):100–110

43. Nichols DA, Brown RD Jr, Thielen KR, Meyer FB, Atkinson JL, Piepgras DG. Endovascular treatment of ruptured posterior circulation aneurysms using electrolytically detachable coils. J Neurosurg 1997;87(3):374–380

44. Birchall D, Khangure M, McAuliffe W, Apsimon H, Knuckey N. Endovascular treatment of posterior circulation aneurysms. Br J Neurosurg 2001;15(1):39–43

45. Pierot L, Boulin A, Castaings L, Rey A, Moret J. Selective occlusion of basilar artery aneurysms using controlled detachable coils: report of 35 cases. Neurosurgery 1996;38(5):948–953 discussion 953–954

46. Jennett B, Bond M. Assessment of outcome after severe brain damage. Lancet 1975;1(7905):480–484

47. Eskridge JM, Song JK. Endovascular embolization of 150 basilar tip aneurysms with Guglielmi detachable coils: results of the Food and Drug Administration multicenter clinical trial. J Neurosurg 1998;89(1):81–86

48. Mukonoweshuro W, Laitt RD, Hughes DG. Endovascular treatment of PICA aneurysms. Neuroradiology 2003;45(3):188–192

49. Yonas H, Agamanolis D, Takaoka Y, et al. Dissecting intracranial aneurysms. Surg Neurol 1977;8:407–415

50. Rabinov JD, Hellinger FR, Morris PP, Ogilvy CS, Putman CM. Endovascular management of vertebrobasilar dissecting aneurysms. AJNR Am J Neuroradiol 2003;24:1421–1428

12

Surgical Treatment of Cerebral Arteriovenous Malformations

ANDREW JEA, MUSTAFA K. BAŞKAYA, AND ROBERTO C. HEROS

Objectives: Upon completion of this chapter, the reader should be able to explain how to select patients for treatment or conservative management and how to develop appropriate treatment strategies that combine embolization, microsurgery, and radiosurgery.

Accreditation: The AANS* is accredited by the Accreditation Council for Continuing Medical Education (ACCME) to sponsor continuing medical education for physicians.

Credit: The AANS designates this educational activity for a maximum of 15 credits in Category 1 credit toward the AMA Physician's Recognition Award. Each physician should claim only those hours of credit that he/she spent in the educational activity.

The Home Study Examination is online on the AANS Web site at: http://www.aans.org/education/books/controversy.asp

* The acronym AANS refers to both the American Association of Neurological Surgeons and the American Association of Neurosurgeons.

Arteriovenous malformations (AVMs) are vascular abnormalities leading to a fistulous connection of arteries and veins without a normal intervening capillary bed. In the cerebral hemispheres, they frequently occur as cone-shaped lesions with the apex of the cone reaching toward the ventricles. Nearly all AVMs are thought to be congenital. Supratentorial location is the most common (90%). The most common presentation of an AVM is intracerebral hemorrhage (ICH). After ICH, seizure is the second most common presentation. Other presentations of AVMs include headache and focal neurological deficits that may be related to steal phenomenon or other alteration in perfusion in the tissue adjacent to the AVM, such as venous hypertension from arterialization of normal draining veins.

In managing unruptured AVMs, it is important to understand the natural history of these vascular malformations. The decision for no treatment or for a single or multimodality treatment paradigm also involves being familiar with the outcomes and risks of each treatment modality—microvascular resection, endovascular embolization, and

stereotactic radiosurgery. Finally, the patient-related factors, such as age, general medical condition, neurological condition, and occupation, must also be taken into consideration before reaching a conclusion. The treatment of AVMs is highly individualized. There is no universal algorithm or protocol to be followed when dealing with these unique problems.

The currently used treatments for AVMs include (1) microsurgical resection only, (2) preoperative endovascular embolization followed by microsurgical resection, (3) stereotactic radiosurgery only, (4) preprocedural endovascular embolization followed by radiosurgical treatment, (5) endovascular embolization only, and (6) observation only. The ultimate goal for all of these modalities is cure for the patient; however, the only way to achieve cure is with complete obliteration of the AVM. Microsurgery is the gold standard for resection of small superficial AVMs against which other methods of treatment must be measured. There is certainly a well-established role for adjunctive endovascular embolization of some AVMs. Clearly, there are specific situations, such as small deep AVMs in eloquent brain structures, where microsurgery should not be used as the primary treatment modality; stereotactic radiosurgery and occasionally embolization (when there is reasonable expectation of complete obliteration by embolization) are the preferred treatment options in these cases. We also make a case for observation in patients with large AVMs in or near critical areas of the brain that are not ideal for surgical resection or radiosurgery. Here, the pursuit of treatment may actually be more harmful to the patient than the natural history of the AVM.

■ Natural History

Several series have evaluated the natural history of AVMs with regard to the risk of hemorrhage. In a series of 168 patients without a history of previous hemorrhage, 18% of patients had subsequent hemorrhage over a mean follow-up of 8.2 years.[1] Annualized hemorrhage rate was 2.2%. In a study reported by Graf et al, hemorrhage risk at 1 year was 2%, at 5 years was 14%, and at 10 years was 31%.[2] A retrospective study of 217 patients with AVMs followed for an average of 10.4 years yielded an annual hemorrhage rate of 3.4%.[3]

An important study by Ondra et al outlined the natural history of AVMs among 160 patients who presented with symptomatic AVMs, which were followed for a mean follow-up of 23.7 years.[4] This study included 160 patients who presented mainly with hemorrhage; they were followed conservatively for an average of 24.7 years. The mean age at presentation was 33 years. The rehemorrhage rate was 4% per year, with an average of 7.7 years for the next hemorrhage to occur. The yearly morbidity rate was 1.7%, and the mortality rate was 1%. This study demonstrated the high morbidity and mortality associated with AVMs regardless of initial mode of presentation including hemorrhage, headache, or seizure.

The only prospective study of the natural history of AVMs resulted in an annual hemorrhage rate of 2.2%. However, follow-up of this group of 139 patients was short at an average of only 1 year.[5] **Table 12-1** summarizes the previously published studies on the natural history of AVMs. Several angioarchitectural factors influence the risk of hemorrhage for AVMs.

■ Surgical Resection

Diagnostic Evaluation

A computed tomography (CT) scan may be used as an initial screening tool for patients presenting with neurological sequelae related to unruptured or ruptured AVMs. This study can be used quickly to determine location of the lesion, acute hemorrhage, hydrocephalus, or areas of encephalomalacia from previous surgery or rupture. A nonenhanced CT may show irregular hyperdense areas frequently associated with calcifications in unruptured AVMs and acute hemorrhage on plain CT scan with ruptured AVMs. With the addition of intravenous contrast material, a CT scan shows the nidus and feeding vessels or dilated draining veins.

Magnetic resonance imaging (MRI) is superior to a CT scan in delineating details of the macro-architecture of the AVM except in the case of acute hemorrhage. These architectural features include exact anatomic relationships of the nidus, feeding arteries, and draining veins as well as topographic relationships between AVM and adjacent brain[6] (**Fig. 12–1A–F**). MRI is sensitive in revealing subacute hemorrhage.[7] The AVM appears as a sponge-like structure, with patchy signal loss, or flow voids, associated with feeding arteries or draining veins on T1-weighted sequences. MRI and angiography in combination provide complementary information that facilitates understanding the three-dimensional structure of the nidus, feeding arteries, and draining veins. Magnetic resonance angiography (MRA) currently cannot replace conventional cerebral angiography. In the case of acute hemorrhage, the hematoma obscures all details of the AVM, making MRA virtually useless. This calls for direct

TABLE 12–1 Natural History Studies for Arteriovenous Malformations

Author (Year)	Type of Study	No. of Patients	Average Years of Follow-Up	Annual Hemorrhage Rate
Brown et al (1996)[1]	Retrospective	168	8.2	2.2%
Graf et al (1983)[2]	Retrospective	71	4.8	2% at 1 year; 14% at 5 years; 31% at 10 years; 6% for the first year after a hemorrhage, then baseline
Crawford et al (1986)[3]	Retrospective	217	10.4	3.4%
Ondra et al (1990)[4]	Retrospective	160	23.7	4%
Mast et al (1997)[5]	Prospective	139	1.0	2.2%

use of cerebral angiography if the characteristics of the hematoma strongly suggest AVM as an etiology.

Complete cerebral angiography with multiple projections is a mandatory step in the preoperative evaluation of a patient with an AVM. Cerebral angiography can localize the nidus, the feeding arteries, and the draining veins. Angiography may assess the flow dynamics within the nidus of the AVM. The search for associated aneurysms is part of the preoperative evaluation. External carotid injections to determine the presence of an external supply are necessary in cases of large-convexity AVMs. It is important that the angiogram be performed close to

the time of surgery, as AVMs can change in size and configuration over time. Vessels that were not seen secondary to compression from a hemorrhage may appear on a follow-up angiogram weeks later.

Many techniques are available for studying the functionality of cortical structures surrounding the AVM. These include the use of positron emission tomography (PET), functional MRI (fMRI), magnetoencephalography, and direct provocative testing of cortical function. Judicious utilization of these techniques will enhance the safety of AVM therapy. Such information may allow the surgeon to tailor treatment modalities to increase

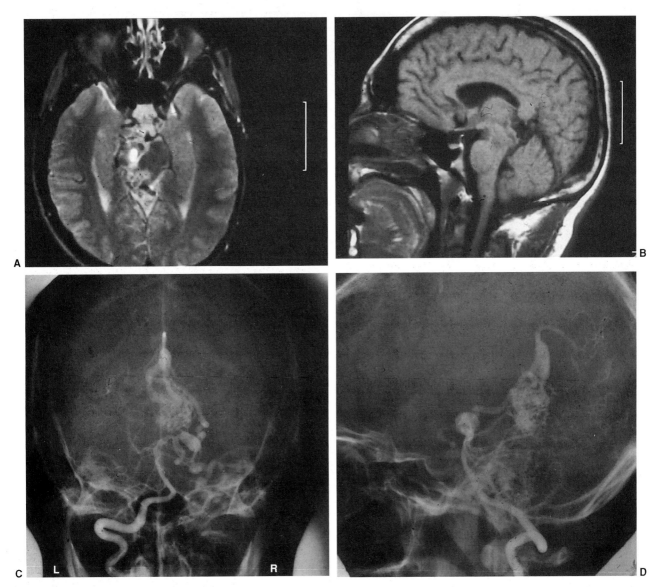

FIGURE 12–1 The role of correct localization of the arteriovenous malformation is shown. On this axial T2-weighted magnetic resonance image (MRI) **(A)**, it is not clear whether this lesion is in the midbrain. Sagittal T1-weighted MRI **(B)** shows that this pial tectal arteriovenous malformation is not located in the midbrain parenchyma. Because of this anatomical location we decided to operate on this patient. The anteroposterior and lateral angiograms **(C, D)** show that this arteriovenous malformation is fed mainly by superior cerebellar artery branches.

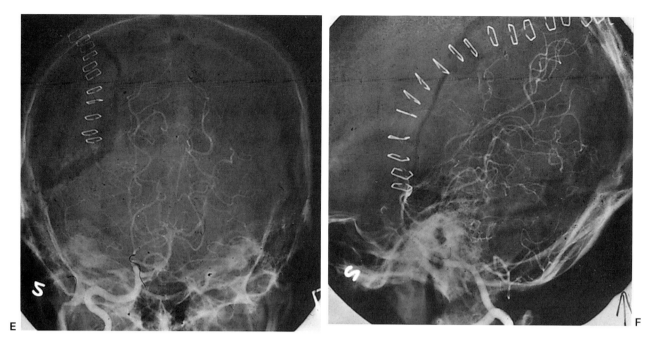

FIGURE 12–1 (continued) The postoperative AP **(E)** and lateral **(F)** angiogram shows complete obliteration.

the margin of safety during treatment and to decrease periprocedural flow-related hemorrhagic or ischemic complications.[8]

Size of Arteriovenous Malformations

In a series of 168 patients followed after presentation without a prior hemorrhage, the size of the AVM was not found to be predictive of future hemorrhage, utilizing a multivariate statistical analysis.[9] However, other studies have found AVMs of small size to be at higher risk of hemorrhage. Spetzler et al compared the feeding artery pressures in small and large AVMs.[10] They found higher feeding artery pressures in the small AVMs and suggested that small AVMs bleed more often than large ones. However, the question of whether this is the case is still controversial.

Draining Veins

Deep drainage has been thought to be an important risk factor for hemorrhage from an AVM. Nataf et al reported a strong correlation between frequency of hemorrhages and presence of deep drainage in AVMs.[11] Arteriovenous malformations with a single draining vein were found to have a higher risk in some studies.[12,13] This can be explained by the fact that impaired drainage through a single vein leads to a high risk of hemodynamic overload and eventual rupture. Impairment in venous drainage caused by stenosis or kinking may also increase the risk of bleeding.[13]

Arteriovenous Malformations and Aneurysms

Prevalence of the association of AVMs with aneurysms varies from 2.7 to 22.7%. This association seems to be correlated with a higher risk of hemorrhage. Brown et al studied 91 patients with unruptured AVMs. Among these, 16 patients had 26 saccular intracranial aneurysms.[14] The researchers found the risk of ICH in patients with co-existing AVM and aneurysm to be 7% at 1 year compared with 3% among those with AVM alone. At 5 years, the risk persisted at 7% per year, while it decreased to 1.7% per year in those with an AVM unassociated with aneurysms. Ninety-six percent of 26 aneurysms were located on an AVM arterial feeder. The significance of intranidal arterial or venous aneurysms, which are quite common in large complex AVMs, is unknown, although it has been suggested that this finding may be associated with an increased risk of hemorrhage.[15]

Indications for Surgical Resection

There are several clear indications for microsurgical resection of AVMs. Arteriovenous malformations with Spetzler–Martin grades I to III on the convexity should generally be resected. The Spetzler–Martin grading system takes into account three factors that greatly affect the surgical resectability of the AVM: size (<3 cm, 1 point; 3–6 cm, 2 points; >6 cm, 3 points), location (non-eloquent cortex, 0 points; eloquent cortex, 1 point), and venous drainage (superficial only, 0 points; deep, 1 point).[16] **Table 12–2** summarizes the methodology for the Spetzler–Martin grading system.

TABLE 12–2 Methodology of Spetzler–Martin Grading of Arteriovenous Malformations

Feature	Characteristic	Points
Size	<3 cm	1
	3–6 cm	2
	>6 cm	3
Venous Drainage	Superficial	0
	Deep	1
Location	Noneloquent cortex	0
	Eloquent cortex	1

However, these are not the only factors that the neurosurgeon must take into account when considering treatment options for an AVM. There are other AVM-related factors, such as the presence of AVM-associated aneurysms and venous restrictive disease, and patient-related factors, such as age, general health, and occupation/avocation. In addition, the specific experience and expertise of the surgeon and the center where treatment is to take place must be taken into account. Each AVM and patient must be considered individually. There is no magic formula to dictate to a physician and surgeon how to proceed in managing a patient. For example, deep venous drainage may actually be an advantage intraoperatively, as the draining veins are hidden away from the surgeon until the last moments of AVM removal. Patients with AVMs that present with major hemorrhage, progressive neurological deterioration, inadequately controlled seizures, intractable headache, or venous restrictive disease should be strongly considered for surgical resection.[17] There is a caveat to operating on ruptured AVMs leading to large intracerebral hemorrhages and significant neurological deficits. These patients should be operated on in a delayed fashion to allow for maximal recovery of neurological function and accurate determination of preoperative neurological status. It is clear that the risk of rebleeding is relatively low (~6% within the first 6 months) during this waiting period. In comparison, the benefits of waiting are great for the patient and surgeon. At the plateau of neurological recovery, the surgeon will then have a true sense of the patient's preoperative neurological condition. What we want to try to avoid is the loss of potential for future neurological recovery by operating early on a patient with intracranial hemorrhage from a ruptured AVM. For example, the patient may be hemiplegic after a hemorrhage from the basal ganglia; significant recovery may occur spontaneously, and it is unfair to the patient to remove the AVM early under the presumption that "He is hemiplegic, I can't make him worse." The surgeon, under this rationale, may turn a reversible hemiplegia into a permanent deficit.

Arteriovenous malformation treatment should be strongly considered in patients with intractable seizures or, in rare cases, intractable headaches, as these symptoms are likely a hindrance to daily living activities. The chance of relieving the symptoms of these patients and giving them a normal life back may outweigh the risks of surgery. Patients with venous restrictive disease may present another strong argument for surgical excision. With the occlusion of venous outflow from the nidus of the AVM, the intranidal hemodynamics begin to change. Acutely, pressure begins to rise in different compartments of the AVM, and chronically, new, fragile venous draining pathways are recruited. These changes are likely to increase the risk of AVM hemorrhage.

Cerebellar and pial brainstem AVMs should also be given strong consideration for surgical resection to prevent the higher risk of bleeding as compared with supratentorial AVMs.[17] A case may also be made for treatment of some basal ganglia and thalamic AVMs, as they carry an annual bleed rate of 11.4%, considerably higher than the average bleeding rate when AVMs in all locations are considered. In addition, morbidity and mortality with each bleed in these locations reach 7.1% and 42.9%, respectively (again, in contrast to the overall mortality rate of AVM hemorrhage of 10%).[18,19]

The above comments about indications are only to suggest that in these cases stronger consideration should be given to treatment as opposed to observation. However, we want to emphasize that all AVMs, whether they have bled or not, causing symptoms or not, should be considered for treatment. The basis for this statement is the well-known fact that, after the first few months of a hemorrhage, the risk of hemorrhage is the same for AVMs that have bled as for those that have not.[4,20] As always, the ultimate recommendation should rest on the balance between the presumed risk of treatment and the risk of future hemorrhage or progressive disability, taking into account the multiple factors discussed and, very specifically, the likely number of years at risk if the AVM is left untreated, which obviously is directly related to the age and general health of the patient.[20]

As emphasized above, decision-making in determining the best management pathway for patients harboring AVMs must include consideration of the patient's age, general health and clinical condition, occupation and lifestyle, location and size of AVM, surgeon's experience, and ethical considerations.[20,21] The patient's age is most important in determining the cumulative risk of AVM rupture during the remainder of the patient's life expectancy. Assuming an annual hemorrhage rate of 2 to 4% and an average life expectancy of 70 years, the cumulative risk (in percentage) of AVM rupture may be estimated by the following formula: 105 minus the patient's age in years.[22,23]

Hence, one may justify a more aggressive approach for surgical treatment in younger patients, as their cumulative risk of hemorrhage is so high. In addition, neurological deficit caused at a young age is generally better tolerated and has a greater chance of recovery. The general health of the patient is important, as a patient with severe comorbid conditions may preclude surgery as a reasonable treatment option. The clinical presentation and neurological condition of a patient will often dictate timing of surgery; for example, the patient may need emergent evacuation of a hematoma caused by a ruptured AVM, or it may be best to wait until the patient has improved to a neurological plateau when AVM resection can be approached electively. The occupation and lifestyle of a patient are important considerations as the neurosurgeon begins to weigh the risks and benefits of treatment of an AVM in a critical area of the brain. For example, a patient who is a pilot and is dependent on his or her sharp visual acuity presenting with an occipital AVM may feel differently about surgical resection with a >50% chance of causing a postoperative hemianopsia than a patient with an AVM in the same location who is a housewife. For obvious reasons, AVM microstructure and surgeon's experience are important factors in determining a treatment strategy. Ethical considerations relate to surgeon's experience and come into play at a point where the surgeon determines if an AVM is operable or inoperable. The latter decision should preferably be made by an experienced cerebrovascular neurosurgeon at a referral center who specializes in AVM surgery. The surgeon should be familiar with the literature as well as his or her own personal experience and should be able to explain to the patient all treatment options with their associated risks and benefits. Importantly, the surgeon should inform the patient clearly and unambiguously of what, in his or her opinion, is the best treatment option, which in certain cases may be no treatment at all.

In general, AVM surgery is elective. As discussed above, we recommend operating on ruptured AVMs that lead to intracranial hemorrhage and significant neurological deficits in a delayed fashion. We have seen many "good" results reported after excision of large AVMs of the thalamus and basal ganglia operated on early after a hemorrhage that rendered the patient hemiplegic. The thinking is that the hemorrhage has already destroyed critical areas of the brain that lead to devastating neurological deficits, and therefore, surgery cannot do further harm to the patient. "Good results" in these instances frequently mean that the patient's neurological condition was the same as before surgery. However, it is possible that the patient's preoperative condition would have changed for the better with time to recover from the ictus. Frequently, the hemorrhage does not destroy functional parts of the brain; instead, the mass from the hemorrhage splays apart gray and white matter, producing a deficit from pressure rather than destruction of critical brain. As the hematoma begins to resolve, these areas of the brain may recover to variable degrees. After a reasonable delay to allow such potential recovery to occur, the surgeon will be in a better position to judge whether, given the degree of the recovery, it may not be preferable to treat the patient with an alternative treatment modality (i.e., radiosurgery) or to recommend conservative therapy.[24]

Outcomes

Microsurgical resection of Spetzler–Martin grades I, II, and III AVMs by experienced surgeons carries high cure rates and low complication rates with immediate elimination of risk of hemorrhage.[25,26] Angiographic cure rate with microsurgery ranges from 94 to 100%. Microsurgery can achieve 100% angiographic obliteration for unruptured convexity AVMs <3 cm with superficial venous drainage.[17] The combined surgical morbidity and mortality for AVMs grade I, II, and III is reported to be less than 10% in several large series.[18,27–35]

In a series of 110 patients harboring grades I to III AVMs taken to the operating room for microsurgical resection, 99% had angiographically confirmed obliteration of the AVM. Two patients (1.8%) required reoperation for residual AVM. Some authors have recommended immediate reoperation for residual malformations following surgical resection.[36] The risk of neurological deterioration in the immediate postop period was 10.9% and declined to 2.7% by 6 months after surgery.[18] In another series of small AVMs, 67 patients underwent microsurgical resection with a surgical outcome of 1.5% morbidity and 0% mortality.[33] Pikus et al reported a series of 19 patients with small AVMs, grades I to III, yielding a 0% rate of morbidity and mortality.[34]

In our series of 311 patients who underwent microsurgical resection alone before 1993 for AVM, grades I to III patients demonstrated 89.9% good outcome, 9.5% significant disability, and 0.5% death.[37] Grades IV and V patients demonstrated 60.7% good outcome, 37.5% significant disability, and 1.8% death. In a follow-up study of 153 consecutive patients with AVMs of all grades with a mean follow-up period of 3.8 years, we looked at the immediate morbidity and mortality rate and compared it to the late morbidity and mortality rate.[28] The overall immediate postoperative of serious morbidity was 24.2%; the serious morbidity at follow-up was 7.8%. The mortality rate at follow-up was 1.3%. There was no history of intracranial hemorrhage in any patient during the follow-up period. At follow-up, 97.8% of patients with grades I to III AVMs were in good or excellent condition, 1.1% experienced a poor outcome, and 1.1% died. In the group of patients with grade IV and V AVMs, 79.0% had good outcome, 17.7% had poor outcome, and 3.2% died. **Table 12–3**[18,26–35,38] and **Table 12–4**[26–32,35,39–41] summarize the microsurgical outcomes from some of the larger published case series for Spetzler–Martin grades I to III and grades IV and V AVMs, respectively.

Completely obliterated AVMs lead to the best outcome in terms of seizure control.[42] After surgical excision, 81%

Table 12–3 Postoperative Outcomes for Grades I to III Arteriovenous Malformations

Author (Year)	No. of Patients	Morbidity and Mortality Rates
Pik et al (2000)[18]	110	10.9% Early morbidity; 2.7% late morbidity
Sisti et al (1993)[33]	67 (small AVMs)	1.5% Combined morbidity and mortality
Pikus et al (1998)[34]	19	0%
Nussbaum et al (1995)[27]	199	9.5% Early morbidity; 0.5% early mortality
Heros et al (1990)[28]	91	1.1% Late morbidity; 1.1% late mortality
Tokunaga et al (2000)[29]	8	0% For grades I and II; 75% early morbidity, 50% late morbidity, and 0% mortality in grade III
Irie et al (2000)[30]	27	0%
Hashimoto et al (2000)[38]	2	0%
Hongo et al (2000)[31]	20	4% Mortality
Russell et al (2002)[35]	35	8.6% Morbidity; 0% mortality
Hartmann et al (2000)[26]	95	5.3% Morbidity; 0% mortality
Hamilton and Spetzler (1994)[32]	71	0%

TABLE 12–4 Postoperative Outcomes for Grades IV and V Arteriovenous Malformations

Author (Year)	No. of Patients	Morbidity and Mortality Rates
Nussbaum et al (1995)[27]	112	37.5% Early morbidity; 1.8% mortality
Heros et al (1990)[28]	62	17.7% Late morbidity; 3.2% late mortality
Tokunaga et al (2000)[29]	4	25% Morbidity; 0% mortality
Irie et al (2000)[30]	4	25% Morbidity; 0% mortality
Hashimoto et al (2000)[38]	3	75% Morbidity; 0% mortality
Hongo et al (2000)[31]	1	100% Mortality
Russell et al (2002)[35]	9	22.2% Morbidity; 11.1% mortality
Hartmann et al (2000)[26]	29	6.9% Morbidity; 0% mortality
Hamilton and Spetzler (1994)[32]	44	21.9% Combined morbidity and mortality for grade IV; 16.7% combined morbidity and mortality for grade V
Hassler and Hejaza (1998)[39]	62	20.5% Combined morbidity and mortality for grade IV; 30.4% combined morbidity and mortality for grade V
Nozaki et al (2000)[40]	32	9% Morbidity; 0% mortality
Jizang et al (2000)[41]	50	26% Early morbidity; 12% late morbidity; 0% mortality

of patients with a history of seizures were seizure free, whereas seizure-free outcome after radiosurgery and embolization was at 43% and 50%, respectively.[43] Heros et al reported a seizure-free survival in patients with AVM experiencing preoperative seizures of 43.6%.[28]

■ Radiosurgery

Indications

Stereotactic radiosurgery can be accomplished with a cobalt X-ray source (gamma knife), with the linear accelerator, or by taking advantage of the Bragg peak effect of heavy radioactive particles produced by a cyclotron.[44] Stereotactic radiosurgery is ideal for small (<3 cm) deep-seated AVMs.[17,18,45,46] Radiosurgery should also be considered for small intrinsic AVMs of the brainstem, thalamus, basal ganglia, and other eloquent areas of the brain, and for patients with operable AVMs but prohibitive major medical problems.

Outcomes

The results of radiosurgery in terms of obliteration rate are hard to evaluate and compare because some series report obliteration rates based only on patients that had late angiography. Other series include obliteration, whether seen by angiography or by MRI. A long-term follow-up study of 118 who underwent first-time radiosurgery only for AVM showed an obliteration rate of 78.0%, good outcome in 75.4%, poor outcome in 11.9%, and mortality in 4.2%.[47] Friedman achieved a 79% obliteration rate in AVMs of less than 10 cm³.[48] For AVMs greater than 10 cm³, the obliteration rate dropped to 47%. Pollock et al reported an overall obliteration rate for 222 patients of 61%; the obliteration rate increased to 83% if only AVMs of less than 4 cm³ in volume were considered.[49] Steinberg et al published an obliteration rate of 100% for AVMs less than 4 cm³ and a 70% obliteration rate for AVMs greater than 3.7 cm in diameter.[50] **Table 12–5**[40,47–53] summarizes the obliteration and complication rates of some large series of stereotactic radiosurgical treatment of AVMs.

Disadvantages

The main disadvantages of radiosurgery are the lack of certainty of obliteration and the delay in complete obliteration in those patients whose AVM is eventually obliterated. During these periods of delay, which may range between 1 and several years, the patient remains at risk for hemorrhage, and the risk is almost the same as if no treatment had occurred (3 to 4% per year). In addition, there is a small but significant risk of neurological

TABLE 12–5 Postradiosurgical Outcomes for Arteriovenous Malformations

Author (Year)	Obliteration Rates	Morbidity and Mortality Rates
Pollock et al (2003)[47]	78.0% By angiography	11.9% Morbidity; 4.2% mortality
Nozaki et al (2000)[40]	N/A	36% Morbidity from rehemorrhage; 0% mortality
Friedman (1999)[48*]	79% (<10 cc); 47% (>10 cc)	N/A
Pollock et al (1998)[49]	61% Overall; 83% (<4 cc) by angiography	N/A
Steinberg et al (1990)[50]	100% (<4 cc); 70% (>3.7 cm in diameter) by angiography	N/A
Stieg et al (2000)[51†]	76% At 3 years	N/A
Inoue et al (2002)[52]	81.3% By angiography	N/A
Shin et al (2002)[53]	84.1% At 3 years; 89.4% at 4 years; 94.7% At 5 years by angiography	N/A

*,†It is not clear that the obliteration rates reported in these two articles were confirmed by angiography or magnetic resonance imaging and angiography.
Abbreviation: N/A, not available.

injury from radiation damage (3 to 10% depending on location).

Radiosurgery is not therapeutically effective for all lesions. Increasing AVM size reciprocally affects radiosurgical obliteration rate.[54] Radiosurgery is not effective in 10 to 15% of even small AVMs.[25] Repeated radiosurgery for previously incompletely obliterated AVMs carries a worse rate for subsequent obliteration than primary radiosurgery.[55] As stated above, there is no definitive evidence to suggest a reduction in the rate of hemorrhage in patients whose lesion is not completely obliterated.[27,28]

A possibility exists that AVMs may reappear after having been totally occluded after radiosurgery, especially in the pediatric population.[56] A summary of factors associated with radiosurgical treatment failure has been compiled and consists of changes in nidus morphology after radiosurgery because of resolution hematoma, recanalization of a previously embolized portion of the AVM, technical errors in treatment planning, large nidus size (>10 cm³), and increasing Spetzler–Martin grade.[57]

Arteriovenous malformations in or adjacent to functional brain tissue have a higher risk of radiation injury.[25,58] There have been rare reports of secondary tumors from radiation exposure from radiosurgery.[51] Other complications include death (<0.2%), radiation injury to brain parenchyma (6.4%), cranial nerve injury (1%), new or worsened seizures (0.8%), and increased

risk of rehemorrhage following radiosurgery in large AVMs and older patients.[57]

Radiosurgery has been praised in terms of its cost effectiveness when used as an alternative to surgical excision of potentially inoperable AVMs. However, we found that in this setting (small AVMs that could be treated either with surgical excision or radiosurgery), microsurgical excision proved to be much more cost effective as compared with radiosurgery when one considers, in a decision-making analysis model, the cost of future hemorrhages on patients treated with radiosurgery.[27]

■ Embolization

Indications

Endovascular embolization can be used to eliminate proximal aneurysms before microsurgery or radiosurgery, particularly if the aneurysms could have been the source of hemorrhage. Embolization can also be used to obliterate deep arterial pedicles that are inaccessible during the early surgical exposure. It can also be used to obliterate the supply from lenticulostriate and thalamoperforating arteries prior to microsurgical resection (**Fig. 12–2A–F**). These small fragile feeding arteries are difficult to access and coagulate with electrocautery, as they retract into the surrounding parenchyma when sectioned. Embolization of superficial feeding arteries is usually not necessary as they can be easily controlled intraoperatively. Progressive, staged reduction in arteriovenous shunting by endovascular embolization may result in gradual restoration of normal cerebral perfusion and vascular reactivity, reducing potential for perioperative complications of brain swelling and hemorrhage with very large high-flow AVMs.[59] Frequently, we use embolization simply to reduce the flow and make surgery safer in AVMs that are either in or adjacent to critical areas of the brain.

Outcomes

Even in experienced hands embolization of AVMs carries significant morbidity and mortality. Deruty et al reported 25% overall morbidity and 8% mortality rates.[60] In the study by Wikholm et al, embolization resulted in severe complications in 6.6%, moderate complications in 15.3%, and mild complications in 17.3% of 150 patients.[61] A meta-analysis of 1246 patients in 32 series showed a minor complication rate of 15%, major complications in 5%, and mortality of 2%.[62] In a series of 36 patients who underwent transarterial embolization of grades IV and V AVMs, 8% morbidity and 8% mortality were seen.[40]

Kwon et al followed 27 patients with >4 cm diameter AVM in eloquent cortex (≥ Spetzler–Martin grade III), that were felt to be inoperable.[63] Eleven patients underwent embolization; 27.3% deteriorated following embolization, and 45.5% experienced hemorrhage following embolization. These results were compared with 16 patients who underwent medical treatment only; 31% of patients under medical treatment deteriorated, and 25% experienced hemorrhage. Palliative embolization of AVMs does not appear to improve clinical results when compared with conservative treatment of AVMs felt to be

inoperable; therefore, it seems unjustified to put these patients through the significant risks of embolization unless the latter has a reasonable chance of resulting in complete obliteration of the AVM.

Occlusion rates after embolization alone has been reported between 5% and 18% in the majority of series.[57,62] Valavanis and Yaşargil have recently reported the highest rate of complete obliteration (40.8%) for AVMs selected for embolization.[64] It is important to know

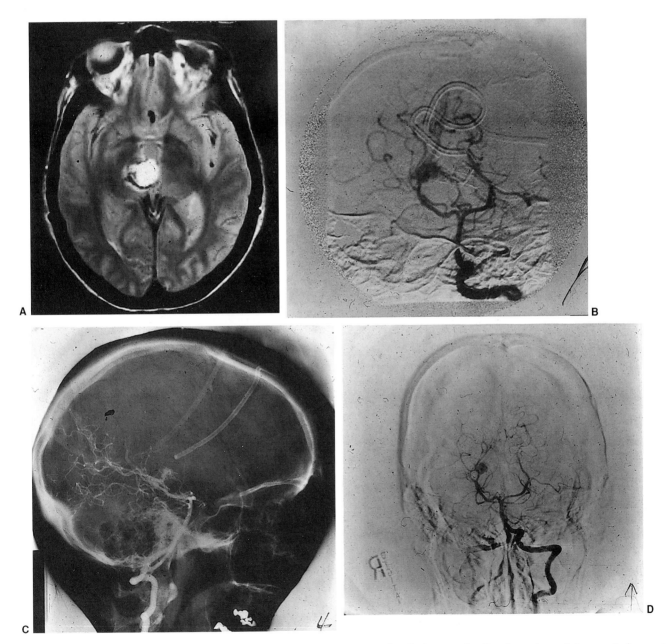

FIGURE 12–2 This figure depicts the role of preoperative embolization to obliterate deep feeders that are not accessible during early surgical exposure. The axial T2-weighted magnetic resonance image (MRI) **(A)** shows an arteriovenous malformation in the right thalamus, which was fed by P2 and posterior thalamoperforating branches of the posterior cerebral artery. Anteroposterior (AP) and lateral vertebral angiography views are shown in **(B, C)**. The postembolization angiogram **(D)** shows elimination of feeders from the posterior thalamoperforating artery.

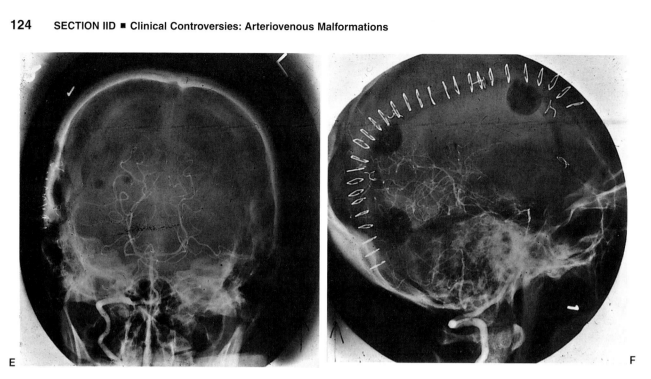

E   F

FIGURE 12–2 (continued) Postoperative AP **(E)** and lateral **(F)** vertebral angiograms show complete excision of the arteriovenous malformation.

that this high rate of obliteration results from careful selection for embolization of those AVMs where it was thought that there was a reasonable chance of complete obliteration by embolization. Vinuela et al reported an obliteration rate of 9.9% in 405 patients with AVMs.[65] Gobin et al reported an obliteration rate of 11.2%.[66] In the previously mentioned studies of Deruty et al and Wikholm et al, obliteration rates of 13% and 13.3% were reported, respectively.[60,61] Debrun et al and Hurst et al published obliteration rates of 5.5% and 15%, respectively.[67,68]

In 32 patients undergoing preoperative silk suture embolization for AVM, 100% embolization was never obtained: >50% obliteration was accomplished in 10 patients, and <50% obliteration was achieved in 22 patients.[69] **Table 12–6**[40,60–68,70,71] summarizes the obliteration and morbidity and mortality rates found in some reports of embolization as a treatment for AVMs.

Disadvantages

Despite some preconceived notions, endovascular procedures are not truly noninvasive, innocuous, or risk-free, as emphasized above. The procedures are frequently long and uncomfortable and may invoke the need for general anesthesia and all its associated risks.[59] Endovascular embolization alone is rarely curative due to a high degree of delayed recanalization. Delayed refilling or recanalization is due to almost completely embolized AVMs rapidly recruiting collateral supply.[59]

TABLE 12–6 Postembolization Outcomes for Arteriovenous Malformation

Author (Year)	Obliteration Rates	Morbidity and Mortality Rates
Deruty et al (1996)[60]	13%	25% Morbidity; 8% mortality
Wikholm et al (1996)[61]	13.3%	6.6% Severe morbidity; 15.3% moderate morbidity; 17.3% mild morbidity
Frizzel and Fisher (1995)[62]	N/A	5% Major morbidity; 15% minor morbidity; 2% mortality
Nozaki et al (2000)[40]	N/A	8% Morbidity; 8% mortality
Kwon et al (2000)[63]	N/A	27.3% Morbidity (45.5% postembolization hemorrhage rate)
Hartmann et al (2002)[70]	N/A	14% Early morbidity; 2% permanent morbidity; 1% mortality
Jahan et al (2001)[71]	N/A	4% Morbidity; 0% mortality
Valavanis and Yasargil (1998)[64]	40.8%	N/A
Vinuela et al (1995)[65]	9.9%	N/A
Gobin et al (1996)[66]	11.2%	N/A
Debrun et al (1997)[67]	5.5%	N/A
Hurst et al (1995)[68]	15%	N/A

Abbreviation: N/A, not available.

Embolization should not be performed for most small- to medium-sized convexity AVMs grades I to III, as they can be surgically resected with minimal blood loss and low morbidity.[17] The risks of embolization include cerebral infarcts from inadvertent obliteration of penetrating arteries or vessels en passage[59] (**Fig. 12–3A–C**) and AVM rupture from occlusion of draining veins before feeding arteries.[17]

The majority of complex AVMs have additional sources of arterial supply—small branches of perforating arteries such as lenticulostriate and anterior choroidal arteries, small leptomeningeal collateral vessels, and tiny deep transmedullary arteries—that are not amenable to embolization.[59] Partially embolized AVMs rapidly and aggressively recruit new sources of arterial supply; indiscriminate embolization may result in occlusion of large cortical vessels, which could have been easily controlled surgically, only to be replaced by collateral flow from many tiny subcortical arteries—thin-walled, fragile, and distended—which are more difficult to control surgically.[59]

Another frequent use of embolization is to reduce the size of large, inoperable AVMs and make them amenable to radiosurgery. However, in many of these

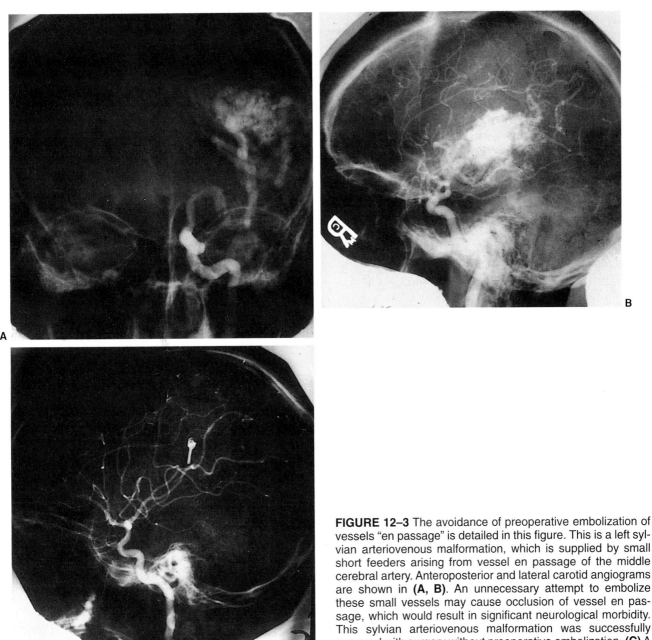

FIGURE 12–3 The avoidance of preoperative embolization of vessels "en passage" is detailed in this figure. This is a left sylvian arteriovenous malformation, which is supplied by small short feeders arising from vessel en passage of the middle cerebral artery. Anteroposterior and lateral carotid angiograms are shown in **(A, B)**. An unnecessary attempt to embolize these small vessels may cause occlusion of vessel en passage, which would result in significant neurological morbidity. This sylvian arteriovenous malformation was successfully removed with surgery without preoperative embolization. **(C)** A postoperative angiogram is shown.

cases, radiosurgery may fail to obliterate the AVM nidus due to delayed recanalization and reappearance of the portion of the nidus that was not included in the radiosurgical target planning.[72] Previous embolization is actually a negative predictor of successful AVM radiosurgery, and some have considered it contraindicated prior to radiosurgery.[49]

■ Observation

Observation alone seems to be the best option for most patients with thalamic, brain stem, and basal ganglia AVMs that are too large for radiosurgery. In addition, it has gradually become apparent to experienced surgeons that almost all grade V and most grade IV AVMs should be left alone unless the patient has a serious progressive deficit or has suffered multiple hemorrhages.[17,28,37,73] In one series, a hemorrhage risk of 1.5% per year for grades IV and V AVMs was lower than that reported for grades I through III.[73] There is no evidence that partial treatment reduces the patient's risk of hemorrhage, again lending support to the option of conservative treatment for grades IV and V AVMs.[73]

■ Conclusion

We have attempted to briefly discuss the various individual treatment modalities and multimodality paradigms for the management of AVMs. We have suggested indications for the major accepted modes of treatment: microsurgery, radiosurgery, and observation. In short, microsurgery with or without preoperative embolization, when felt to carry acceptable morbidity by an experienced surgeon, should be considered the primary form of treatment for Spetzler–Martin grades I, II, and III AVMs. For small, deep AVMs where an experienced surgeon estimates that the morbidity of surgery would be too high, stereotactic radiosurgery should be considered. In general, large AVMs in or near critical areas of the brain (grades IV and V) should be observed; there is currently no reasonable treatment with acceptable rates of complications for these lesions. Simply stated, there is little role for endovascular embolization as a cure for AVM because those AVMs that can frequently be obliterated completely are usually the ones that can be surgically removed with less morbidity. Embolization may be used as an adjunct to microsurgery, as discussed above, or for palliation for intractable symptoms, particularly progressive deficits felt to be because of "steal" or venous hypertension in patients with large, high-flow AVMs. Sometimes, we use embolization palliatively to reduce flow in hopes of helping patients who suffer from intractable epilepsy or headaches or who have had

multiple hemorrhages; this is particularly the case when there are angiographic features thought to increase the risk of hemorrhage, such as intranidal aneurysms, direct fistulae, or venous outlet obstruction.

With cerebral AVMs, it is important to keep in mind that the treatment is most frequently aimed at preventing hemorrhage in the future. Rarely, we treat a cerebral AVM to improve symptomatology such as intractable seizures or a progressive neurological deficit from "steal," venous hypertension, etc. In this context, it must be kept in mind that the risk of hemorrhage is essentially the same in a patient with an arteriovenous malformation that has never bled as in that presented by a patient with arteriovenous malformations that have bled in the past (more than 6 months).[20] In other words, in general, the risk of hemorrhage of an arteriovenous malformation whether it has bled or not is ~3 to 4% per year. After hemorrhage, the risk is ~6% during the first 6 months, but then it settles down to about the same 3 to 4% per year risk as hemorrhage of AVMs that have never bled. This risk of hemorrhage from an unruptured AVM is considerably greater than from incidental aneurysms, a fact that is not widely recognized. Granted, the morbidity of aneurysmal subarachnoid hemorrhage is significantly higher than the morbidity of hemorrhage from an AVM, but still, the latter is significant (about a 10% risk of death and about a 30% risk of serious neurological morbidity from each hemorrhage from an AVM). With these considerations in mind, we consider treatment of patients harboring cerebral AVMs whenever possible with acceptable risks, whether they have bled or not in the past.[20]

As emphasized previously, each patient with an AVM must be approached individually considering a multitude of factors including the size, configuration, and location of the AVM, the age, health and occupation of the patient, and the skill and experience of the treating team. As stated previously, the ideal treatment for cerebral AVMs is microsurgical excision, which eliminates immediately the risk of future hemorrhage. Therefore, in general, we recommend surgical excision of the AVM in patients who are relatively young and in good health provided that the treatment could be accomplished with relatively low risk. As stated above, this is the case with practically all patients with Spetzler–Martin grades I and II AVMs and with most patients with grade III AVMs. As a result of an analysis of our own series,[28] as well as others from the literature, we have concluded that the treatment of grade V AVMs carries an unacceptable risk, and therefore, we rarely recommend treatment of these lesions. The same is the case with the majority of grade IV AVMs, although by careful selection, we have kept the risk of operating on patients with grade IV AVMs to an acceptable level (serious morbidity and mortality of 12.2%).[28] When we use embolization, we use it specifically for the purpose of making the overall treatment plan of preoperative embolization and surgical excision safer; that is, when we consider the risk of embolization, which is not small as discussed before, we must be convinced that the combined risk of preoperative embolization and surgery is smaller than the risk would be if we undertook surgical excision without embolization. Additionally, we discuss with our endovascular colleagues very carefully the aim of preoperative embolization, which is simply to make the surgery safer. Generally, this entails occluding deep feeding pedicles that are inaccessible during the early surgical stages. There is no point in taking the risk of occluding endovascularly feeding pedicles to which the surgeon has immediate access upon exposure of the AVM; for example, cortical middle cerebral branches in a superficial AVM. Another aim of preoperative embolization is to significantly decrease flow in AVMs that are adjacent to critical areas of the brain, which then allows the surgeon to work at the very margin of the AVM with a considerably reduced risk of hemorrhage and damage to critical brain. We do not feel that embolization simply for the sake of reducing flow and making the surgery quicker and easier is justified under most circumstances, given the risk of embolization, except in the rare high-flow AVM where there is a risk of "perfusion breakthrough" from sudden occlusion of the shunt by removal of the AVM.[74] We believe that there are few indications for primary treatment of an AVM by embolization without subsequent surgical excision. As discussed before, simply reducing the flow to an AVM without obliterating it completely by embolization not only appears to not reduce the risk of future hemorrhage, but it is likely that it increases it. Clearly, there are AVMs that can be occluded completely with embolization, but, as discussed before, these are usually AVMs that can be readily excised with minimal risk, and in general, we prefer the latter tactic because the risk is lower than the risk of embolization with these AVMs. Of course, there are patients that because of their age or comorbidities may be best treated by embolization to completely occlude their AVM if this is possible and the AVM is too large for radiosurgery. There are other indications for embolization simply to reduce the flow of the AVM, such as in patients that present with a steal, or with intractable headaches due to dilated dural feeders, or in patients who have particular features such as aneurysms or direct fistulae that make us presume a higher risk of hemorrhage if left untreated. We have also used "palliative" embolization in patients with large, unresectable AVMs that present with accumulating deficits from multiple hemorrhages, but we are not sure that we alter favorably the natural history in these patients.

Radiosurgery is a most welcome addition to our armamentarium for treating cerebral AVMs. We recommend radiosurgery to patients who have a relatively small AVM (generally <3 cm, although we may stretch that limit size to 3.5 or 4 cm in some circumstances) and have AVMs located in critical areas of the brain where the surgical morbidity would be unacceptable. For patients with small AVMs in accessible areas of the brain, we recommend microsurgical excision given its very low risk and immediate elimination of the risk of hemorrhage, as discussed above. However, in elderly patients or in patients with significant comorbidities, radiosurgery may be considered under these circumstances. One treatment paradigm that we have not been enthusiastic about is that of using preoperative embolization to "reduce the size of the AVM" so that it then becomes amenable to radiosurgery. We remain unconvinced that those parts of the AVM that appear to be completely obliterated by the embolization in the immediate post-embolization angiogram remain, in fact, occluded and without risk of hemorrhage, and therefore, when we recommend radiosurgery, we recommend including all of the AVM, whether embolized or not, in the field. That limits our indications for radiosurgery to relatively small AVMs, and in these cases, there seems to be no reason to use embolization given the fact that, as discussed, embolization does not reduce the risk of future hemorrhage unless it results in complete obliteration of the malformation and, clearly, there is a substantial risk to embolization.

As suggested, we recommend no treatment at all to most patients with grade V AVMs, and we recommend treatment only to selected patients with grade IV AVMs.

■ References

1. Brown RD Jr, Weiber DO, Torner JC, O'Fallon WM. Incidence and prevalence of intracranial vascular malformations in Olmsted County, Minnesota, 1965 to 1992. Neurology 1996;46:949–952
2. Graf CJ, Perret GE, Torner JC. Bleeding from cerebral arteriovenous malformations as part of their natural history. J Neurosurg 1983;58:331–337
3. Crawford PM, West CR, Chadwick DW, et al. Arteriovenous malformations of the brain: the natural history in unoperated patients. J Neurol Neurosurg Psychiatry 1986;49:1–10
4. Ondra SL, Troupp H, George ED, et al. The natural history of symptomatic arteriovenous malformations of the brain: a 24 year follow-up assessment. J Neurosurg 1990;73:387–391
5. Mast H, Young WL, Koennecke HC, et al. Risk of spontaneous hemorrhage after diagnosis of cerebral arteriovenous malformation. Lancet 1997;350:1065–1068
6. Leblanc R, Levesque M, Comair Y, Ethier R. Magnetic resonance imaging of cerebral arteriovenous malformations. Neurosurgery 1987;21:15–20
7. Smith HJ, Strother CM, Kikuchi Y, et al. MR imaging in the management of supratentorial intracranial AVMs. AJR Am J Roentgenol 1988;150:1143–1153
8. Bambakidis NC, Sunshine JL, Faulhaber PF, Tarr RW, Selman WR, Ratcheson RA. Functional evaluation of arteriovenous malformations. Neurosurg Focus 2001;11(5):Article 2
9. Lunsford LD, Kondziolka D, Flickinger JC, et al. Stereotactic radiosurgery for arteriovenous malformations. J Neurosurg 1991;75:512–524

10. Spetzler RF, Hargraves RW, McCormick PW, Zambramski JM, Flom RA, Zimmerman RS. Relationship of perfusion pressure and size to risk of hemorrhage from arteriovenous malformations. J Neurosurg 1992;76:918–923

11. Nataf F, Meder JF, Roux FX. Angioarchitecture associated with haemorrhage in cerebral arteriovenous malformations: a prognostic statistical model. Neuroradiology 1997;39:52–58

12. Albert P, Saldago H, Polaoina M, Trujillo F, Ponce de Leon A, Durand F. A study on the venous drainage of 150 cerebral arteriovenous malformations as related to haemorrhagic risks and size of the lesion. Acta Neurochir (Wien) 1990;103:30–34

13. Miyasaka Y, Yada K, Ohwada T, Kitahara T, Kurata A, Irikura K. An analysis of the venous drainage system as a factor in hemorrhage from arteriovenous malformations. J Neurosurg 1992;76:239–243

14. Brown RD, Weibers DO, Forbes GS. Unruptured intracranial aneurysms and arteriovenous malformations: frequency of intracranial hemorrhage and relationship of lesions. J Neurosurg 1990;73:859–863

15. Turjman F, Massoud TF, Vinuela F, Sayre JW, Gugliemi G, Duckwiler G. Correlation of the angioarchitectural features of cerebral arteriovenous malformations with clinical presentation of hemorrhage. Neurosurgery 1995;37(5):856–860

16. Spetzler RF, Martin NA. A proposed grading system for arteriovenous malformations. J Neurosurg 1986;65:476–483

17. Tew JM Jr, Lewis AI. Honored guest presentation: management strategies for the treatment of intracranial arteriovenous malformations. Clin Neurosurg 2000;46:267–284

18. Pik JH, Morgan MK. Microsurgery for small arteriovenous malformations of the brain: results in 110 consecutive patients. Neurosurgery 2000;47(3):571–575

19. Kinouchi H, Mizoi K, Takahashi A, Ezura M, Yoshimoto T. Combined embolization and microsurgery for cerebral arteriovenous malformation. Neurol Med Chir (Tokyo) 2002;42(9):372–378

20. Heros RC, Tu Y-K. Is surgical therapy needed for unruptured arteriovenous malformations? Neurology 1987;37:279–286

21. Heros RC. Treatment of arteriovenous malformations: gamma knife surgery. J Neurosurg 2002;97(4):753–754

22. Brown RD Jr. Simple risk predictions for arteriovenous malformation hemorrhage. Letter. Neurosurgery 2000;46:1024

23. Kondziolka D, McLaughlin MR, Kestle JR. Simple risk predictions for arteriovenous malformation hemorrhage. Neurosurgery 1995;37:851–855

24. Ogilvy CS, Stieg PE, Awad I, et al. Recommendations for the management of intracranial arteriovenous malformations: a statement for healthcare professionals from a special writing group of the Stroke Council, American Stroke Association. Circulation 2001;103(21):2644–2657

25. Barrow DL. Controversies in neurosurgery: microsurgery versus radiosurgery for arteriovenous malformations—the case for microsurgery. Clin Neurosurg 2000;46:285–294

26. Hartmann A, Stapf C, Hofmeister C, et al. Determinants of neurological outcome after surgery for brain arteriovenous malformation. Stroke 2000;31(10):2361–2364

27. Nussbaum ES, Heros RC, Camarata PJ. Surgical treatment of intracranial arteriovenous malformations with an analysis of cost-effectiveness. Clin Neurosurg 1995;42:348–369

28. Heros RC, Korosue K, Diebold PM. Surgical excision of cerebral arteriovenous malformations: late results. Neurosurgery 1990;26(4):570–577

29. Tokunaga K, Kinugasa K, Meguro T, et al. Curative treatment of cerebral arteriovenous malformations by embolisation using cellulose acetate polymer followed by surgical resection. J Clin Neurosci 2000;7(Suppl 1):1–5

30. Irie K, Nagao S, Honma Y, et al. Treatment of arteriovenous malformation of the brain—preliminary experience. J Clin Neurosci 2000;7(Suppl 1):24–29

31. Hongo K, Koike G, Isohe M, et al. Surgical resection of cerebral arteriovenous malformation combined with pre-operative embolization. J Clin Neurosci 2000;7(Suppl 1):88–91

32. Hamilton MG, Spetzler RF. The prospective application of a grading system for arteriovenous malformations. Neurosurgery 1994;34:2–7

33. Sisti MB, Koder A, Stein BM. Microsurgery for 67 intracranial arteriovenous malformations less than 3 cm in diameter. J Neurosurg 1993;79:653–660

34. Pikus HJ, Beach ML, Harbaugh RE. Microsurgical treatment of arteriovenous malformations: analysis and comparison with stereotactic radiosurgery. J Neurosurg 1998;88:641–646

35. Russell SM, Woo HH, Joseffer SS, Jafar JJ. Role of frameless stereotaxy in the surgical treatment of cerebral arteriovenous malformations: technique and outcomes in a controlled study of 44 consecutive patients. Neurosurgery 2002;51(5):1108–1118

36. Batjer HH. Treatment decisions in brain AVMs: the case for and against surgery. Clin Neurosurg 2000;46:319–325

37. Heros RC, Morcos J, Korosue K. Arteriovenous malformations of the brain: surgical management. Clin Neurosurg 1993;40:139–173

38. Hashimoto H, Iida J, Hironaka Y, Sakaki T. Surgical management of cerebral arteriovenous malformations with intraoperative digital subtraction angiography. J Clin Neurosci 2000;7(Suppl 1):33–35

39. Hassler W, Hejazi N. Complications of angioma surgery: personal experience in 191 patients with cerebral angiomas. Neurol Med Chir (Tokyo) 1998;38:238–244

40. Nozaki K, Hashimoto N, Miyamoto S, Kikuchi H. Resectability of Spetzler-Martin grade IV and V cerebral arteriovenous malformations. J Clin Neurosci 2000;7(Suppl 1):78–81

41. Jizang Z, Shuo W, Jingsheng L, et al. Combination of intraoperative embolization with surgical resection for treatment of giant cerebral arteriovenous malformations. J Clin Neurosci 2000;7(Suppl 1):54–59

42. Kida Y, Kobayashi T, Tanaka T, et al. Seizure control after radiosurgery on cerebral arteriovenous malformations. J Clin Neurosci 2000;7(Suppl 1):6–9

43. Hoh BL, Chapman PH, Loeffler JS, Carter BS, Ogilvy CS. Results of multimodality treatment for 141 patients with brain arteriovenous malformations and seizures: factors associated with seizure incidence and seizure outcomes. Neurosurgery 2002;51(2):303–309

44. Heros RC, Korosue K. Radiation treatment of cerebral arteriovenous malformations. N Engl J Med 1990;323:127–129

45. Pollock BE, Lunsford LD, Kondziolka D, Bissonette DJ, Flickinger JC. Stereotactic radiosurgery for postgeniculate visual pathway arteriovenous malformations. J Neurosurg 1996;84:437–441

46. Sasaki T, Kurita H, Saito I, et al. Arteriovenous malformations in the basal ganglia and thalamus: management and results in 101 cases. J Neurosurg 1998;88:285–292

47. Pollock BE, Gorman DA, Coffey RJ. Patient outcome after arteriovenous malformation radiosurgical management: results based on a 5- to 14-year follow-up study. Neurosurgery 2003;52:1291–1297

48. Friedman WA. Radiosurgery versus surgery for arteriovenous malformations: the case for radiosurgery. Clin Neurosurg 1999;45:18–20

49. Pollock BE, Flickinger JC, Lundsford LD, Maitz A, Kondziolka D. Factors associated with successful arteriovenous malformation radiosurgery. Neurosurgery 1998;42:1239–1247

50. Steinberg GK, Fabricant JI, Marks MP, et al. Stereotactic heavy-charged-particle Bragg-peak radiation for intracranial arteriovenous malformations. N Engl J Med 1990;3232:96–101

51. Stieg PE, Friedlander RM, Loeffler JS, Alexander E III. Arteriovenous malformations: indications for stereotactic radiosurgery. Clin Neurosurg 2000;47:242–248

52. Inoue HK, Ohye C. Hemorrhage risks and obliteration rates of arteriovenous malformations after gamma knife radiosurgery. J Neurosurg 2002;97(Suppl 5):474–476
53. Shin M, Kawamoto S, Kurita H, et al. Retrospective analysis of a 10-year experience of stereotactic radiosurgery for arteriovenous malformation in children and adolescents. J Neurosurg 2002;97:779–784
54. Friedman WA, Bova FJ. Linear accelerator radiosurgery for arteriovenous malformations. J Neurosurg 1992;77:832–841
55. Foote KD, Friedman WA, Ellis TL, Bova FJ, Buatti JM, Meeks SL. Salvage retreatment after failure of radiosurgery in patients with arteriovenous malformations. J Neurosurg 2003;98(2):337–341
56. Lindqvist M, Karlsson B, Guo WY, Kihlstrom L, Lippitz B, Yamamoto M. Angiographic long-term follow-up data for arteriovenous malformations previously proven to be obliterated after gamma knife radiosurgery. Neurosurgery 2000;46(4):803–808
57. Fleetwood IG, Steinberg GK. Arteriovenous malformations. Lancet 2002;359(9309):863–873
58. Friedman WA, Bova FJ, Mendenhall WM. Linear accelerator radiosurgery for arteriovenous malformations: the relationship of size to outcome. J Neurosurg 1995;82:180–189
59. Martin NA, Khanna R, Doberstein C, Bentson J. Therapeutic embolization of arteriovenous malformations: the case for and against. Clin Neurosurg 2000;46:295–318
60. Deruty R, Pelissou-Guyotat I, Amat D, et al. Complications after multidisciplinary treatment of cerebral arteriovenous malformations. Acta Neurochir (Wien) 1996;138:119–131
61. Wikholm G, Lundqvist C, Svendsen P. Embolization of cerebral arteriovenous malformations: part I—technique, morphology, and complications. Neurosurgery 1996;39:448–459
62. Frizzel RT, Fisher WS. Cure, morbidity, and mortality associated with embolization of brain arteriovenous malformations: a review of 1246 patients in 32 series of a 35-year period. Neurosurgery 1995;37:1031–1040
63. Kwon O, Han DH, Han MH, Chung YS. Palliatively treated cerebral arteriovenous malformations: follow-up results. J Clin Neurosci 2000;7(Suppl 1):69–72
64. Valavanis A, Yasargil MG. The endovascular treatment of brain arteriovenous malformations. Adv Tech Stand Neurosurg 1998;24:131–214
65. Vinuela F, Duckwiler G, Gugliemi G. Intravascular embolization of brain arteriovenous malformations. In: Macinunas RJ, ed. Endovascular Neurological Intervention. Park Ridge, IL: American Association of Neurological Surgeons; 1995:189–199
66. Gobin YP, Laurent A, Merienne L, et al. Treatment of brain arteriovenous malformations by embolization and radiosurgery. J Neurosurg 1996;85:19–28
67. Debrun GM, Aletich V, Ausman JI, et al. Embolization of the nidus of brain arteriovenous malformations with n-butyl cyanoacrylate. Neurosurgery 1997;40:112–121
68. Hurst RW, Berenstein A, Kupersmith MJ, et al. Deep central arteriovenous malformations of the brain: the role of endovascular treatment. J Neurosurg 1995;82:190–195
69. Dehdashti AR, Muster M, Reverdin A, et al. Preoperative silk suture embolization of cerebral and dural arteriovenous malformations. Neurosurg Focus 2001;11(5):Article 6
70. Hartmann A, Pile-Spellman J, Stapf C, et al. Risk of endovascular treatment of brain arteriovenous malformation. Stroke 2002;33:1816–1820
71. Jahan R, Murayama Y, Gobin YP, et al. Embolization of arteriovenous malformations with Onyx: clinicopathological experience in 23 patients. Neurosurgery 2001;48:984–997
72. Pollock BE, Kondziolka D, Lunsford LD, Bissonette D, Flickinger JC. Repeat stereotactic radiosurgery of arteriovenous malformations: factors associated with incomplete obliteration. Neurosurgery 1996;38:318–324
73. Han PP, Ponce FA, Spetzler RF. Intention-to-treat analysis of Spetzler-Martin grades IV and V arteriovenous malformations: natural history and treatment paradigm. J Neurosurg 2003;98:3–7
74. Spetzler RF, Wilson CB, Weinstein P, et al. Normal perfusion pressure breakthrough theory. Clin Neurosurg 1978;25:651–672

13

Endovascular Treatment of Arteriovenous Malformations

GARY M. NESBIT, GEORGE LUH, RAYMOND TIEN, AND STANLEY L. BARNWELL

Objectives: Upon completion of this chapter, the reader should recognize the indications for AVM embolization and the endovascular techniques used for safe and effective nidus occlusion.

Accreditation: The AANS* is accredited by the Accreditation Council for Continuing Medical Education (ACCME) to sponsor continuing medical education for physicians.

Credit: The AANS designates this educational activity for a maximum of 15 credits in Category 1 credit toward the AMA Physician's Recognition Award. Each physician should claim only those hours of credit that he/she spent in the educational activity.

The Home Study Examination is online on the AANS Web site at: http://www.aans.org/education/books/controversy.asp

* The acronym AANS refers to both the American Association of Neurological Surgeons and the American Association of Neurosurgeons.

The treatment of brain arteriovenous malformations (AVMs) is a complex task that requires close cooperation between the neurosurgeon, neuroradiologist, radiation therapist, and critical care specialist. Each individual case must have a clearly defined goal, based on its estimated natural history and risk of hemorrhage or other neurological sequelae and the risks of the therapeutic plan. The endovascular treatment of AVMs, with its benefits and risks, must be carefully integrated into the overall decision-making process. Since the first reported case in 1960, remarkable advances have been made in endovascular therapy that have improved both safety and efficacy. Advances in catheter design, particulate, liquid, coil-based embolic material, and imaging techniques have all contributed to this improved safety profile; however, the increased capability yields increased complexity and clinical responsibility. The goal of this chapter is to provide insight into the endovascular treatment of AVMs to hopefully provide order to this array of treatment options. To this end, we will discuss the indications, treatment strategies, techniques, and complications of endovascular therapy in the treatment of brain AVMs.

■ Indications and Treatment Strategies

Not all AVMs that can be treated necessarily need treatment. An understanding of the natural history of the disease and the risk of treatment is crucial when counseling patients about treatment options. The characteristics of the AVM, patient age, comorbidities, and psychosocial factors are all important to consider when developing a treatment plan. The patient and family's expectations of treatment must be clearly understood, as they must understand the risks of the various stages of treatment and the entire treatment plan.

The prevalence of brain AVMs, based on autopsy studies, is ~0.15%,[1,2] with the majority, 64 to 80%, of AVMs presenting before 40 years of age.[3] Symptoms of AVMs include headache, seizures and epilepsy, focal neurological deficit, and intracranial hemorrhage. Headaches are quite common in patients with AVMs; they are the most common symptom leading to discovery of an AVM. Headaches and a variety of neurological deficits can occur that are unrelated to previous hemorrhage.[2,3] These symptoms can be caused by decreased tissue perfusion, venous hypertension, and mass effect from dilated veins. Seizures can occur in from 28 to 67% of patients. Although the risk of bleeding is lower in patients with seizures than in patients with previous hemorrhage, it is higher than in those without seizures.

Hemorrhage is the most common single presenting symptom, occurring in over 50% of patients,[4,5] with the estimated overall risk of hemorrhage from a brain AVM discovered incidentally or from evaluation of seizure or other nonhemorrhagic symptoms ranging from 2 to 4% per year.[6-8] Each bleeding episode carries approximately a 10% mortality rate and a 30 to 50% morbidity rate due to persistent neurologic deficits,[9] and the risk of rebleeding ranges from 6 to 18% in the first year but decreases to 2% per year after 10 years.[7,10]

Morphologic factors that increase the risk for AVM hemorrhage include intranidal aneurysms, restricted venous outflow, deep venous drainage, previous hemorrhage, small AVM size, diffuse AVM morphology, and higher feeding artery pressures.[11] A more recent study has found that deep location and large size (>3 cm) were independent predictors of future hemorrhage.[12] Also, hemorrhage at presentation did not necessarily predict higher subsequent hemorrhage risk. This study emphasized that the factors present at the time of initial hemorrhage are not necessarily the same factors that predict future hemorrhage. For example, small AVMs are thought to be more prone to hemorrhage, but this may be because small AVMs tend to present with hemorrhage, though they are less likely than large AVMs to cause other symptoms, such as seizures. It is beyond the scope of this chapter to discuss in detail the natural history of AVMs, but an important point to remember is that the natural history of many patients is benign, and observation alone may be a reasonable option.[13]

There are four main indications for endovascular embolization of brain AVMs: complete obliteration for cure, presurgical treatment, preradiosurgical treatment, and palliative flow reduction. Each of these indications carries a different decision algorithm and risk profile as the goals for each are quite distinct.

Complete occlusion of the AVM nidus by endovascular embolization alone is uncommon; reports of persistent cure rates in the literature vary from 5 to 32%.[14,15] This relatively low rate reflects the varied approaches to AVM treatment at various centers, as many reports in the literature include the entire experience of AVM treatment, including embolization as an adjunct to surgery and radiosurgery rather than focusing on only those

attempted for cure. The recanalization of AVMs angiographically "cured" by embolization has been reported; however, the permanency of occlusion is, at least partially, influenced by the embolization material used.[16-18] Particulate embolization with polyvinyl alcohol (PVA) has been shown to be effective in controlling intraoperative bleeding; however, vessels embolized with PVA alone tend to recanalize after a few weeks.[19-22] Although recanalization of "cured" AVMs with liquid embolic agents (**Fig. 13–1**), such as *n*-butyl cyanoacrylate (*n*-BCA), has also been reported, the incidence is much lower than with PVA.[15,23,24] In comparison, complete surgical excision has nearly a 100% cure rate but carries a higher morbidity and mortality rate, and case reports of AVM recurrence after "complete" surgical excision do exist.[25-27] Therefore, the use of endovascular embolization as the sole treatment modality for brain AVMs should only be considered in select cases with appropriate angio-architecture and perhaps be reserved for patients with relative contraindications to surgery or radiosurgery.

Presurgical embolization is the most widely used application for endovascular therapy of brain AVMs and is undertaken to reduce the surgical risks of uncontrollable hemorrhage and to improve surgical visualization. Clearly defined goals must be set, and open communication between the neurosurgeon and interventional neuroradiologist is critical in planning the course of therapy. Often, the easiest vessels to embolize are also the easiest to control during surgery and may not require embolization. Conversely, the more difficult vessels to embolize may be critical to successful surgical cure, and despite the increased risk, embolization is necessary in such situations. In considering presurgical embolization the combined risk of embolization and surgery must be less than that of the surgery performed without an embolization. Presurgical embolization is usually directed toward associated aneurysms, surgically inaccessible feeding pedicles, high-flow arteriovenous fistulae, and general reduction in flow within and the size of the nidus.

Aneurysms occur in 7 to 46% of patients with AVMs, and 40 to 75% of these aneurysms occur on feeding arteries[28-30] probably related to vasculo-dynamic responses to increased flow. Whether or not to treat these aneurysms remains controversial,[30-32] as studies indicate that the majority of feeding artery aneurysms will regress after removal of the AVM.[28,29] In the largest review to date, Meisel et al[30] evaluated 662 patients with AVMs and concluded that feeding artery aneurysms do not need to be treated prior to AVM treatment, and that after 3.5 years a 50% reduction in aneurysm size was noted in more than 50% of the cases. Persistent AVM occlusion with time was necessary to observe the size decrease, which raises the question as to the long-term effects of aneurysm shrinkage with partial AVM occlusion

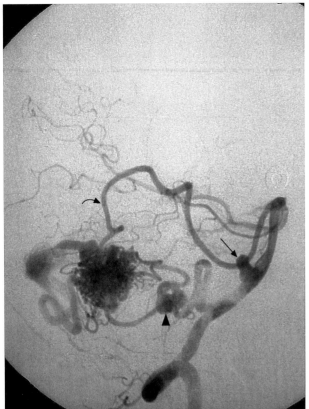

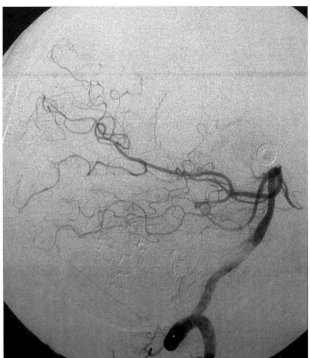

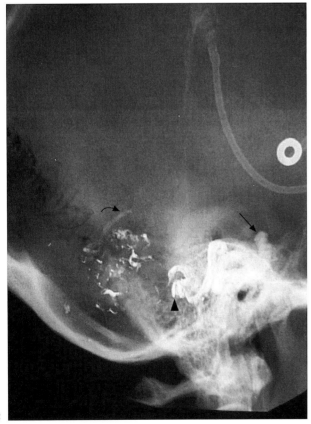

FIGURE 13–1 Angiographic obliterative embolization with *n*-butyl cyanoacrylate (*n*-BCA) in an arteriovenous malformation (AVM) with subarachnoid and intracerebellar hemorrhage. **(A)** Lateral right vertebral angiogram. Enlarged right posterior inferior cerebellar artery (PICA) with an origin aneurysm (arrow) and pedicle aneurysm (arrowhead) supplying a 2.5-cm AVM. The superior cerebellar artery (SCA; curved arrow) also provides supply. Based on the hemorrhage location the pedicle aneurysm was thought to have ruptured. Embolization of the PICA proximal to the aneurysm and the SCA just above the AVM resulted in complete obliteration of the AVM nidus and pedicle aneurysm on the postembolization angiogram **(B)** and radiograph of glue cast **(C)**. Arrows and arrowhead correlate with same locations.

because the residual nidus will eventually recruit collaterals and pedicle flow will increase. Another study showed that following AVM treatment with less than 50% reduction in AVM size, no proximal feeding artery aneurysms had decreased in size, and two had enlarged and bled.[32] The question remains as to the long-term hemorrhage risk of these residual aneurysms, those that have either remained stable and that have decreased in size. There is no question that if a patient presents with hemorrhage that is thought to be caused by a feeding-artery aneurysm rather than the AVM, then the aneurysm should be treated and should be secured prior to attempting embolization of the AVM. Endovascular treatment of a ruptured feeding artery aneurysm can be a key adjunctive therapy, especially if it has a favorable configuration for endovascular embolization and is located anatomically too proximal to the AVM nidus to be reached by the neurosurgeon through a single craniotomy.

The occlusion of deep or surgically inaccessible feeding arteries is of critical benefit to a successful surgical cure. In fact, embolization of the superficial feeding arteries without treatment of the deep feeding arteries may lead to increased flow from these vessels and make the surgery much more difficult and dangerous than if no embolization was performed at all. Lenticulostriate, thalamoperforator, periventricular, choroidal, or deep posterior cerebral artery feeders are the most difficult to control at surgery and would be the best target vessels for endovascular embolization (**Fig. 13–2**). Unfortunately, these vessels are also often the most difficult to embolize and may carry too high of a collateral neurological risk due to the supply of normal structures en route to the AVM. Nonetheless, these vessels are often critical and require a coordinated effort between the endovascular and surgical specialist for the overall therapeutic plan.

On the other hand, embolization of surgically accessible superficial feeding pedicles is often performed with the goal of reduction of the nidal flow and overall size prior to surgery. Even though these pedicles can be clipped at surgery, the ability to embolize significant portions of the nidus via these pedicles can significantly reduce the surgical morbidity. Martin et al compared various aspects of preoperative embolization, including the degree of flow reduction and nidus occlusion, to the ease of surgical excision in 18 patients. They found that the only significant postembolization result that predicted easier, safer, and quicker surgical excision was nidus size reduction greater than 66%.[31] This usually requires embolization of the majority of pedicles, surgically accessible or not.

Preoperative graded flow reduction to reduce normal perfusion pressure breakthrough is another useful application of endovascular therapy.[31,33–35] Large AVMs with significant intranidal arteriovenous shunting have high-flow velocities and low pressure in the feeding arteries. The feeding artery branches supplying normal brain tissue adjacent to the AVM will also have low pressure within them. Local cerebral perfusion to normal brain tissue adjacent to the AVM is further decreased by relatively high shunt-induced venous pressures. The decreased perfusion pressure to the normal brain tissue adjacent to the AVM also results in decreased blood flow. This state of low perfusion pressure and low blood flow results is maximally vasodilated vessels that eventually lose their ability to autoregulate for changes in blood flow and pressure. A sudden decrease in high-flow arteriovenous shunting through the AVM, from either complete embolization or surgical resection, results in an abrupt increase in pressure in the feeding artery and its normal branches. Decreased flow through the AVM also decreases the high venous pressures that were present prior to treatment. These features combine to cause increased local arterial and brain perfusion pressure, and the lack of cerebrovascular compensation from the loss of autoregulation can result in cerebral edema and catastrophic hemorrhage, known as normal perfusion pressure breakthrough.

Numerous articles in the literature have reported edema and hemorrhage into surrounding brain tissue following abrupt hemodynamic changes precipitated by sudden removal of the high-flow arteriovenous shunting through the AVM.[36–38] Certain angiographic characteristics of the AVM that might predispose to perfusion pressure breakthrough include large nidus size with high shunt flow; poor opacification of vessels to the normal surrounding brain; extensive collateral flow from other vascular territories ("sump effect") including the external carotid arteries; and clinical symptoms of progressive or fluctuating, nonepileptogenic neurological deficits.[38,39] Staged AVM embolization (**Fig. 13–3**) is a recommended method to gradually reduce the degree of arteriovenous shunting, thereby gradually increasing the pedicle pressure, reducing the venous outflow pressure, and improving the local cerebral autoregulatory function. Staged embolization usually consists of occlusion of a certain portion of the AVM, often a single vascular distribution, with second or third embolization sessions after a few days to a few weeks. The actual time between stages is controversial; however, most interventionists separate them by at least 1 week to reestablish compensatory autoregulation. Following the staged embolization, complete surgical resection of the AVM can proceed with a reduction in the risk of normal perfusion pressure breakthrough and its devastating sequelae.

Radiosurgery is an important alternative to surgical resection in the treatment of certain brain AVMs. Arteriovenous malformations located in areas of the brain that are surgically inaccessible due to the involvement of significantly eloquent tissue or are morphologically too

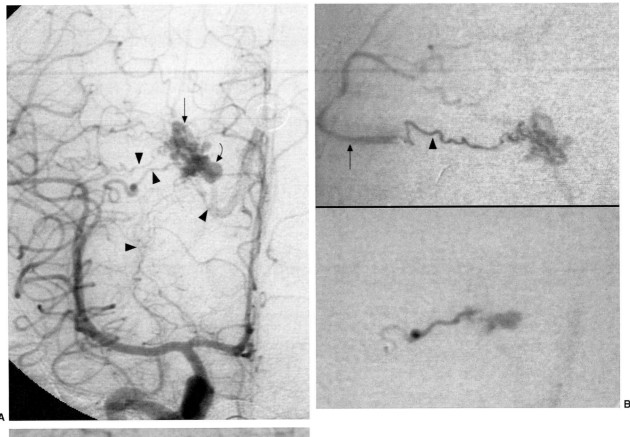

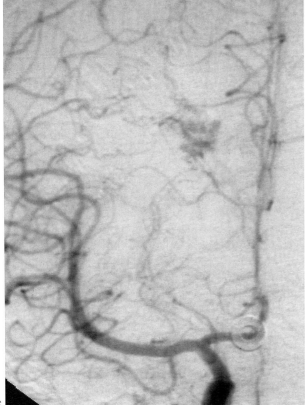

FIGURE 13–2 Embolization of deep perforating artery, arteriovenous fistula, and varix in an arteriovenous malformation (AVM) with intraventricular hemorrhage. **(A)** Anteroposterior (AP) right internal carotid angiogram. A small, deep AVM nidus (arrow) with varix (curved arrow), the most likely source of hemorrhage, is being supplied by (arrowheads, bottom to top) lenticulostriate, sylvian perforators, and a peripheral perforator. The lenticulostriate is small and has too many normal branches en route. The sylvian branches were approached, and on the AP super-selective angiograms **(B)** only the lower branch (arrowhead) was appropriately engaged; the upper branch resulted in reflux into the middle cerebral artery (MCA; arrow). This vessel was embolized with a wedged injection and occlusion of the lower supply and varix as shown on the postembolization angiogram **(C)**. The surgeon was able to clip the lateral perforating vessels (arrowheads) prior to engaging the AVM, which had completely thrombosed at surgery the following day.

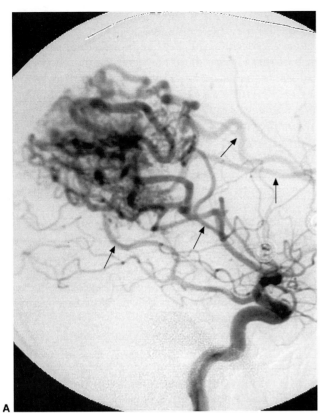

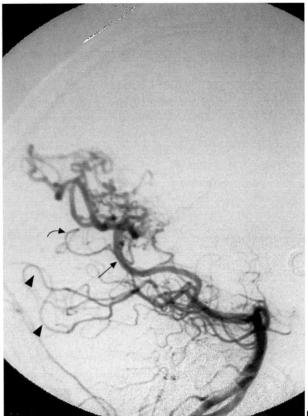

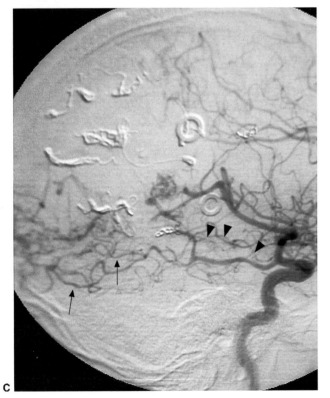

FIGURE 13–3 Staged embolization of a large parietal AVM with intraparenchymal hemorrhage. Lateral right internal carotid **(A)** and left vertebral artery **(B)** angiograms demonstrate supply from multiple right middle cerebral, anterior cerebral, and posterior cerebral artery branches (arrows). The slower filling of the normal branches (curved arrow) near the AVM compared with the occipital branches (arrowheads) indicates poor perfusion. The anterior and posterior cerebral branches were embolized at the first stage, followed by the middle cerebral branches 1 week later, the day prior to surgery. On the postembolization carotid angiogram **(C)**, note the hyperemia (arrows) in the previous region of poor perfusion, indicating some perfusion pressure breakthrough. The patient suffered no sequelae from this and had an uneventful resection. The anterior choroidal supply (arrowheads) could not be adequately engaged due to its small size.

dangerous for surgical resection are often considered for radiosurgery. This technique has up to an 80% cure rate with low morbidity and mortality in AVMs less than 3 cm in diameter; however, the efficacy and safety significantly decreases in AVMs greater than 3 cm and in AVMs with intranidal fistulas.[24,40] One study suggested that embolization prior to radiosurgery may be beneficial to reduce AVM nidus size and therefore radiosurgical target volume—to eliminate high-risk AVM features, such as intranidal aneurysms, that might predispose to hemorrhage during the 2- to 3-year delay before the radiation-induced AVM obliteration occurs—and to eliminate high-flow intranidal fistulas, which may be refractory to radiation therapy.[41] However, for small AVMs it is unclear whether or not embolization prior to radiosurgery shows any benefit compared with radiosurgery alone. Studies show that for small AVMs, the overall cure rates are similar for embolization prior to radiosurgery compared with radiosurgery alone.[40,41] For medium-sized AVMs (3 to 6 cm) there may be some benefit to preradiosurgical embolization. The risks of preradiosurgical embolization for large AVMs (>6 cm) appear to outweigh the benefits. In fact, the benefits of radiosurgery in the treatment of large AVMs are highly suspect, and embolization has little effect upon this outcome. Attempts at nidus size reduction with embolization to decrease the size of the radiation focus have yielded limited results; although, as with embolization for obliterative cure, treatment with liquid agents in this setting is more effective than particles. Nonetheless, there does not appear to be any significant protective effect from hemorrhage during the latent period between radiosurgery and radiation-induced AVM obliteration from preradiosurgical embolization in these large lesions. In addition, recanalization of previously embolized portions of the AVM nidus can be a source of incomplete AVM obliteration following radiosurgery.[24]

Palliative flow reduction by partial AVM embolization in patients with intractable headaches or epilepsy has been successfully performed in select cases.[15,42] Embolization of external carotid artery branches or posterior cerebral artery branches may be helpful in patients with headaches refractory to other therapies. However, the patient needs to understand that any palliative effects of partial AVM embolization may only be temporary due to the eventual recruitment of collaterals, and their symptoms must be of enough significance to warrant the risks of such treatment.

■ Techniques of Embolization

The techniques used in the endovascular treatment of AVMs are beyond the scope of this chapter; however, they consist of access to the cerebral vasculature, navigation to

specific site(s) for embolization, assessment of risk of embolization at the site(s), and injection of the embolic material to occlude the AVM and/or feeding pedicle. In each of these areas, there has been continued improvement in materials and techniques, and using assessment of risk and efficacy based on older literature is limited.

Guidesheaths and guide catheters, often not considered important to the overall success of therapy, can play a critical role in many patients. These devices have improved, providing more stability proximally in conjunction with more safety distally. Techniques, such as coaxial-introducer catheters, to minimize vascular damage, and arteriotomy closure devices have decreased the access complications at the puncture site and in the cervical region. Microcatheter and microguidewire technology has also dramatically improved with softer over-the-wire catheters and hydrophilic flow-directed devices that can be used in combinations of over-the-wire and flow-directed techniques to safely navigate to a more distal location in much less time.

Improvements in imaging with higher spatial and temporal resolution digital subtraction angiography and three-dimensional angiography[43] have also dramatically improved the ability to detect the higher-risk aspects of the AVM and subtle normal branches. Provocative testing with barbiturates and improved evoked potentials has also improved the safety profile of selecting appropriate locations and pedicles for embolization.

Although particulate embolization with PVA and coils has not changed dramatically, improvements in the liquid embolic arena have been seen.[19] The liquid agent n-butyl cyanoacrylate (n-BCA) has been available for over a decade and has provided a more permanent occlusion and potential improved outcomes with presurgical embolization.[44–46] The only liquid embolic agent approved in the United States for the presurgical embolization of AVMs is TRUFILL (n-BCA; Cordis Endovascular, Miami Lakes, FL). It is a liquid adhesive that polymerizes into a solid material upon contact with blood fluids or tissue via an ionic mechanism and is similar, but purer and more consistent, to the older product, Histoacryl, available in Europe. It is usually mixed with ethiodized oil as a radiopaque polymerizing retardant and can be mixed with tantalum powder for added radiopacity. This material can provide for a more thorough nidus penetration and pedicle occlusion compared with PVA, although in the randomized trial comparing the two there was little difference in AVM dimension reduction (79.4% in the n-BCA group and 86.9% in the PVA group) or in the number of pedicles treated despite a 16.8% lower fluoroscopy time in the n-BCA group was seen.[47] No differences in the surgical resection time, need for transfusion, or final Glasgow outcome scores were seen, although there was a significant decrease in postresection hematoma (2 of 42 in the n-BCA group and 8 of 45 in the PVA group). Although *n*-BCA is widely used, some technical disadvantages exist, which include the variable viscosity and polymerization time with varied concentrations of *n*-BCA and ethiodized oil and *n*-BCA's lack of cohesiveness. It also carries a small, but real risk of adherence to catheters or in vessels due to the adhesive nature of the material.

Another liquid agent that has currently completed study is ethylene–vinyl copolymer (EVOH), also known as Onyx (MicroTherapeutics Inc., Irvine, CA). This material, dissolved in dimethylsulfoxide (DMSO), precipitates into a soft material that is more cohesive than adhesive and has a consistent viscosity compared with *n*-BCA. The recently completed randomized trial comparing Trufill *n*-BCA and Onyx is currently being analyzed; we await results. Anecdotally, in our experience in this trial we found certain advantageous handling characteristics of Onyx, such as it's cohesiveness. Disadvantages of Onyx include having to use DMSO as a solvent, and an inability to vary the injection rate of Onyx.

■ Complications of Endovascular Arteriovenous Malformation Treatment

The procedural adverse events reported in the literature include the complications associated with cerebral angiography or catheterization of the intracranial vasculature—allergic reaction, cerebral ischemia or infarction, arterial injury such as dissection and puncture site hematoma, or contrast material nephropathy; complications associated with the embolization—cerebral infarction, catheter entrapment, pulmonary embolism, and arterial injury or rupture; and complications associated with the AVM—feeding pedicle, nidal or venous rupture, neurologic deficits, and normal perfusion pressure breakthrough.[48–57] The morbidity in the more recent case series is from 5.6 to 19%, with a major morbidity of 2.0 to 8.7% and a mortality of 0 to 3.7%.[41,56,57] In the more rigorous *n*-BCA versus PVA Trial,[47] the incidence of stroke and preoperative hemorrhagic complications was 13% in the *n*-BCA group and 19.2% in the PVA group, although most of the events resulted in only minor neurological sequelae.

■ Conclusion

The treatment of brain arteriovenous malformations (AVMs) is a complex task that requires input from the entire multidisciplinary team. Each case must have clearly defined goals, and the endovascular treatment of AVMs must be carefully integrated into the overall decision-making process. Advances in catheter design,

embolic material, and imaging techniques have all contributed to an improved safety profile, and endovascular treatment plays a critical role in overall safe and effective management of a majority of brain AVMs. Further advances should only increase the safety and efficacy profile of this sometimes curative and often adjunctive therapy.

■ References

1. Deruty R, Pelissou-Guyotat I, Mottolese C, Bascoulergue Y, Amat D. The combined management of cerebral arteriovenous malformations. Experience with 100 cases and review of the literature. Acta Neurochir (Wien) 1993;123:101–112
2. Wilkins RH. Natural history of intracranial vascular malformations: a review. Neurosurgery 1985;16:421–430
3. Jellinger K. Vascular malformations of the central nervous system: a morphological overview. Neurosurg Rev 1986;9:177–216
4. The AVM Study Group. Arteriovenous malformations of the brain in adults. N Engl J Med 1999;340:1812–1818
5. Hofmeister C, Stapf C, Hartmann A, et al. Demographic, morphologic and clinical characteristics of 1289 patients with brain arteriovenous malformation. Stroke 2000;31:1307–1310
6. Mohr J. Neurological manifestations and factors related to therapeutic decisions. In: Wilson C, Stein B, ed. Intracranial Arteriovenous Malformations. Baltimore: Williams and Wilkins; 1984:12–23
7. Graf C, Perret G, Torner J. Bleeding from cerebral arteriovenous malformations as part of their natural history. J Neurosurg 1983;58:331–337
8. Ondra SL, Troupp H, George ED, Schwab K. The natural history of symptomatic arteriovenous malformations of the brain: a 24-year follow-up assessment. J Neurosurg 1990;73:387–391
9. Hartmann A, Mast H, Mohr JP, et al. Morbidity of intracranial hemorrhage in patients with cerebral arteriovenous malformation. Stroke 1998;29(5):931–934
10. Kagetsu NJ. Natural history of symptomatic brain AVM's. J Neurosurg 1991 Aug;75(2):338–339
11. Pollock BE. The role of embolization in combination with stereotatic radiosurgery in the management of pial and dural arteriovenous malformations. In: Connors JJ, Wojak JC, eds. Interventional Neuroradiology: Strategies and Practical Techniques. Philadelphia: WB Saunders; 1999:267–275
12. Stefani MA, Porter PJ, terBrugge KG, et al. Large and deep brain arteriovenous malformations are associated with risk of future hemorrhage. Stroke 2002;33:1220–1224
13. Batjer HH. Treatment decisions in brain AVMs: the case for and against surgery. Clin Neurosurg 2000;46:319–325
14. Berenstein A, Lasjaunias P. Surgical Neuroangiography: Endovascular Treatment of Cerebral Lesions. Berlin: Springer-Verlag 1992;4:148–150
15. Wikholm G, Lundqvist C, Svendsen P. The Goteborg cohort of embolized cerebral arteriovenous malformations: a 6 year follow-up. Neurosurgery 2001;49(4):799–805
16. Nakstad PH, Bakke SJ, Hald JK. Embolization of intracranial arteriovenous malformations and fistulas with polyvinyl alcohol particles and platinum fiber coils. Neuroradiology 1992;34:348–351
17. Purdy PD, Batjer HH, Risser RC, Samson D. Arteriovenous malformations of the brain: choosing embolic materials to enhance safety and ease of excision. J Neurosurg 1992;77:217–222
18. Wikholm W. Role of transarterial embolization in the management of cerebral arteriovenous malformations. Acta Radiol Suppl 1996;(404):1–25.

19. Khayata MH, Dean BL, Spetzler RF. Materials and embolic agents for endovascular treatment. Neurosurg Clin N Am 1994;5(3):475–484.

20. Fournier D, Terbrugge K, Rodesch G, Lasjaunias P. Revascularization of brain arteriovenous malformations after embolization with bucrylate. Neuroradiology 1990;32:497–501

21. Wallace RC, Flom RA, Khayata MH, et al. The safety and effectiveness of brain arteriovenous malformation embolization using acrylic and particles: the experiences of a single institution. Neurosurgery 1995;37:606–618

22. Gruber A, Mazal PR, Bavinzski G, Killer M, Budka H, Richling B. Repermeation of partially embolized cerebral arteriovenous malformations: a clinical, radiologic, and histologic study. AJNR Am J Neuroradiol 1996;17:1323–1331

23. Sorimachi T, Koike T, Takeuchi S, et al. Embolization of cerebral arteriovenous malformations achieved with polyvinyl alcohol particles: angiographic reappearance and complications. AJNR Am J Neuroradiol 1999;20:1323–1328

24. Kwon Y, Jeon SR, Kim JH, et al. Analysis of the causes of treatment failure in gamma knife radiosurgery for intracranial arteriovenous malformations. J Neurosurg 2000;93(3):104–106

25. Hino A, Fujimoto M, Iwamoto Y, Takahashi Y, Katsumori T. An adult case of recurrent arteriovenous malformation after "complete" surgical excision: a case report. Surg Neurol 1999;52(2):156–158

26. Gabriel EM, Sampson JH, Wilkins RH. Recurrence of a cerebral arteriovenous malformation after surgical excision. J Neurosurg 1996;84(5):879–82

27. Freudenstein D, Duffner F, Ernemann U, Rachinger J, Grote E. Recurrence of a cerebral arteriovenous malformation after surgical excision. Cerebrovasc Dis 2001;11(1):59–64

28. Stapf C, Mohr JP, Pile-Spellman J, et al. Concurrent arterial aneurysms in brain arteriovenous malformations with haemorrhagic presentation. J Neurol Neurosurg Psychiatry 2002;73(3):294–298

29. Westphal M, Grzyska U. Clinical significance of pedicle aneurysms on feeding vessels, especially those located in infratentorial arteriovenous malformations. J Neurosurg 2000;92(6):995–1001

30. Meisel HJ, Mansmann U, Alvarez H, Rodesch G, Brock M, Lasjaunias P. Cerebral arteriovenous malformations and associated aneurysms: analysis of 305 cases from a series of 662 patients. Neurosurgery 2000;46(4):793–800

31. Martin NA, Khanna R, Doberstein C, Bentson J. Therapeutic embolization of arteriovenous malformations: the case for and against. Clin Neurosurg 2000;46:295–318

32. Redekop G, TerBrugge K, Montanera W, Willinsky R. Arterial aneurysms associated with cerebral arteriovenous malformations: classification, incidence, and risk of hemorrhage. J Neurosurg 1998;89(4):539–546

33. Duckwiler G, Dion J, Vinuela F, Jabour B, Martin N, Bentson J. Intravascular microcatheter pressure monitoring: experimental results and early clinical evaluation. AJNR Am J Neuroradiol 1990;11(1):169–175

34. Nornes H, Grip A. Hemodynamic aspects of cerebral arteriovenous malformations. J Neurosurg 1980;53(4):456–464

35. Spetzler RF, Hargraves RW, McCormick PW, Zabramski JM, Flom RA, Zimmerman RS. Relationship of perfusion pressure and size to risk of hemorrhage from arteriovenous malformations. J Neurosurg 1992;76(6):918–923

36. Drake CG. Cerebral arteriovenous malformations: considerations for and experience with surgical treatment in 166 cases. Clin Neurosurg 1979;26:145–208

37. Luessenhop AJ, Rosa L. Cerebral arteriovenous malformations. Indications for and results of surgery, and the role of intravascular techniques. J Neurosurg 1984;60(1):14–22

38. Spetzler RF, Martin NA, Carter LP, Flom RA, Raudzens PA, Wilkinson E. Surgical management of large AVM's by staged embolization and operative excision. J Neurosurg 1987;67(1):17–28

39. Spetzler R, Wilson C, Weinstein P, Mehdorn M, Townsend J, Telles D. Normal perfusion pressure breakthrough theory. Clin Neurosurg 1978;25:651–672

40. Friedman WA, Bova FJ, Mendenhall WM. Linear accelerator radiosurgery for arteriovenous malformations: the relationship of size to outcome. J Neurosurg 1995;82(2):180–189

41. Gobin YP, Laurent A, Merienne L, et al. Treatment of brain arteriovenous malformations by embolization and radiosurgery. J Neurosurg 1996;85(1):19–28

42. Lundqvist C, Wikholm G, Svendsen P. Embolization of cerebral arteriovenous malformations: Part II—Aspects of complications and late outcome. Neurosurgery 1996;39(3):460–467

43. Jafar JJ, Davis AJ, Berenstein A, et al. The effect of embolization with N-butyl cyanoacrylate prior to surgical resection of cerebral arteriovenous malformations. J Neurosurg 1993;78:60–69

44. DeMeritt JS, Pile-Spellman J, Mast H, et al. Outcome analysis of preoperative embolization with N-butyl cyanoacrylate in cerebral arteriovenous malformations. AJNR Am J Neuroradiol 1995;16(9):1801–1807

45. Valavanis A, Yasargil MG. The endovascular treatment of brain arteriovenous malformations. Adv Tech Stand Neurosurg 1998;24:131–214

46. Prestigiacomo CJ, Niimi Y, Setton A, Berenstein A. Three-dimensional rotational spinal angiography in the evaluation and treatment of vascular malformations. AJNR Am J Neuroradiol 2003;24(7):1429–1435

47. n-BCA Trail investigators. N-butyl cyanoacrylate embolization of cerebral arteriovenous malformations: results of a prospective, randomized, multi-center trial. AJNR Am J Neuroradiol 2002;23(5):748–755

48. Berenstein A, Lasjaunias P. Surgical Neuroangiography: Endovascular Treatment of Cerebral Lesions. Berlin: Springer-Verlag; 1992;4:1–344

49. Barnwell S, Dowd C, Higashida R, Halback V, Hieshima G. Endovascular therapy for cerebral arteriovenous malformations. In: Apuzzo M, ed. Brain Surgery. New York, NY: Churchill Livingstone; 1993:1225–1250

50. Lownie S. Clinical and technical complications of endovascular therapy in the central nervous system. Semin Intervent Radiol 1993;10:243–253.

51. Nakstad PH, Nornes H. Superselective angiography, embolisation and surgery in treatment of arteriovenous malformations of the brain. Neuroradiology 1994;36:410–413

52. Frizzel RT, Fisher WS. Cure, morbidity, and mortality associated with embolization of brain arteriovenous malformations: a review of 1246 patients in 32 series over a 35-year period. Neurosurgery 1995;37(6):1031–1040

53. Qureshi AI, Luft AR, Sharma M, Guterman LR, Hopkins LN. Prevention and treatment of thromboembolic and ischemic complications associated with endovascular procedures: part II—clinical aspects and recommendations. Neurosurgery 2000;46(6):1360–1376

54. Fogarty-Mack P, Pile-Spellman J, Hacein-Bey L, et al. The effect of arteriovenous malformations on the distribution of intracerebral arterial pressures. AJNR Am J Neuroradiol 1996;17:1443–1449

55. Pelz DM, Lownie SP, Fox AJ, Hutton LC. Symptomatic pulmonary complications from liquid acrylate embolization of brain arteriovenous malformations. AJNR Am J Neuroradiol 1995;16:19–26

56. Wikholm G, Lundqvist C, Svendsen P. Embolization of cerebral arteriovenous malformations: part I, techniques, morphology, and complications. Neurosurg 1996 Sept;39(3):448–459

57. Debrun G, Vinuela F, Fox A, Drake CG. Embolization of cerebral arteriovenous malformations with bucrylate. J Neurosurg 1982;56(5):615–627

14

Radiosurgical Treatment of Arteriovenous Malformations

DOUGLAS KONDZIOLKA, L. DADE LUNSFORD, AND JOHN C. FLICKINGER

Objectives: Upon completion of this chapter, the reader should recognize the indications for selecting radiosurgery over other treatment options and the results expected from this therapy.

Accreditation: The AANS* is accredited by the Accreditation Council for Continuing Medical Education (ACCME) to sponsor continuing medical education for physicians.

Credit: The AANS designates this educational activity for a maximum of 15 credits in Category 1 credit toward the AMA Physician's Recognition Award. Each physician should claim only those hours of credit that he/she spent in the educational activity.

The Home Study Examination is online on the AANS Web site at: http://www.aans.org/education/books/controversy.asp

* The acronym AANS refers to both the American Association of Neurological Surgeons and the American Association of Neurosurgeons.

Patients and doctors have to choose between different management options for arteriovenous malformations (AVM); hence, controversy is common. Interpretation of the available literature (the science), together with physician judgment (the art), allows doctors to make clinical decisions with patients. The choices may be controversial in some instances and agreed upon by all in others. In this chapter, we discuss controversies associated with AVM radiosurgery, particularly in relation to patient selection and technique.

Successful AVM radiosurgery is dependent upon achievement of the outcome of complete AVM nidus obliteration that leads to elimination of the future hemorrhage risk.[1-3] In achieving this goal, there should be no morbidity or mortality from hemorrhage or radiation-induced brain injury. When these outcomes can be achieved with a high likelihood, a strong case can be made *for* radiosurgery. If clinical or angiographic factors argue *against* the achievement of these goals, then other strategies should be considered. Physicians who make an argument for radiosurgery cite one or more of the following: (1) that radiosurgery is an effective therapy

required for the management of deep-brain AVMs; (2) that radiosurgery is an effective therapy for residual AVMs after subtotal resection; (3) that radiosurgery is worthwhile in an attempt to lower management risks for AVMs in functional brain locations; (4) because embolization does not cure most AVMs, additional therapy such as radiosurgery may be required; (5) microsurgical resection may not be the best choice for some patients depending on their general health; and (6) reduced cost. Radiosurgery is the first and only biologic AVM therapy; it represents the beginning of future cellular approaches to vascular malformation diseases. For this reason, the future of radiosurgery may be impacted positively by the development of other biologic strategies such as brain protection or endothelial sensitization.

■ Decision Making

Those who make an argument against the use of radiosurgery argue the following points: (1) that radiosurgery does not always work especially when only partial AVM obliteration is achieved[4]; (2) that brain hemorrhage may occur during the time it takes for radiosurgery to work; (3) that radiation-related morbidity may cause functional neurological deficits; (4) that there may exist "long-term" problems after brain irradiation[5]; and (5) that resection may be a more cost-effective treatment over the long term.[6] Though all these points can be argued, most neurosurgeons agree that the role of radiosurgery is greatest for patients with small-volume, deep-brain AVMs.[2,7–9] It has a lesser role for patients with larger and surgically accessible AVMs. In between these two extremes, there exists much debate. The role of radiosurgery for patients with small yet accessible AVMs is growing steadily.[10] For patients with large-volume yet deeply located AVMs, multimodality management often is required. Thus, whether radiosurgery should be considered in the management of an individual patient depends upon the factors of AVM volume, brain location, prior hemorrhage history, patient age, and surgical resectability. These factors have been studied in detail by different groups toward predicting successful AVM outcomes or reasons for radiosurgery failure.[3,11–14] The factors of AVM obliteration and radiosurgical morbidity on decision making are addressed in further detail later in this chapter.

■ Case Illustrations

Case 1

A 20-year-old woman sustained a brain hemorrhage caused by an arteriovenous malformation in the region of the angular gyrus (**Fig. 14–1A–D, 1F, 1G**). The arguments for the use of radiosurgery are the location of the AVM within a critical brain area and that its overall size made it suitable for radiosurgery. However, because she had sustained a hemorrhage that caused neurological deficits, resection was considered because any potential deficits were already present. An argument against radiosurgery is the chance for hemorrhage during the latency to obliteration. The expected obliteration rate for an AVM of this size would be ~80% after a single procedure. Four years after radiosurgery, a small persistent nidus was identified on the vertebral angiogram (**Fig. 14-1E**). A second radiosurgery was performed that was followed by complete AVM obliteration.

Case 2

A 45-year-old man presented with headaches. They were caused by a temporal lobe arteriovenous malformation supplied by the middle cerebral artery. An aneurysm just proximal to the arteriovenous malformation was also identified (**Fig. 14–2A,B**). An argument for the use of

radiosurgery is the small AVM volume, thus allowing radiosurgery as an alternative to resection or embolization. Arguments against the role of radiosurgery include the resectability of the AVM in this location (with relatively low risk) and the sustained hemorrhage risk during the radiosurgery latency interval. Management of the proximal aneurysm via intraoperative clipping is a strong argument for resection. This patient underwent radiosurgery; his 2-year angiogram showed complete AVM obliteration and elimination of the aneurysm.

Case 3

A 22-year-old woman suffered an intracerebral hemorrhage from an AVM located in the posterior limb of the left internal capsule. The hemorrhage caused hemiparesis, which had improved to a level of only mild arm weakness (**Fig. 14–3A,B**). She underwent radiosurgery because of the critical brain location of the malformation, its small and suitable size for radiosurgery, and the belief that this approach represented the lowest overall management risk. An argument could be made against radiosurgery because the patient had already sustained one hemorrhage and remained at a higher risk for a second bleed. However, the potential morbidity of resection appeared to outweigh this risk. Two years after radiosurgery, complete obliteration of the malformation was documented.

Case 4

A 40-year-old woman sustained an intraventricular and subarachnoid hemorrhage from a left parietal arteriovenous malformation. Symptoms from her intraventricular hemorrhage resolved. The case for radiosurgery included the critical brain location of the malformation and its suitable size. The argument against radiosurgery was that there remained a continued risk of rebleeding prior to nidus obliteration, and that the nidus was superficial in location and suitable for resection. However, the good functional status of the patient and the critical brain location were stronger arguments for radiosurgery (**Fig. 14–4A–E**). Three years following radiosurgery complete obliteration of the malformation was confirmed. She remains active with no new neurological deficits.

■ Why Does Radiosurgery Work?

Radiosurgery is effective because single-fraction irradiation causes significant injury to the endothelial cells of blood vessels that compose the AVM.[8,15–17] Stereotactic definition of the AVM target ensures that these radiobiological effects are limited to the malformation. Conformal radiosurgery allows irradiation of only a small volume of surrounding normal tissue in the region of radiation dose fall-off.[2,18] Dose-prescription formulae are used to help select an appropriate radiation dose depending on imaging and clinical factors.[19,20]

The immediate effect of radiosurgery is to damage the endothelial cells of the AVM vessels. The release of tissue-specific cytokines common to other forms of radiation-induced injury is likely to mediate such acute effects. Inflammatory cells mediate tissue repair in response to irradiation. Later, chronic inflammation consists of the ingrowth of granulation tissue that contains

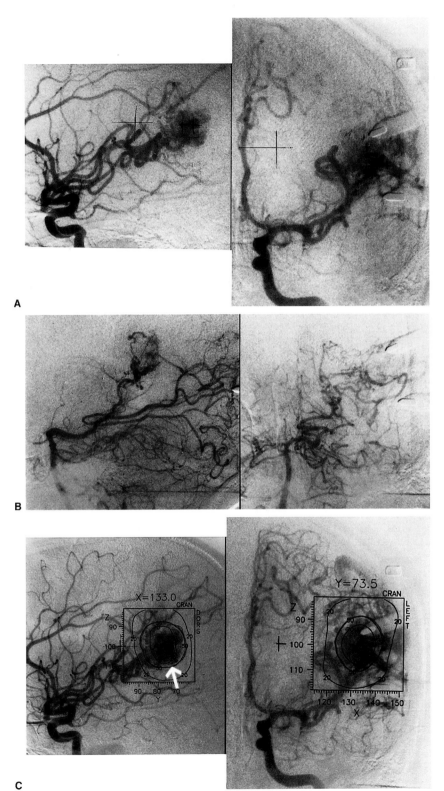

FIGURE 14–1 (A) Left carotid angiogram of a 20-year-old student who presented with hemorrhage shows a parietal lobe arteriovenous malformation (AVM). The vertebral artery supply is shown in **(B)**. The radiosurgery dose plan is shown in **(C)** (volume 5.8 cc); the arrow points to a circle indicating the 50% isodose. (*Continued on pages 142 and 143.*)

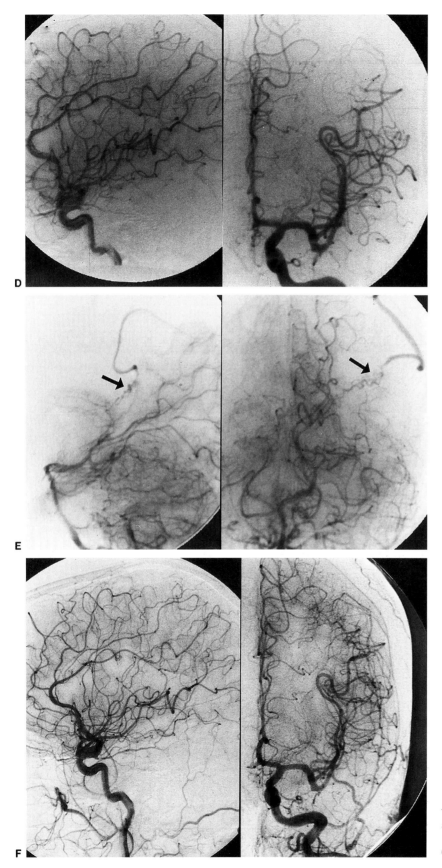

FIGURE 14–1 (*Continued*) Four years later the carotid **(D)** and vertebral **(E)** angiograms show a small remaining nidus (arrow). Following repeat radiosurgery, angiogram **(F)** show complete obliteration.

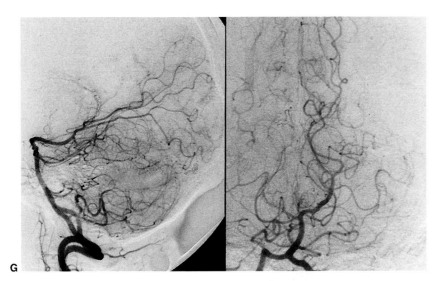

FIGURE 14–1 (*Continued*) angiogram (**G**) show complete obliteration.

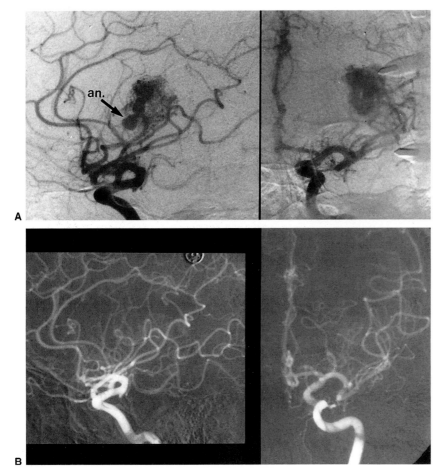

FIGURE 14–2 Angiograms before radiosurgery showing a left temporal lobe arteriovenous malformation (AVM) with a proximal aneurysm (top). His 2-year angiogram showed obliteration of the AVM and the aneurysm (bottom).

fibroblasts and new capillaries. These events may explain the delayed imaging changes sometimes observed after radiosurgery (as in Case 4 above). Szeifert et al identified the presence of actin-producing fibroblasts, so-called myofibroblasts, that are hypothesized to exert contractile properties and facilitate AVM obliteration.[21] It is common that contrast-enhanced magnetic resonance imaging (MRI) studies at this late stage after obliteration show enhancement of the obliterated AVM. This finding does not indicate a "patent" AVM, but, we believe, a marker

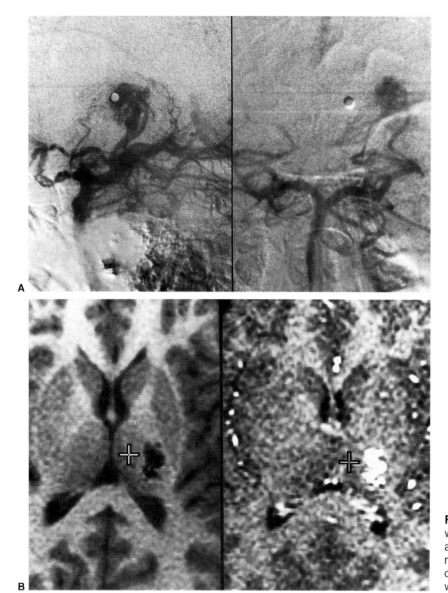

FIGURE 14–3 (Top) Angiograms in a young woman who sustained a hemorrhage from an internal capsule arteriovenous malformation (middle). Complete obliteration was confirmed on angiography after 2 years with no new neurological deficits.

for the newly formed capillary network within the scarred AVM tissue remnant. Several reports have noted the rare, late finding of cyst formation at the AVM site, which probably represents expansion of the extracellular fluid space within the fibrosis.[5,22] Radiosurgery may affect seizure control through irradiation of epileptogenic tissue or through correction of abnormal hemodynamic conditions.[23–25]

■ Results of Stereotactic Radiosurgery

Clinical Experience

At the University of Pittsburgh, 805 AVM patients had gamma knife radiosurgery during a 13-year interval. The mean patient age was 36 years (range 2 to 82). Prior intracranial hemorrhage was reported in 49% of patients ($n = 395$), headaches in 42%, and seizures in 29%. The wide variety of different clinical presentations ensures discussion of the different treatment options in all patients. All referred vascular malformation cases are discussed at a weekly conference attended by neurosurgeons, neuroradiologists, and radiation oncologists. Intravascular embolization was performed in 138 patients (17%) before radiosurgery. Eighty-one patients (11%) had already undergone one or more surgical procedures prior to radiosurgery. For some of these patients, the goal of surgery had been AVM resection, while in others the goal of surgery was hematoma removal. The mean AVM volume was 3.0 ml (range 0.03 to 24 ml). The 50% isodose was used as the margin isodose in 74% of patients. Only 0.7% of patients were treated below the 50% isodose.

The Spetzler–Martin grading system was used to classify all AVMs according to size, critical location, and venous drainage. As noted above, the most commonly referred patient was one with a small-volume, deeply located AVM (grade III, $n = 307$, 38%). The most infrequent patient had an AVM ($n = 23$, 2.8%) that was small, superficial, and noncritical in location (grade I). In such patients, we first recommend a resection unless the patient has a medical contraindication or refuses that recommendation. Fourteen percent of patients ($n = 113$) had a grade VI AVM. The AVM was located totally within the parenchyma of the brainstem or thalamus. The mean

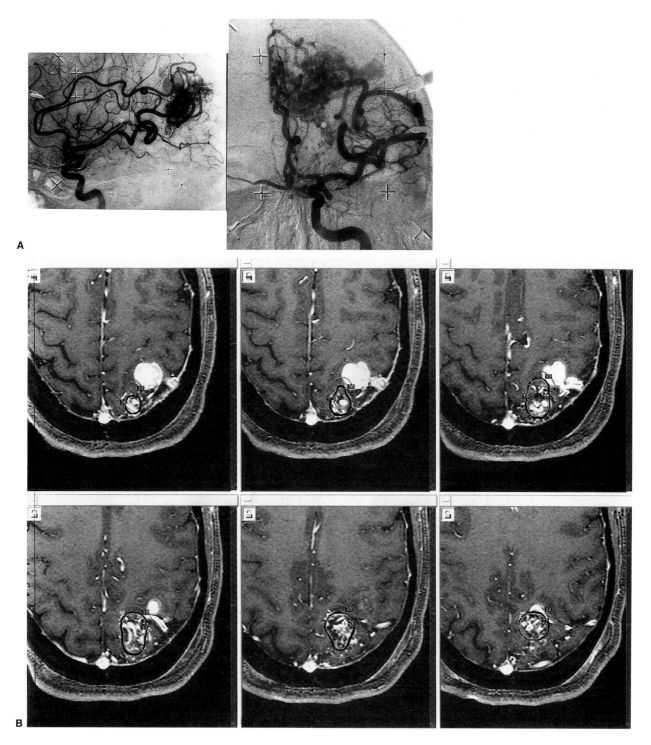

FIGURE 14–4 (A) Anterior–posterior and lateral angiograms showing a left parietal arteriovenous malformation (AVM) in a 40-year-old woman. The radiosurgery dose plan is shown on the MRI scan in **(B)** and the angiogram in **(C)**. (*Continued on page 146.*)

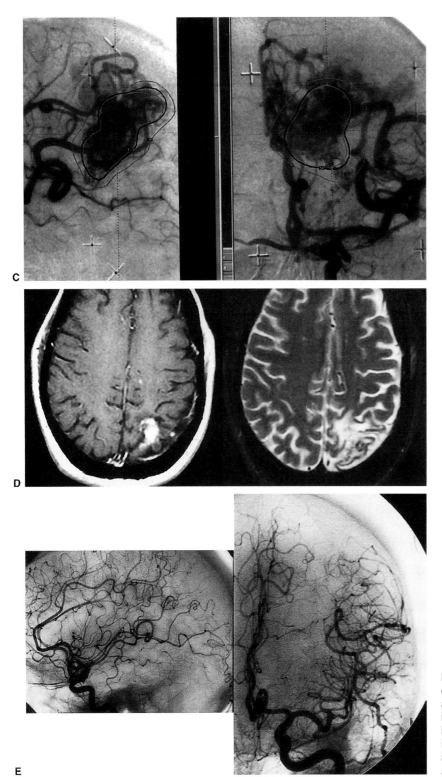

FIGURE 14–4 (*Continued*) The radiosurgery dose plan is shown on the MRI scan in **(B)** and the angiogram in **(C)** (dark line = 50% isodose line to AVM margin). Three years later, the MRI showed no flow-void signal, indicating AVM obliteration **(D)**. Repeat angiography at 3 years confirmed complete AVM obliteration **(E)**.

dose delivered to the AVM margin was 20 Gy, and the mean maximum dose was 37 Gy. Although there is no such thing as an "inoperable" AVM, we consider an AVM to be associated with an acceptably high risk for resection when located completely within the parenchyma of the brainstem, thalamus, or basal ganglia. In our series, 50 patients had brainstem AVMs, 81 had thalamic AVMs, and 38 had basal ganglia malformations.

When radiosurgery did not lead to complete AVM obliteration, further discussion occurred over the merits of repeat radiosurgery or resection. Fifty-two patients underwent repeat radiosurgery for persistent AVM nidus after at least 3 years had elapsed since the first procedure. If after 3 to 4 years, a residual AVM nidus *with* early venous drainage remains, then a second radiosurgical procedure should be performed.[26] We do not recommend additional management for patients who harbor only an early draining vein as this feature resolves over an additional observation interval.[27] In addition, we know of no patient who sustained a later hemorrhage when only an early draining vein was present. Some patients will have an angiogram that shows some abnormal appearing vessels in the region of the irradiated AVM, without early venous drainage. This fine vascular blush may indicate the neocapillary network within the scarred malformation. Such findings also require no additional therapy.

Retreatment is associated with a 70% probability of obliteration.[4,28] At the second procedure, only the small remnant need be irradiated, usually at a dose higher than the first dose delivered (especially if the initial AVM was large and the remnant is small, depending on location).

How Arteriovenous Malformation Obliteration Affects Decision Making

Whether an AVM can be successfully obliterated depends on whether proper stereotactic nidus definition can be performed followed by delivery of an adequate radiosurgery dose.[29] A complete analysis of 197 AVM patients with up to a 3-year angiographic follow-up showed an overall complete obliteration rate of 72% after a single procedure. These results were stratified by volume. In 20 of 197 patients (10%) the targeted AVM nidus failed to obliterate totally. The most important reason for lack of complete obliteration was improper targeting.[28] An additional 35 patients (18%) had a residual AVM that was not included in the original treatment volume. Many of these patients then underwent a second radiosurgery procedure. Important obliteration factors were identified in this study: incomplete imaging-definition of the AVM, reappearance of AVM after initial compression by hematoma, and recanalization of a previously embolized nidus. We and others advocate the use of multimodality imaging (MRI, magnetic resonance angiography [MRA], and conventional stereotactic angiography) to obtain the best results.[30,31] For the smallest AVM (less than 1.3 ml), 90% of patients had complete obliteration (45 of 50), and 98% had obliteration of the target (49 of 50). For AVMs between 1.4 and 3 ml, 41 of 49 patients had complete obliteration (84%), and 47 of 49 had obliteration of the included target (96%). These data indicate that the radiosurgical dose will achieve our goal with a high likelihood if we can accurately tailor it to the entire lesion margin.

In a separate analysis of our data, we reported a multivariate analysis of AVM obliteration as related to dose and volume.[29] A clear dose response up to 25 Gy was identified. We concluded that large AVMs have low obliteration rates because of the combination of lower treatment doses used and the greater problems encountered with target definition. A recent analysis of 95 patients with thalamic or basal ganglia AVMs found similar obliteration rates when stratified by volume; overall, 80% of patients were cured after a single procedure. Thus, AVM volume means not only that more tissue exists to undergo obliteration but that also there may be additional challenges in stereotactic targeting.

Pikus et al argued that the high rate of complete microsurgical resection in their 72-patient AVM series (99%) with 8% rate of new permanent neurological deficits substantiated their belief that resection was better than radiosurgery for small AVMs.[32] However, only three of their patients (4%) had AVMs in the basal ganglia, thalamus, or brainstem. Porter et al constructed a decision analysis model based on obliteration estimates and morbidity rates for resection and radiosurgery.[6] They concluded that resection conferred a clinical benefit because of early protection from hemorrhage. Radiosurgery became a superior treatment if the surgical morbidity rate exceeded 12%. They did not factor the use of second stage or repeat radiosurgery into their model, choosing to leave patients with subtotally obliterated AVMs "unprotected" for the rest of their expected life. This outcome is rare because most patients achieve complete obliteration but may require more than one procedure. Thus, how obliteration data are used and from where such data are obtained (brain locations) are of paramount importance to the decision to use different techniques.

How Radiosurgery Morbidity Affects Decision Making

Immediate postradiosurgery complications are rare; thus, many patients and physicians choose radiosurgery because of rapid return to activities and employment. Postradiosurgery seizures are rare when we administer therapeutic levels of anticonvulsant medication to patients with supratentorial lobar AVMs. One must consider the chance for delayed morbidity after radiosurgery that corresponds with the time course for AVM obliteration. We found that the rate of developing any postradiosurgery imaging change between 2 and 7 years after radiosurgery is 30%.[12] We believe that the majority of these changes are hemodynamic or inflammatory. Most do not cause neurological symptoms. Symptomatic imaging changes are found in 10%. These changes resolve in half the patients within 3 years of onset as compared with a 95% resolution rate in patients with asymptomatic imaging findings.

There are several ways to predict in advance the chance for adverse radiation effects. A multivariate analysis of imaging changes with various radiosurgical parameters found that the only significant independent correlation was the total volume of tissue that received greater than or equal to 12 Gy.[11] Symptomatic imaging changes were correlated with the volume that received this dose and with location (brainstem vs. nonbrainstem). Although radiosurgery may seem to be the only viable treatment option for intraparenchymal brainstem AVMs, a higher risk must be expected.

Finally, the persistent risk of hemorrhage during the obliteration latency interval remains one of the strongest arguments against radiosurgery in some cases. Although Karlsson et al reported protection from rehemorrhage in the interval prior to complete obliteration, neither the Pittsburgh nor University of Florida series identified such a benefit.[13,14,33] In our experience, the hemorrhage rate after radiosurgery remains the same as the hemorrhage rate before radiosurgery until the AVM obliterates. We have never observed a bleed after obliteration.

Options for Large Arteriovenous Malformations: Staged Volume Radiosurgery and Embolization

We now consider prospective staged radiosurgery for larger AVMs (volume staging) especially for patients who present with hemorrhage and who are not suitable for resection. With this approach, the AVM volume is divided into components to allow radiosurgery of smaller volumes at higher, more effective, and more tolerable doses. Forty-six patients have now undergone staged radiosurgery at our center. Irradiation of an entire large AVM at a low dose (below 15 Gy to the AVM margin) has such a low obliteration rate that it is probably not worthwhile. We separate the AVM radiosurgeries by 4 to 6 months to allow repair of sublethal deoxyribonucleic acid damage in normal brain.[34] There is evidence to suggest that even incompletely obliterated AVMs may become easier to resect after a period of several years. Perhaps prophylactic staged radiosurgery may facilitate eventual resection of AVMs previously considered untreatable.[35] This approach is new and outcomes are being evaluated currently.

In the past, we used endovascular embolization to reduce the volume of the AVM nidus in preparation for eventual radiosurgery, usually 4 to 6 weeks later. In some patients, this strategy proved effective and permanent occlusion of the embolized portion and the irradiated portion was the result. We continue to perform embolization if there is a high likelihood of significant volume reduction following that procedure. Embolization must also be performed with a reasonable risk-to-benefit ratio. If our neurointerventional team does not believe that significant feeding artery and nidus occlusion is likely, we consider a staged radiosurgery approach.

■ Summary

Arteriovenous malformation radiosurgery has been in practice for over 30 years and is now a common method to manage properly selected patients with brain AVMs. The techniques have been refined along with our understanding of the expected response. It is this understanding of expected outcomes that should allow a rational discussion of the pertinent issues for management of patients with AVMs. Some patients will require multimodality approaches. All AVM patients should seek to understand whether stereotactic radiosurgery is an appropriate option for their problem.

■ References

1. Friedman W, Bova F. Linear accelerator radiosurgery for arteriovenous malformations. J Neurosurg 1992;77:832–841
2. Lunsford LD, Kondziolka D, Flickinger J, et al. Stereotactic radiosurgery for arteriovenous malformations of the brain. J Neurosurg 1991;75:512–524
3. Pollock B, Flickinger JC, Lunsford LD, Maitz A, Kondziolka D. Factors associated with successful arteriovenous malformation radiosurgery. Neurosurgery 1998;42:1239–1247
4. Maesawa S, Flickinger JC, Kondziolka D, Lunsford LD. Repeated radiosurgery for incompletely obliterated arteriovenous malformations. J Neurosurg 2000;92:961–970
5. Yamamoto M, Jimbo M, Hara M, et al. Gamma knife radiosurgery for arteriovenous malformations: long-term follow-up results focusing oncomplications occurring more than 5 years after irradiation. Neurosurgery 1996;38:906–914
6. Porter P, Shin A, Detsky A, et al. Surgery versus radiosurgery for small, operable cerebral arteriovenous malformations: a clinical and cost comparison. Neurosurgery 1997;41:757–766
7. Betti O, Munari C, Rosler R. Stereotactic radiosurgery with the linear accelerator: treatment of arteriovenous malformations. Neurosurgery 1989;24:311–321
8. Colombo F, Benedetti A, Pozza F, et al. Linear accelerator radiosurgery of cerebral arteriovenous malformations. Neurosurgery 1989;24:833–840
9. Yamamoto Y, Coffey R, Nichols B, et al. Interim report on the radiosurgical treatment of cerebral arteriovenous malformations. J Neurosurg 1995;83:832–837
10. Pollock BE, Lunsford LD, Kondziolka D, et al. Patient outcomes after stereotactic radiosurgery for "operable" arteriovenous malformations. Neurosurgery 1994;35:1–8
11. Flickinger JC, Kondziolka D, Pollock B, et al. Complications from arteriovenous malformation radiosurgery: multivariate analysis and risk modeling. Int J Radiat Oncol Biol Phys 1997;38:485–490
12. Flickinger JC, Kondziolka D, Maitz A, et al. Analysis of neurological sequelae from radiosurgery of arteriovenous malformations: how location affects outcome. Int J Radiat Oncol Biol Phys 1998;40:273–278

13. Friedman W, Blatt D, Bova F, et al. The risk of hemorrhage after radiosurgery for arteriovenous malformations. J Neurosurg 1996;84:912–919

14. Karlsson B, Lindquist C, Steiner L. Effect of gamma knife surgery on the risk of rupture prior to AVM obliteration. Minim Invasive Neurosurg 1996;39:21–27

15. Flickinger JC, Kondziolka D, Lunsford LD, et al. A multi-institutional analysis of complication outcomes after arteriovenous malformation radiosurgery. Int J Radiat Oncol Biol Phys 1999;44:67–74

16. Schneider B, Eberhard D, Steiner L. Histopathology of arteriovenous malformations after gamma knife radiosurgery. J Neurosurg 1997;87:352–357

17. Wu A, Lindner G, Maitz A, et al. Physics of gamma knife approach on convergent beams in stereotactic radiosurgery. Int J Radiat Oncol Biol Phys 1990;18:941–949

18. Kondziolka D, Lunsford LD. Intraparenchymal brainstem radiosurgery. Neurosurg Clin N Am 1993;4:469–479

19. Flickinger JC. An integrated logistic formula for prediction of complications from radiosurgery. Int J Radiat Oncol Biol Phys 1989;17:879–885

20. Flickinger JC, Lunsford LD, Kondziolka D. Dose prescription and dose volume effects in radiosurgery. Neurosurg Clin N Am 1992;3:51–59

21. Szeifert GT, Kemeny AA, Timperley W, et al. The potential role of myofibroblasts in the obliteration of arteriovenous malformations after radiosurgery. Neurosurgery 1997;40:61–66

22. Hara M, Nakamura M, Shiokawa Y, et al. Delayed cyst formation after radiosurgery for cerebral arteriovenous malformation: two case reports. Minim Invasive Neurosurg 1998;41:40–45

23. Gerszten PC, Adelson PD, Kondziolka D, et al. Seizure outcome in children treated for arteriovenous malformations after gamma knife radiosurgery. Pediatr Neurosurg 1996;24:139–144

24. Huang CF, Somaza S, Lunsford LD, et al. Radiosurgery in the management of epilepsy associated with arteriovenous malformations. 2nd International Stereotactic Radiosurgery Society Meeting, Boston, Massachusetts, June 1995. Radiosurgery 1996;1:195–200

25. Steiner L, Lindquist C, Adler JR, et al. Clinical outcome of radiosurgery for cerebral arteriovenous malformations. J Neurosurg 1992;77:1–8

26. Karlsson B, Kihlstrom L, Lindquist C, et al. Gamma knife surgery for previously irradiated arteriovenous malformations. Neurosurgery 1998;42:1–6

27. Karlsson B, Lindquist M, Lindquist C, et al. Long-term angiographic outcome of arteriovenous malformations responding incompletely to gamma knife surgery. 2nd International Stereotactic Radiosurgery Society Meeting, Boston, Massachusetts, June 1995. Radiosurgery 1996;1:188–194

28. Pollock BE, Kondziolka D, Lunsford LD, et al. Repeat stereotactic radiosurgery of arteriovenous malformations: factors associated with incomplete obliteration. Neurosurgery 1996;38:318–324

29. Flickinger JC, Pollock BE, Kondziolka D, et al. A dose-response analysis of arteriovenous malformation obliteration after radiosurgery. Int J Radiat Oncol Biol Phys 1996;36:873–879

30. Friedman W, Bova F, Mendenhall W. Linear accelerator radiosurgery for arteriovenous malformations: the relationship of size to outcome. J Neurosurg 1995;82:180–189

31. Kondziolka D, Lunsford LD, Kanal E, et al. Stereotactic magnetic resonance angiography for targeting in arteriovenous malformation radiosurgery. Neurosurgery 1994;35:585–591

32. Pikus H, Beach ML, Harbaugh R. Microsurgical treatment of arteriovenous malformations: analysis and comparison to stereotactic radiosurgery. J Neurosurg 1998;88:641–646

33. Pollock BE, Flickinger JC, Lunsford LD, et al. Hemorrhage risk after radiosurgery for arteriovenous malformations. Neurosurgery 1996;38:652–661

34. Firlik A, Levy E, Kondziolka D, Yonas H. Staged volume radiosurgery and resection: a new treatment for a giant arteriovenous malformation. Neurosurgery 1998;43:1223–1228

35. Steinberg G, Chang S, Levy R, et al. Surgical resection of large incompletely treated intracranial arteriovenous malformations following stereotactic radiosurgery. J Neurosurg 1996;84:920–928

15

Surgical Treatment of Intracranial Dural Arteriovenous Fistulas

Y. JONATHAN ZHANG, C. MICHAEL CAWLEY, JACQUES E. DION, AND DANIEL LOUIS BARROW

Objectives: Upon completion of this chapter, the reader should be able to classify dural arteriovenous fistulas, explain their clinical features, and identify the surgical techniques used to obliterate them.

Accreditation: The AANS* is accredited by the Accreditation Council for Continuing Medical Education (ACCME) to sponsor continuing medical education for physicians.

Credit: The AANS designates this educational activity for a maximum of 15 credits in Category 1 credit toward the AMA Physician's Recognition Award. Each physician should claim only those hours of credit that he/she spent in the educational activity.

The Home Study Examination is online on the AANS Web site at: http://www.aans.org/education/books/controversy.asp

* The acronym AANS refers to both the American Association of Neurological Surgeons and the American Association of Neurosurgeons.

A dural arteriovenous fistula (DAVF), also known as a dural arteriovenous malformation (DAVM), is an abnormal arteriovenous connection that occurs solely within the leaflets of the dura mater, usually within or near the walls of a dural sinus. A truly unique patho-anatomic entity, DAVFs only gained wide recognition and had their pathophysiology and clinical behaviors gradually elucidated in the past two decades. No longer angiographic curiosities, DAVFs can present with a wide spectrum of symptomatology, and their natural history may range from very benign with spontaneous resolution to highly dangerous with frequent life-threatening intracranial hemorrhage.

The past two decades also witnessed important advances in endovascular techniques for treatment of DAVF as safety, technical feasibility, and outcome continue to improve. The effectiveness, risks, and complications of these techniques are undergoing continuous reassessment as experience and technology evolve. Yet, neurosurgical treatment continues to provide safe and effective definitive management for various intracranial

DAVFs in different locations. Not infrequently, surgical therapy may be a safer and more efficacious option for a particular lesion. We review the anatomy, indications, general principles, techniques, and outcome of neurosurgical management of selected intracranial DAVFs.

■ Classification of Intracranial Dural Arteriovenous Fistulas

Dural arteriovenous fistulas have been classified according to location, hemodynamics, associated dural sinus thrombosis, and their venous drainage pattern, which are related to their clinical manifestations[1-4] and responses to treatment modalities. Individual symptomatology is dependent on lesion location, while the clinical behavior (benign vs. aggressive) is dependent upon the pattern of fistulous venous drainage. Borden et al have devised a simple and well-accepted classification scheme.[1] Type I has drainage only into a dural sinus or meningeal veins. Type II has drainage into a dural sinus and leptomeningeal veins. Type III has drainage into leptomeningeal veins only. Those DAVFs with leptomeningeal venous drainage (Borden types II and III) are associated with an aggressive natural history and high incidence of hemorrhagic and progressive neurological complications. Those DAVFs draining exclusively into a dural sinus (Borden type I) are associated with a benign natural history.

In a review of the literature on the distribution and clinical courses of 377 DAVFs, Awad and Little found 62.6% occurring in the transverse-sigmoid sinus area, 11.9% in the cavernous sinus area, 8.4% in the tentorial incisural area, 7.4% in the convexity-sagittal sinus area, 5.8% in the orbital-anterior falx area, and 3.7% in the sylvian-middle fossa region.[5] The ratio of aggressive to benign behavior was 1:8.8 for transverse-sigmoid sinus location, 1:6.5 for cavernous sinus location, 31:1 for tentorial-incisural location, 1:1 for convexity-sagittal sinus location, 2.1:1 for orbital-anterior falx location, and 2.5:1 for sylvian-middle fossa location. The presence of aggressive behavior (mostly resulting in stroke, hemorrhage, dementia, and blindness) is usually related to the presence of leptomeningeal venous drainage, echoing the findings of Borden et al[1,6] There are anecdotal reports of DAVFs located in the clivus, in the inferior petrosal sinus, in the deep venous sinuses, and in the torcular areas. Additionally, a small group of patients may harbor and present with multiple DAVFs.

■ Pathophysiology and Natural History

The vascular tree is a remarkably dynamic system that can adjust to many normal and abnormal factors with remodeling and flow alteration. There are normal dural arteriovenous connections that may adapt with dilation and/or flow reversal secondary to venous hypertension. Frequently, venous abnormalities, congenital or acquired, can be identified accompanying DAVFs. These include aplasia, stenosis, and partial or complete thrombosis. Such flow restriction may be further complicated by other hormonal and metabolic factors that eventually lead to an inappropriate remodeling process of the original normal channels, forming pathological DAVFs.[7] As the lesions progress, the venous hypertension may congest normal leptomeningeal drainage causing flow reversal and formation of venous varices because the intracranial venous system is valveless and potentially bidirectional. It is noted that such pathological leptomeningeal venous hypertension is the source of significant neurological complications.[8]

Davies et al studied the natural history of benign (Borden type I) and aggressive (Borden types II and III)

DAVFs.[9,10] Only 2% of the untreated patients with type I DAVFs presented with hemorrhage or progressive neurological deficits. In contrast, 39% of type II and 79% of type III patients presented with these aggressive symptoms. Without treatment, 81% of the patients with Borden type I DAVFs were improved or cured. However, in the untreated patients with Borden types II and III lesions, there was an intracranial hemorrhage rate of 19.2% per patient year, a nonhemorrhagic neurological deficit rate of 10.2% per patient year, and a mortality rate of 19.3% per patient year. More disturbingly, 18% of patients who were treated with partial embolization and who demonstrated persistent retrograde leptomeningeal venous drainage experienced recurrent intracranial hemorrhage or a new neurological deficit.[9–11] Therefore, the presence of retrograde leptomeningeal venous drainage is an overwhelming prognosticating factor for aggressive intracranial DAVFs and their unfavorable natural courses.

■ Clinical Features

The symptoms of DAVFs are secondary to the increased blood flow and resultant intracranial venous hypertension. If the fistulous volume is low with good venous outflow, there may be no symptoms other than a bruit in those DAVFs close to the temporal bone. As venous hypertension and congestion develop with progressive shunting from the fistula, additional symptoms and complications emerge. In the region of the cavernous sinus and orbits, local signs and symptoms make up the majority of clinical presentation. In other locations, the symptomatology may be more general. When a high-flow fistula develops, increased intracranial pressure may occur, with associated symptoms of headache and papilledema, simulating pseudotumor cerebri. Moreover, when venous hypertension is borne by a leptomeningeal vein, the risks of intraparenchymal and subarachnoid hemorrhage are extremely high.[2,4,5,8,12] A venous aneurysm in the context of DAVFs may have the highest rupture tendency of all intracranial aneurysmal lesions. Rarely, a dilated venous varix can present as a local mass lesion, especially in crowded locations such as the posterior fossa near the brain stem and cranial nerves.[13]

Another clinical problem seen with high-volume fistulas that drain extensively through the leptomeningeal veins is the ischemic parenchymal changes and resultant gliosis and necrosis secondary to chronic venous hypertension and congestion. Patients with such problems may present with seizures, dementia, or other focal neurological deficits.[14–17] More intriguingly, patients with rare DAVFs in the region of the foramen magnum may have leptomeningeal venous drainage through lower dependent medullary veins. Venous hypertension in these plexuses can cause myelopathy with neurologic deficits many segments below the level of fistula.[18–20]

■ Overview of Dural Arteriovenous Fistulas Treatment Options and Indications

Following the diagnosis of a DAVF, the clinician faces a wide variety of management options. An expectant therapeutic approach is possible in many cases and may be safer than any attempt at lesion obliteration. In other instances, palliative treatment of the lesion aiming at controlling the associated symptoms such as pain, ophthalmoplegia, or pulsatile tinnitus is undertaken. In some lesions, secondary manifestations such as increased intracranial pressure and papilledema may require more urgent intervention than the DAVF itself. Lesion obliteration through a variety of feasible approaches may be entertained as definitive treatment for certain DAVFs when aggressive clinical behaviors are anticipated. In each case, the therapeutic strategy should be highly individualized and guided to improve symptoms or to prevent catastrophic consequences of the lesion natural history.

A given therapeutic attitude can never be generalized to all DAVFs in view of the highly variable clinical manifestations and possibilities of natural course. Treatment options for DAVFs, in general, include expectant observation, carotid compression, endovascular transarterial and/or transvenous embolization, and microsurgical disconnection. Conventional radiotherapy and stereotactic radiosurgery as alternative therapeutic options for some DAVFs have been reported. However, there needs to be better characterization of optimal dosimetry, time response, and effectiveness of lesion obliteration, as well as radiation safety or protection to adjacent eloquent neural structures.

Noninvasive options, including observation and carotid compression, are suitable for lesions without aggressive clinical or angiographic features, i.e., leptomeningeal venous drainage. Close clinical follow-up is important in these management strategies, and patients should be educated to report any significant changes in their symptoms. Some changes in symptoms, including sudden resolution of a usual symptom like bruit, may signify the transformation of a previously benign DAVF to an aggressive lesion with cortical venous drainage replacing dural outflow. Once an aggressive venous drainage pattern develops, endovascular or surgical intervention should be strongly considered.

As experience and technology evolve, endovascular therapy has been used to manage an increasing proportion of intracranial DAVFs safely and with good results. However, transarterial embolization alone has limited effectiveness in treating lesions that have a plethora of arterial feeders with numerous channels from multiple sources, particularly when many of the feeding arteries are very small in diameter and stem directly off pial trunks.[21–23] Such circumstances are usually encountered in lesions located in the tentorial-incisura and anterior fossa-falx.

Many "angiographic cures" by transarterial embolization should be viewed as suspect or temporary, because lesions have been shown to recanalize, or acquire alternate arterial supply. Transvenous embolization, especially in combination with adjuvant transarterial embolization to reduce fistulous inflow, has become the favored approach for endovascular therapy of intracranial DAVFs.[22–25] Percutaneous transvenous therapy of intracranial DAVFs can be performed only when a venous drainage pouch that is separate from veins draining normal brain tissue can be identified and accessed by a microguidewire–microcatheter system. When transvenous embolization is limited to the venous outlet immediately distal to the fistula nidus, and functional drainage can be preserved, embolization with platinum coils can provide safe and effective treatment. However, venous outflow occlusion without obliteration of the arteriovenous shunt itself may result in increased venous hypertension in other channels and in hemorrhage or worsened clinical symptomatology.[24,26,27] Open microsurgical fistula disconnection is indicated in cases of endovascular failure or technical infeasibility. Occasionally, direct surgical exposure of the dural sinus can provide the transvenous entry for endovascular obliteration of certain DAVFs by sinus packing when venous access is complicated by severe stenosis or bifocal occlusion of the sinus.

■ Surgical Techniques for Managing Intracranial Dural Arteriovenous Fistulas

Simple feeding arterial ligation, like stand-alone transarterial embolization, has a very low clinical and radiographical cure rate.[28] The partially treated fistulas usually continue to fill and may recruit new arterial supply and alter venous draining patterns, eventually evolving into more dangerous lesions. Thus, surgical ligation of feeding branches is not advisable in the modern management of DAVFs. Objectives of surgical intervention include complete physical interruption of arterialized leptomeningeal venous connections. Recently, some authors have reported good results with simple microsurgical disconnection of pathological leptomeningeal venous outflow flush with the dural leaflet.[29–33] Such a strategy shares the same philosophy with transvenous embolization technique, which is to occlude the venous outlet at the nidus without an interval venous segment between the occlusion and the nidus. Usually, in DAVFs with retrograde leptomeningeal venous drainage, these veins no longer contribute to the venous drainage from normal brain tissue, and occlusion of the venous side of the fistula can be performed without risk of venous infarction. Surgical excision of the pathological dura may be associated with significant blood loss and neurological complications.[34,35]

Debates over the optimal strategy continue, and only long-term follow-up of treated patients will demonstrate the efficacy of each procedure. The safety of open surgical approaches may be enhanced by preoperative adjuvant transarterial embolization so as to decrease flow through the DAVFs and control many of the external carotid supply channels to these lesions.[36–39] Moreover, superselective angiography may provide detailed information about the precise location and angioarchitecture of the lesion. Intraoperative angiography and the occasional open coil-induced thrombosis of arterialized venous aneurysms or the cavernous sinus have further improved the effectiveness of neurosurgical treatment. With meticulous attention to detail, experienced neurosurgeons have achieved good results with limited morbidity.[21,29–33,36,38,40–42]

■ Transverse and Sigmoid Sinus Dural Arteriovenous Fistulas

Improvements of endovascular techniques and a better understanding of the pathophysiology of these lesions have increased the number of treatment options. The type of treatment (surgical vs. endovascular) and the route of attack (arterial vs. venous) depend on whether the involved sinuses remain patent or have thrombosed. Once treatment is deemed necessary, occlusion of the sinus by either endovascular or surgical routes, as described by Mullan,[43] can safely eliminate the majority of these lesions. When the fistula nidus is located in a segment of isolated sinus from the thromboses, open surgical exposure of the dural sinus can provide venous access for intraoperative endovascular sinus occlusion.[33,36,37,40,42]

The operative exposure requires the patient to be in a lateral or prone position. A small rectangular skin flap is made over the transverse sinus, with optional intraoperative stereotaxis guidance, and a fringe of the occipital muscles is undermined using electrical cautery. A burrhole or a small rectangular channel of bone is drilled away over the sinus, packing continuously with bone wax to achieve meticulous hemostasis. The exposed sinus wall is covered instantly with prothrombotic materials, like Gelfoam™ (Pfizer, Inc., New York, New York) or Surgicel™ (Johnson & Johnson, New Brunswick, New Jersey), and suction pressure is applied through saline-soaked cotton. In this manner, the entire extent of the transverse sinus can be exposed with only minor hemorrhage. Then, sinus occlusion can proceed with endovascular techniques. After the sinus is occluded, intraoperative angiography should confirm the obliteration of all retrograde leptomeningeal venous flow and the fistula itself. If there are cortical veins draining independently from the fistulous wall, these will need to be interrupted flush with the sinus wall after opening the dura.

When success is measured by the extent to which the lesion is eliminated, such combined therapy offers the best results with 68% complete angiographic obliteration, compared with 41% for embolization alone and 33% for surgery alone.[28] Long-term clinical and angiographic follow-up is important for patients with residual filling or persistent symptoms.

■ Tentorial Incisura Dural Arteriovenous Fistulas

Dural arteriovenous malformations of the tentorial incisura demonstrate an unfavorable natural history. These lesions are frequently associated with retrograde leptomeningeal venous drainage through the perimesencephalic system into the vein of Galen and carry a high risk of hemorrhage, almost always in the form of subarachnoid hemorrhage.[12,44,45] Venous hypertension of the brain stem structures, which normally drain through such venous plexuses, can cause other focal neurological deficits. Typically, there is a plethora of arterial feeders from a myriad of meningeal arteries, converging into a pathological region of the tentorial leaflet at the incisura, where there are numerous arteriovenous communications instead of a single shunt. The small caliber of the feeding branches and frequent presence of dural branches arising from the distal posterior cerebral and superior cerebellar arteries make transarterial embolization difficult to perform; the lack of an adjacent large dural sinus makes transvenous access equally difficult. Complete lesion obliteration frequently requires open surgical treatment, usually in combination with preparatory arterial embolization from external carotid branches.

We have adopted a venous disconnection technique, which evolved from earlier dural excision methods.[32] The procedure is performed via a subtemporal approach, taking care to preserve any normal bridging veins. Arterialized veins connecting the tentorium to the temporal lobe are coagulated and divided. The portion of tentorium with obvious DAVF involvement is extensively bipolar coagulated. The tentorium is carefully incised to expose the inferior surface, and any arterialized venous connection with the cerebellum and brain stem is carefully coagulated and divided. At the incisural border, meningeal branches of the posterior cerebral and superior cerebellar arteries can be similarly discon-nected. Intraoperative angiography is performed to con-firm the efficacy of obliteration. Some authors advocate direct puncture and open coil-embolization of any resid-ual giant venous aneurysms.[34] The minimum goal of sur-gical therapy should be to eliminate the leptomeningeal venous drainage, and thus the major risk of hemorrhage. Residual arteriovenous shunting should be closely followed with serial postoperative angiograms. In a meta-analysis of the English literature,[28] combined therapy demon-strated the best success rate in lesion obliteration (89%), compared with either surgical treatment alone (78%) or endovascular therapy alone (25%).

▪ Anterior Fossa-Falx Dural Arteriovenous Fistulas

Feeding vessels typically arise from the anterior or posterior ethmoidal arteries and less commonly from the anterior falcine artery in anterior fossa-falx DAVFs. The ethmoidal arteries are usually branches of the ophthalmic artery and cannot be embolized without significant risk of complications involving the visual system. Therefore, surgical obliteration is the preferred method of treatment for anterior fossa DAVFs. These lesions drain overwhelmingly through lep-tomeningeal venous channels with a very high incidence of venous varices and aneurysms, thus accounting for an aggressive natural course and high risk of intracerebral hemorrhage.[46,47]

Surgical obliteration is performed through a low frontal craniotomy with minimal brain retraction. If a large intraparenchymal hematoma is present, it should be evacuated initially to allow brain relaxation and safe mobilization of the frontal pole. In most cases, the lesion consists of simple fistulous connections between the feeding arteries and the pial veins without a significant dural nidus. Microsurgical occlusion of the vascular con-nection between the dura of the cribriform plate area and the arterialized pial veins is curative without the need for further resection of the dysplastic lep-tomeningeal veins. Intraoperative angiography is useful to confirm the obliteration of the fistula. Success rates of over 95% for surgical intervention have been reported in the literature.[28]

▪ Cavernous Sinus Dural Arteriovenous Fistulas

Endovascular methods are the primary means of manag-ing cavernous sinus DAVFs. Dural arteriovenous fistulas in this region present little risk of hemorrhage due to the unusual presence of leptomeningeal venous drainage.

Transvenous embolization is the preferred treatment once intervention is indicated, although transarterial embolization is a reasonable alternative if all fistulous feeders are from the external carotid system. There are a variety of transvenous access approaches to the cavernous sinus, including direct percutaneous puncture of the superior ophthalmic vein[48] and cavernous sinus[49] through the superior orbital fissure. Endovascular failure is very rare; thus, surgery seldom is required.

▪ Other Rare Dural Arteriovenous Fistulas

Dural arteriovenous fistulas involving the convexity-superior sagittal sinus and the middle fossa dura (usually the sphenoparietal and superior petrosal sinuses) with variable leptomeningeal venous drainage pattern are rare. Arterial supplies usually arise from the middle meningeal artery and other external carotid branches, thus permitting transarterial embolization to reduce shunt inflow. Combined with arterial embolization, transvenous therapy usually can achieve sinus occlusion to cure the fistula radiographically. When venous access is complicated by sinus thrombosis, surgical exposure of the involved sinus using techniques similar to the above for transverse sinus fistulas can be applied. Microsurgical leptomeningeal venous disconnection can be performed as well.[39,41,42] Intraoperative angiography is valuable to document the resolution of fistula.

Another rare location for DAVFs is in the region of the foramen magnum. These lesions may drain directly into the pontine or spinal medullary venous circulation. Dural arteriovenous fistulas located in the posterior fossa are so unusual that they have not been well characterized in the literature. However, when retrograde leptomeningeal venous drainage develops with ensuing venous hyperten-sion, the natural course of these lesions is expected to be poor. The safety and feasibility of transarterial emboliza-tion are limited by the multitude of small arterial feeders arising directly from the vertebral arteries. Transvenous routes of endovascular obliteration are limited by the pre-dominance of leptomeningeal venous drainage as opposed to dural sinus outflow. Open surgical oblitera-tion of such DAVFs is feasible and effective. This is approached via a posterior far-lateral craniocervical expo-sure with upper cervical laminectomy and suboccipital craniotomy. The pathological dura with fistula is exposed and extensively coagulated, and the vertebral artery is controlled. Once the dura is opened, the leptomeningeal venous connection is identified and may be clip-ligated flush with the dura. Intraoperative evoked potential mon-itoring for the appropriate spinal cord segments and brain stem may add safety to the venous disconnection. An intraoperative angiogram may be helpful to confirm obliteration of the DAVF; however, injection of all possible feeders may not be technically possible in the operating room, and a postoperative angiogram may be necessary.

■ Conclusion

Continued careful clinical analysis of patients with intracranial DAVFs will expand our knowledge about such lesions and about the risks and effectiveness of various treatment modalities. Endovascular techniques will continue to improve and likely will have greater application in the management of intracranial DAVFs. Today, open surgical treatment, accompanied by adjunctive endovascular and intraoperative angiographic techniques, remains useful, safe, and effective for selected lesions, especially for DAVFs of the tentorial-incisura and anterior fossa region. Multidisciplinary cerebrovascular teams with experience in the recognition and management of intracranial dural arteriovenous fistulas, and with expertise in the subtleties of various diagnostic and treatment modalities, can deliver the best care for patients with such challenging pathology.

■ References

1. Borden JA, Wu JK, Shucart WA. A proposed classification for spinal and cranial dural arteriovenous fistulous malformations and implications for treatment. J Neurosurg 1995;82:166–179

2. Brown RD, Wiebers DO, Nichols DA. Intracranial dural arteriovenous fistulae: angiographic predictors of intracranial hemorrhage and clinical outcome in nonsurgical patients. J Neurosurg 1994;81:531–538

3. Chung SJ, Kim JS, Kim JC, et al. Intracranial dural arteriovenous fistulas: analysis of 60 patients. Cerebrovasc Dis 2002;13:79–88

4. Cognard C, Gobin YP, Pierot L, et al. Cerebral dural arteriovenous fistulas: clinical and angiographic correlation with a revised classification of venous drainage. Radiology 1995;194:671–680

5. Awad IA, Little JR, Akrawi WP, et al. Intracranial dural arteriovenous malformations: factors predisposing to an aggressive neurological course. J Neurosurg 1990;72:839–850

6. Davies MA, ter Brugge K, Willinski R, et al. The validity of classification for the clinical presentation of intracranial dural arteriovenous fistulas. J Neurosurg 1996;85:830–837

7. Gibbons GH, Dzau VJ. The emerging concept of vascular remodeling. N Engl J Med 1994;330:1431–1438

8. Bederson JB. Pathophysiology and animal models of dural arteriovenous malformations. In: Awad IA, Barrow DL, eds. Dural Arteriovenous Malformations. Park Ridge, IL: American Association of Neurological Surgeons; 1993: 23–33

9. Davies MA, Saleh J, ter Brugge K, et al. The natural history and management of intracranial dural arteriovenous fistulae. Part 1: Benign lesions. Intervent Neuroradiol 1997;3:295–302

10. Davies MA, ter Brugge K, Willinski R, et al. The natural history and management of intracranial dural arteriovenous fistulae. Part 2: aggressive lesions. Intervent Neuroradiol 1997;3:303–311

11. Duffau H, Lopes M, Janosevic V, et al. Early rebleeding from intracranial dural arteriovenous fistulas: report of 20 cases and review of the literature. J Neurosurg 1999;90:78–84

12. Lasjaunias P, Chiu M, ter Brugge K, et al. Neurological manifestation of intracranial dural arteriovenous malformations. J Neurosurg 1986;64:724–730

13. Ito M, Sonokawa T, Mishina H, et al. Dural arteriovenous malformation manifesting as tic douloureux. Surg Neurol 1996;45:370–375

14. Datta NN, Rehman SU, Kwok JC, et al. Reversible dementia due to dural arteriovenous fistula: a simple surgical option. Neurosurg Rev 1998;21:174–176

15. Matsuda S, Waragai M, Shinotoh H, et al. Intracranial dural arteriovenous fistula (DAVF) presenting progressive dementia and parkinsonism. J Neurol Sci 1999;165:43–47

16. Tanaka K, Morooka Y, Nakagawa Y, et al. Dural arteriovenous malformation manifesting as dementia due to ischemia in bilateral thalami. A case report. Surg Neurol 1999;51:489–493

17. Yamakami I, Kobayashi E, Yamaura A. Diffuse white matter changes caused by dural arteriovenous fistula. J Clin Neurosci 2001;8:471–475

18. Bret P, Salzmann M, Bascoulergue Y, et al. Dural arteriovenous fistula of the posterior fossa draining into the spinal medullary veins–an unusual cause of myelopathy: case report. Neurosurgery 1994;35:965–968

19. Reinges MH, Thron A, Mull M, et al. Dural arteriovenous fistulae at the foramen magnum. J Neurol 2001;248:197–203

20. Versari PP, D'Aliberti G, Talamonti G, et al. Progressive myelopathy caused by intracranial dural arteriovenous fistula: report of two cases and review of the literature. Neurosurgery 1993;33:914–918

21. Barnwell SL, Halbach VV, Dowd CF, et al. A variant of arteriovenous fistulas within the wall of dural sinuses. Results of combined surgical and endovascular therapy. J Neurosurg 1991;74:199–204

22. Halbach VV, Higashida RT, Hieshima GB, et al. Transvenous embolization of dural fistulas involving the transverse and sigmoid sinuses. AJNR Am J Neuroradiol 1989;10:385–392

23. Urtasun F, Biondi A, Casasco A, et al. Cerebral dural arteriovenous fistulas: percutaneous transvenous embolization. Radiology 1996;199:209–217

24. Roy D, Raymond J. The role of transvenous embolization in the treatment of intracranial dural arteriovenous fistulas. Neurosurgery 1997;40:1133–1144

25. Yu J, Ling F, Zhang P. Treatment of cerebral dural arteriovenous fistula targeting drainage vein or sinus. Zhonghua Wai Ke Za Zhi 2001;39:669–671 [Chinese Journal of Surgery]

26. Dawson RC III, Joseph GJ, Owens DS, et al. Transvenous embolization as the primary therapy for arteriovenous fistulas of the lateral and sigmoid sinuses. AJNR Am J Neuroradiol 1998;19:571–576

27. Olteanu-Nerbe V, Uhl E, Steiger HJ, et al. Dural arteriovenous fistulas including the transverse and sigmoid sinuses: results of treatment in 30 cases. Acta Neurochir (Wien) 1997;139:307–318

28. Lucas CP, Zabramski JM, Spetzler RF, et al. Treatment of intracranial dural arteriovenous malformations: a meta-analysis from the English language literature. Neurosurgery 1997;40:1119–1132

29. Collice M, D'Aliberti G, Arena O, et al. Surgical treatment of intracranial dural arteriovenous fistulae: role of venous drainage. Neurosurgery 2000;47:56–67

30. Hoh BL, Choudhri TF, Connolly ES Jr, et al. Surgical management of high-grade intracranial dural arteriovenous fistulas: leptomeningeal venous disruption without nidus excision. Neurosurgery 1998;42:796–805

31. Thompson BG, Doppman JL, Oldfield EH. Treatment of cranial dural arteriovenous fistulae by interruption of leptomeningeal venous drainage. J Neurosurg 1994;80:617–623

32. Tomak PR, Cloft HJ, Kaga A, et al. Evolution of the management of tentorial dural arteriovenous malformations. Neurosurgery 2003;52:750–762

33. Ushikoshi S, Houkin K, Kuroda S, et al. Surgical treatment of intracranial dural arteriovenous fistulas. Surg Neurol 2002;57:253–261

34. Mullan S. Surgical therapy: indications and general principles. In Awad IA, Barrow DL, eds. Dural Arteriovenous Malformations. Park Ridge, IL: American Association of Neurological Surgeons; 1993: 213–229

35. Sundt TM, Piepgras DG. The surgical approach to arteriovenous malformations of the lateral and sigmoid dural sinuses. J Neurosurg 1983;59:32–39

36. Goto K, Sidipratomo P, Ogata N, et al. Combining endovascular and neurosurgical treatments of high-risk dural arteriovenous fistulas in the lateral sinus and the confluence of the sinuses. J Neurosurg 1999;90:289–299

37. Kasai K, Iwasa H, Yamada N, et al. Combined treatment of a dural arteriovenous malformation of the lateral sinus using transarterial and direct lateral sinus embolisation. Neuroradiology 1996;38: 494–496

38. Pelz DM, Lownie SP, Fox AJ, et al. Intracranial dural arteriovenous fistulae with pial venous drainage: combined endovascular-neurosurgical therapy. Can J Neurol Sci 1997;24:210–218

39. Pierot L, Visot A, Boulin A, et al. Combined neurosurgical and neuroradiological treatment of a complex superior sagittal sinus dural fistula: technical note. Neurosurgery 1998;42:194–197

40. Endo S, Kuwayama N, Takaku A, et al. Direct packing of the isolated sinus in patients with dural arteriovenous fistulas of the transverse-sigmoid sinus. J Neurosurg 1998;88:449–456

41. Houdart E, Saint-Maurice JP, Chapot R, et al. Transcranial approach for venous embolization of dural arteriovenous fistulas. J Neurosurg 2002;97:280–286

42. Kawaguchi S, Sakaki T, Morimoto T, et al. Surgery for dural arteriovenous fistula in superior sagittal sinus and transverse sigmoid sinus. J Clin Neurosci 2000;7(Suppl 1):47–49

43. Mullan S. Reflection upon the nature and management of intracranial and intraspinal vascular malformations and fistulae. J Neurosurg 1994;80:606–616

44. Picard L, Bracard S, Islak C, et al. Dural fistulae of the tentorium cerebelli. J Neuroradiol 1990;17:161–181

45. Vinuela F, Fox AJ, Pelz DM, et al. Unusual clinical manifestations of dural arteriovenous malformations. J Neurosurg 1986;64:554–558

46. Halbach VV, Higashida RT, Hieshima GB, et al. Dural arteriovenous fistulas supplied by ethmoidal arteries. Neurosurgery 1990;26:816–823

47. Martin NA, King WA, Wilson CB, et al. Management of dural arteriovenous malformations of the anterior cranial fossa. J Neurosurg 1990;72:692–697

48. Benndorf G, Bender A, Campi A, et al. Treatment of a cavernous sinus dural arteriovenous fistula by deep orbital puncture of the superior ophthalmic vein. Neuroradiology 2001;43:499–502

49. Teng MM, Lirng JF, Chang T, et al. Embolisation of carotid cavernous fistula by means of direct puncture through the superior orbital fissure. Radiology 1995;194:705–711

16

Endovascular Treatment of Dural Arteriovenous Fistulas

YASUNARI NIIMI, ALEJANDRO BERENSTEIN, AVI SETTON, AND MARK J. KUPERSMITH

Objectives: Upon completion of this chapter, the reader should be able to identify the transarterial and transvenous embolization techniques that can be used to treat dural arteriovenous fistulas at various intracranial and spinal locations.

Accreditation: The AANS* is accredited by the Accreditation Council for Continuing Medical Education (ACCME) to sponsor continuing medical education for physicians.

Credit: The AANS designates this educational activity for a maximum of 15 credits in Category 1 credit toward the AMA Physician's Recognition Award. Each physician should claim only those hours of credit that he/she spent in the educational activity.

The Home Study Examination is online on the AANS Web site at: http://www.aans.org/education/books/controversy.asp

* The acronym AANS refers to both the American Association of Neurological Surgeons and the American Association of Neurosurgeons.

■ General Considerations

Dural arteriovenous fistulas (DAVFs) are arteriovenous shunts supplied by dural feeding arteries and usually occur within or near the dural sinuses in various locations. They can secondarily recruit pial or transosseous cutaneous feeders. Most adult lesions are considered as acquired, and the most well-accepted triggering factor for development is sinus thrombosis, which can be idiopathic or due to trauma, tumor,[1] surgery, infection, or hypercoagulability secondary to hormonal influence.[2–5] Angiography for these lesions frequently shows evidence of partial or complete sinus thrombosis with various degrees of outflow restriction of the venous drainage of the normal brain or the fistulas themselves. However, the inciting factor leading to the development of DAVFs is frequently undetected, suggesting that other unidentified factors must be present.

Dural arteriovenous fistulas can present with a variety of symptoms, which are mostly related to the direction of the abnormal venous drainage and disturbance of normal venous drainage of the brain, spinal cord, or orbit.[6] Cognard et al and Borden et al proposed classifications of DAVFs based on venous drainage. Borden et al classified DAVFs into three types. Type I DAVFs drain into the dural sinus in an antegrade fashion. Type II DAVFs drain into the venous sinus with retrograde drainage into subarachnoid veins. Type III DAVFs drain into the subarachnoid veins.[7] Cognard et al proposed a similar but more detailed classification. They classified DAVFs into five types: type I, located in the main sinus with antegrade flow; type II, in the main sinus with reflux into the sinus (IIa), cortical vein (IIb), or both (IIa+b); type III, with direct cortical venous drainage without venous ectasia; type IV, with direct cortical venous drainage with venous ectasia; and type V, with spinal venous drainage.[8] These classifications correlate well with clinical symptomatology and prognosis.[9]

Venous hypertension is the most important etiologic factor and can be focal or global. Focal venous hypertension can develop due to primary pial (cortical or perimedullary) venous drainage of the fistula[10] or secondary reflux to pial veins from the sinus due to sinus outflow restriction. Venous hypertension can cause venous rupture at any point of the cortical venous drainage resulting in intracerebral or subarachnoid hemorrhage, seizures, venous infarcts, or focal neurological deficits due to venous ischemia. Focal ectasia and stenosis of draining veins are the frequent findings in those cases presenting with hemorrhage and commonly seen in the tentorial-incisural, or anterior cranial fossa DAVFs. Spinal cord venous hypertension due to perimedullary venous drainage in posterior fossa DAVFs or spinal DAVFs can cause progressive myelopathy. Orbital signs and congestion associated with cavernous sinus DAVFs are attributed to focal venous hypertension of the ophthalmic venous system. Global venous hypertension can also occur due to functional outflow restriction of the venous drainage of the entire brain secondary to the arteriovenous (AV) shunting and dural sinus thrombosis or maldevelopment of the normal venous system. It can cause dementia or decreased mental activities and papilledema due to increased intracranial pressure.[6,9,11,12–14] This type of global cerebral dysfunction and papilledema can be reversible by closing the fistulas with preservation of the patency of the deep venous system.[3]

Other mechanisms of a functional disturbance in the venous system include venous mass effect, which can cause cranial neuropathy or optic neuropathy, and thrombosis such as of the ophthalmic vein, which causes retinal and choroidal hemorrhage and dysfunction, and sudden proptosis in cases with cavernous sinus DAVFs.[15] Pulsatile tinnitus is another symptom due to high-flow venous drainage conducting to the auditory apparatus. A disturbance in the arterial circulation can rarely cause symptoms; Lasjaunias described cranial nerve palsy that developed from a possible arterial steal phenomenon.[6]

The prognosis of untreated DAVFs is poor if there is primary or secondary pial venous drainage but is usually benign if there is only drainage into the dural sinus without pial venous reflux[16–18] The spinal DAVFs usually have a poor prognosis due to progressive myelopathy if they are not treated.[19] It is important to recognize that DAVFs are a dynamic disease and the direction of evolution is unpredictable. They can increase or decrease in flow or even disappear depending on the location; or they may reroute their venous drainage due to progression of venous or sinus thrombosis. Although the disappearance of cranial bruit or symptoms may indicate favorable spontaneous thrombosis of the AV shunting, it can also reflect further thrombosis of the sinus with development of pial venous drainage, which places the patient at risk for hemorrhage, cerebral infarcts, and seizures.[18,20] Changes in the symptoms, therefore, should be carefully evaluated with contrast magnetic resonance imaging

(MRI) and, if necessary, with angiography for development of pial venous drainage.[19]

Although the classification of DAVFs based on venous drainage correlates well with the symptomatology, for consideration of treatment strategies, a classification based on the location of the lesion is preferred and facilitates comparison between surgical and endovascular approaches. We discuss angiographic features, symptomatology, indications, and techniques for endovascular treatment of DAVFs. Pediatric and spinal DAVFs are discussed separately, because they have distinct angiographic features, natural history, and treatment methods from adult intracranial DAVFs.

Pretherapeutic angiographic evaluation should address the location of the AV shunts, arterial supply, flow characteristics through the fistula, venous drainage, and existence and extent of thrombosis of cortical veins or dural sinuses, as well as the drainage of the normal brain. Evaluation of the venous phase of the cerebral circulation before and after endovascular treatment is especially important to assess the etiology of the symptoms and clinical findings and to predict their improvement after treatment.

Endovascular treatment for DAVFs can be performed by transarterial, transvenous, or a combined approach. For transarterial embolization, liquid embolic agents such as n-butyl cyanoacrylate (NBCA) are the most effective in penetrating to the fistula site and permanently occluding the shunt. For optimal transarterial embolization using a liquid agent, the tip of the microcatheter has to be wedged into the feeder beyond the supply to the normal tissue to obtain flow control and penetration of the agent into the venous side.[21] Particulate agents such as polyvinyl alcohol (PVA) tend to result in proximal occlusion and recanalization of the fistulas either by collateral vessels to the fistula sites or recanalization of the embolized vessel itself.[22] In general, particulate agents are a less-definite material but can be used for palliative embolization or if distal catheterization adequate for liquid agents is not possible. A cautionary comment for arterial embolization concerns the use of coils. It is important not to place coils in the proximal portion of the arterial feeders because it is rarely curative; it excludes the future transarterial access and facilitates development of inaccessible collateral supply to the fistulas. Coils in the arterial route are only used to protect normal vessels prior to liquid embolization.[22] For transvenous embolization, coils are generally used to occlude the venous side of the fistulas. If the internal jugular vein is not available for the transvenous embolization of a sinus, transcranial approach to the sinus may be possible.[23] It is important to evaluate the feasibility of the occlusion of the affected portion of the sinus on the pretherapeutic angiogram. If there is venous drainage of the normal brain to the sinus, that segment of the sinus should not be occluded. Transvenous coil embolization is occasionally possible without occlusion of the sinus if the DAVF drains into a venous lake that is separated from the sinus.[24]

Conventional radiotherapy for DAVFs was reported with some success before the development of endovascular embolization and refined surgical techniques. Radiosurgery for selected DAVFs has been recently reported with or without combination with transarterial embolization[25–28]; however, we have no experience with radiosurgery and thus are not discussing it in this review.

■ Transverse-Sigmoid Dural Arteriovenous Fistulas

Transverse-sigmoid sinus region DAVFs are the most common type of DAVFs found in Western countries. They are supplied by multiple dural branches to the transverse and sigmoid sinuses from the external carotid, internal carotid, and vertebral arteries. Venous outflow restriction due to thrombosis of the sigmoid or transverse sinus is common and results in cortical venous drainage that can cause hemorrhage,[29] seizure, or venous infarction.[30] If there is no cortical venous drainage, patients usually present with only bruit, which is the most common symptom. Spontaneous thrombosis of the fistulas in this location has not been documented.

The existence of cortical venous drainage is an absolute indication for treatment even for asymptomatic patients, because the natural history is poor if untreated. If bruit is the only symptom for those who do not have cortical venous drainage, the indication for treatment is relative. In this situation, the treatment plan can be chosen from conservative observation, partial treatment with preservation of the sinus patency, or complete obliteration with occlusion of the draining sinus. This decision should be made depending on the patient's age, tolerability for bruit, and reliability of the patient for follow-up visits. For those patients who tolerate the noise and have no cortical venous drainage, we favor conservative observation. If treatment is demanded by the patient because of intolerance of bruit, the patient should be treated without sinus occlusion even if the treatment results in only partial obliteration of the fistulas. Once conservative observation is chosen, the patient should be closely monitored with periodic clinical examination and contrast-enhanced MRI. If there is MRI evidence of initiation or progression of sinus thrombosis and development of cortical venous drainage, the patient should undergo cerebral angiography. If cortical venous drainage is confirmed by angiography, the patient should be treated prior to the development of hemorrhage or neurological symptoms.

Embolization is the premier mode of treatment and can be performed by transarterial, transvenous, or a combined approach with a high rate of total obliteration of the DAVFs. Transarterial embolization is favored for small lesions because patency of the sinus can be preserved. This approach is also the first choice and is frequently curative for those lesions draining to the isolated sinus with cortical venous drainage due to sinus thrombosis proximal and distal to the fistula site (**Fig. 16–1**). For extensive lesions with multiple feeders and multiple fistula sites, a transvenous or a combined approach is favored because complete cure is difficult by transarterial embolization alone.[31,32] If transvenous embolization is considered for complete obliteration of the fistulas, it is essential to identify and avoid occlusion of the junction between the vein of Labbé and the transverse sinus. It is also important to preserve the venous drainage of the cerebellum to the sinus (**Fig. 16–2**), which is especially relevant when occlusion of a long segment of the sinus or medial transverse sinus is planned. Once feasibility of sinus occlusion is confirmed, the technique for sinus obliteration is relatively simple. Even if the distal sinus is not opacified on the angiographic study, it is usually possible to reach the fistula site either through the contralateral sinus or through the nonopacified or thrombosed segment of the sinus with gentle guidewire and catheter manipulation.[33] If sinus occlusion is not feasible, a combined approach with transvenous occlusion of the feasible part of the sinus and transarterial embolization for the remaining fistulas is considered. Recanalization of the occluded sinus with stenting to redirect the venous drainage from cortical veins to the sinus combined with additional transarterial embolization to decrease the shunt is theoretically a reasonable option.[34] However, long-term patency of the recanalized sinus is currently not known.

Good results can be usually obtained by endovascular treatment for DAVFs in this location; therefore, the indications for surgery have become limited to only exceptional cases in which both transarterial and transvenous approaches are not feasible or failed.

■ Cavernous Dural Arteriovenous Fistulas

Dural arteriovenous fistulas involving the cavernous sinus are characterized by wide variation in their angioarchitecture, which is reflected in the variety of clinical symptoms and findings and also influences treatment strategies. Fistula sites can be at the dural membrane of one (**Fig. 16–3**) or both cavernous sinuses (**Fig. 16–4**). Unilateral fistulas can receive unilateral or bilateral supply from dural branches of the ICA or ECA and can drain either unilaterally or bilaterally.[35] The pattern of venous

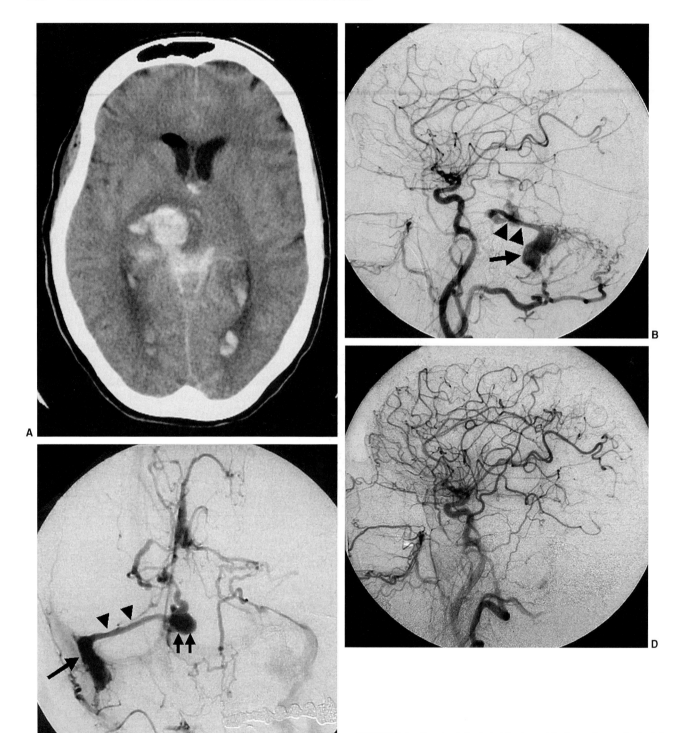

FIGURE 16–1 A 59-year-old woman presented with right cerebellar hematoma and subarachnoid hemorrhage. On the next day, the patient experienced another intracerebral hematoma in the right thalamus. **(A)** A noncontrast computerized tomography (CT) image after the second hemorrhage shows a right thalamic hematoma. **(B)** A lateral view of the right common carotid angiogram demonstrates dural arteriovenous fistulas (DAVFs) to the isolated right sigmoid sinus (arrow) draining predominantly to the superior petrosal sinus (arrowheads) with reflux to the cortical veins. **(C)** An anteroposterior view of the late-arterial phase of the right occipital angiogram demonstrates DAVFs to the isolated sigmoid sinus (arrow) refluxing to the superior petrosal sinus (arrowheads), then to the multiple cortical veins. There is a venous ectasia (two arrows) at the junction between the superior petrosal sinus and the perimesencephalic vein, indicating venous outflow restriction. **(D)** A lateral view of the right common carotid angiogram after two transarterial embolizations demonstrates complete occlusion of the DAVFs. The patient had no further hemorrhage.

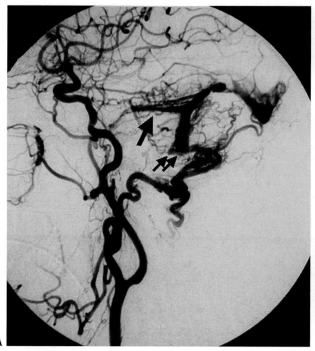
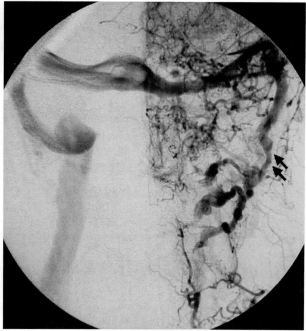

FIGURE 16–2 A 67-year-old woman presented with a 1-year history of headaches and pulsatile bruit. **(A)** A lateral view of the left common carotid angiogram shows the left sigmoid sinus dural arteriovenous fistulas supplied by transmastoid branches of the occipital artery, middle meningeal artery, posterior auricular artery, and the basal tentorial artery from the internal carotid artery. The venous drainage is through the opposite transverse and sigmoid sinuses as well as reflux to the left superior petrosal sinus (arrow) and cortical veins on the surface of the temporal lobe and cerebellar hemisphere. The left sigmoid sinus is occluded (two arrows). **(B)** An antero-posterior view of the left common carotid angiogram shows evidence of venous hypertension of the left cerebellar hemisphere and the occipitotemporal lobe. The left sigmoid sinus is occluded (two arrows) with collateral venous drainage to the paravertebral veins.

drainage can be anterior to the ophthalmic venous system, posterior to the superior or inferior petrosal sinus, lateral and superior to the sylvian vein, inferior through the foramen ovale to the pterygoid plexus, medial through the coronary sinuses to the opposite cavernous sinus, or in more than one direction and pattern. Bilateral fistulas have a higher incidence of cortical venous drainage as compared with unilateral shunts. Thrombosis of some draining veins is a frequent observation, and the symptoms and clinical findings are closely related to the pattern of venous drainage. The anterior venous drainage to the ophthalmic vein causes exophthalmos, chemosis, conjunctival injection, restricted extraocular muscular movements, increased intraocular pressure, and visual loss from optic nerve or retinal/choroidal dysfunction, or even hemorrhages.[18,29,36] An acute exacerbation of eye and orbital problems can occur spontaneously or after treatment. This is usually due to progressive thrombosis of the ophthalmic venous system or anterior cavernous sinus that causes increased orbital congestion and intraocular pressure.[37,38] This condition is usually self-limited if the DAVF is closed, but supportive measures may be necessary to preserve vision. In the case of spontaneous exacerbation, emergent angiography should be performed with intent to embolize if there are any remaining fistulas, to decrease the venous hypertension. The postero-inferior drainage causes cranial nerve paralysis[39,40] and pulsatile tinnitus. Although the cortical venous drainage can potentially cause intracranial hemorrhage, seizure, or neurological deficits due to focal venous hypertension of the brain, they are unusual for cavernous DAVFs, probably because of multiple drainage pathways of the cavernous sinus.

The first choice of treatment is embolization by a transarterial, a transvenous, or a combined approach. Those with minor symptoms without cortical venous drainage can be treated with manual carotid compression,[41] medical therapy, or conservative observation without intervention, which sometimes leads to thrombosis of the shunts.[36] It is important to verify that there is no carotid artery stenosis before initiating manual carotid compression. Surgical interventions are rarely necessary, due to the high success rate of endovascular treatment. However, surgical ligation of the origin of the cortical venous drainage can be simply performed and effective when endovascular treatment fails.

During transarterial embolization, special attention should be paid not to compromise the cranial nerve

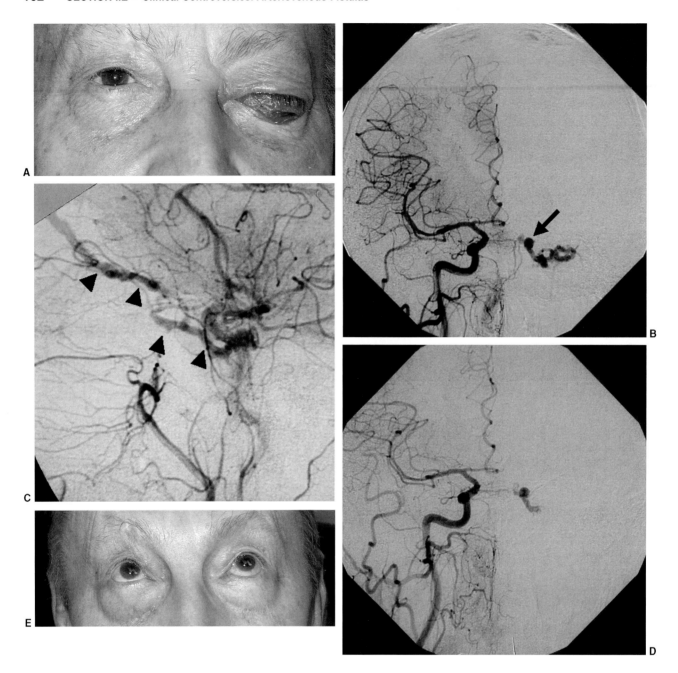

FIGURE 16–3 A 67-year-old right-handed man presented with progressive visual loss, exophthalmos, and chemosis of the left eye over the last 3 weeks. The patient had subjective bruit for the last few months. Despite maintaining normal intraocular pressure by medication, progressive visual loss and retinal hemorrhage were detected. **(A)** A clinical photograph before treatment shows significant proptosis and chemosis of the left eye. **(B)** An anteroposterior view of the right common carotid angiogram demonstrates the left cavernous dural arteriovenous fistulas (DAVFs) supplied by C5 branches of the right internal carotid artery and ascending pharyngeal artery branches crossing the midline. The venous drainage is predominantly to the dilated left superior ophthalmic vein (arrow). **(C)** The midarterial phase of the left common carotid angiogram in the lateral view demonstrates the left cavernous DAVFs supplied by small C5 branches of the internal carotid artery and the accessory meningeal artery and ascending pharyngeal artery branches, draining to the left superior ophthalmic vein (arrowheads). **(D)** An anteroposterior view of the right common carotid angiogram after the embolization shows residual shunts to the left cavernous sinus from the right C5 branches with partial opacification of the left superior ophthalmic vein with increased stagnation of contrast material. **(E)** The patient was further treated with manual compression of the left carotid artery with complete resolution of the symptoms. In this clinical photograph taken 4 months after the embolization, complete resolution of the exophthalmos and chemosis can be seen.

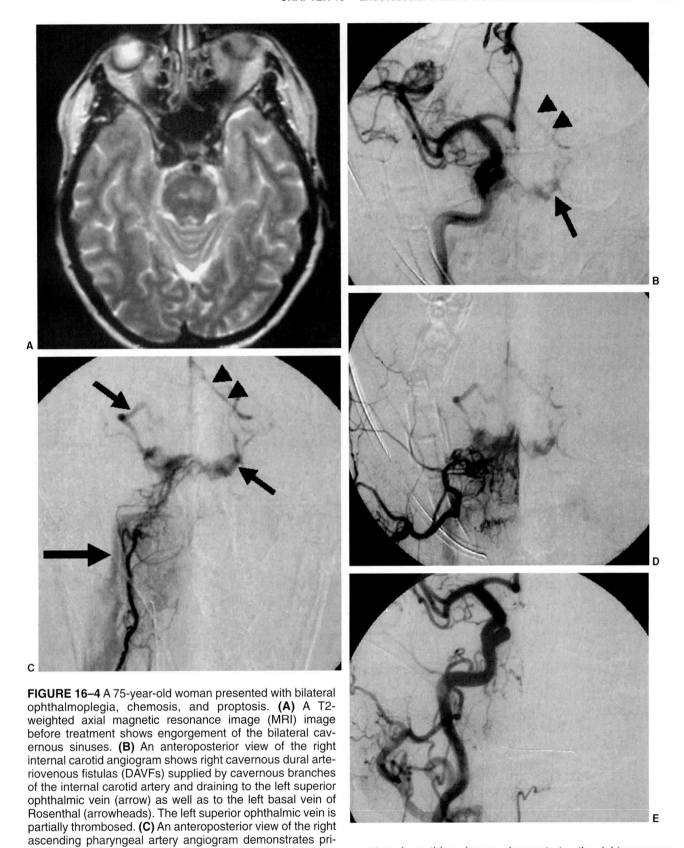

FIGURE 16–4 A 75-year-old woman presented with bilateral ophthalmoplegia, chemosis, and proptosis. **(A)** A T2-weighted axial magnetic resonance image (MRI) image before treatment shows engorgement of the bilateral cavernous sinuses. **(B)** An anteroposterior view of the right internal carotid angiogram shows right cavernous dural arteriovenous fistulas (DAVFs) supplied by cavernous branches of the internal carotid artery and draining to the left superior ophthalmic vein (arrow) as well as to the left basal vein of Rosenthal (arrowheads). The left superior ophthalmic vein is partially thrombosed. **(C)** An anteroposterior view of the right ascending pharyngeal artery angiogram demonstrates primarily the right cavernous DAVFs draining to bilateral superior ophthalmic veins (small arrows), right inferior petrosal sinus (large arrow), and the left basal vein of Rosenthal (arrowheads). **(D)** An anteroposterior view of the right distal

external carotid angiogram demonstrates the right cavernous DAVFs supplied by the artery of foramen rotundum and accessory meningeal artery. **(E, F)** An anteroposterior view of the right common (E) and left internal

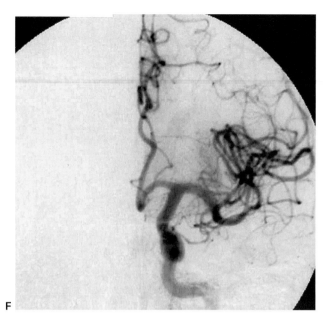

FIGURE 16–4 (*Continued*) **(F)** carotid angiogram after transarterial embolization demonstrates no visualization of remaining DAVFs. A left external carotid angiogram also did not show any residual DAVFs (not shown). The patient had significant decrease in intraocular pressure and chemosis in both eyes after embolization. Ophthalmoplegia also partially improved.

vascular supply and to prevent the migration of embolic agents into the cerebral circulation through anastomosis between the external carotid artery (ECA) and the internal carotid artery (ICA).[42] Partial treatment may be warranted to eliminate cortical venous drainage, decrease noise, or improve cranial nerve dysfunction in some situations, such as in elderly patients with significant risk factors for extensive embolization and anesthesia.

Transvenous embolization has a high cure rate and is preferred by some authors.[43] Catheterization of the cavernous sinus is frequently possible through the inferior petrosal sinus even if it is not opacified on the pretreatment angiogram. For selected cases with inferior petrosal sinus occlusion, superior ophthalmic vein approach via the facial vein through the transfemoral venous approach or direct puncture of the superior ophthalmic vein,[44–46] or direct puncture of the middle cerebral vein[47] or petrosal vein[48] by craniotomy, can be an option to catheterize the cavernous sinus. The disadvantage of transvenous embolization with coils is the need to obliterate a major portion of one or both cavernous sinuses, which may cause new or worsening of cranial nerve paralysis. It is important to first close the junction with the cortical veins so as not to create or increase cortical venous drainage by occluding the extracranial outflow from the sinus. Compartmentalization of the cavernous sinus may make the appropriate transvenous embolization difficult.[49] Combined transarterial and transvenous embolization can be useful for complex lesions.

■ Superior Sagittal Sinus/Torcular Dural Arteriovenous Fistulas

These DAVFs can present with only headaches,[50] but many of them present with hemorrhage, difficult-to-control seizures, or dementia due to venous hypertension associated with direct cortical venous drainage, or reflux to cortical veins from the superior sagittal sinus. Arteriovenous fistulas in this location usually receive bilateral meningeal feeders. Transbony supply from the scalp arteries and anterior cerebral artery supply may also be present. Transarterial embolization is the first choice of treatment, and angiographic cure can be expected if lesions are not extensive (**Fig. 16–5**). For extensive lesions with multiple fistulas along the long segment of the superior sagittal sinus (SSS) and torcula, complete cure is more difficult and palliative transarterial embolization to control the venous hypertension is performed. Transvenous embolization of the SSS often necessitates occlusion of a segment of the superior sagittal sinus, for which careful analysis of the pretreatment cerebral angiogram is important to evaluate the availability of collateral venous drainage to drain the normal brain. Cases with paramedian DAVFs draining into a venous lake separated from the superior sagittal sinus can be cured without sacrificing the sinus either by transarterial or transvenous embolization (**Fig. 16–6**).

Surgical skeletonization of the sinus can be performed for selected cases in which effective treatment cannot be performed by transarterial or transvenous embolization.[50]

Complete occlusion of extensive DAVFs involving the torcular herophili is usually difficult by any modality of treatment. Palliative transarterial embolization is usually the only treatment option, often with limited success. The ability to preserve important venous structures by application of the rapidly advancing stent technology should allow successful treatment of these DAVFs.

■ Anterior Cranial Fossa Dural Arteriovenous Fistulas

Most of these DAVFs present with intracerebral hematoma or subarachnoid hemorrhage because the fistulas drain to the olfactory vein or the parasagittal cortical vein, and then to the proximal superior sagittal sinus.[51,52] Feeders usually originate from anterior or posterior ethmoidal arteries arising from the ophthalmic artery. An additional less-significant supply may originate from the distal internal maxillary artery. The first choice of treatment is surgical ligation of the draining vein

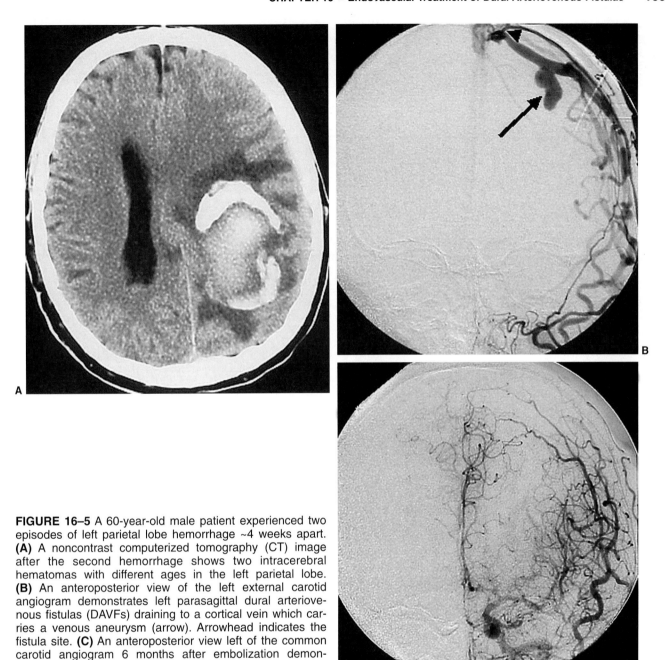

FIGURE 16–5 A 60-year-old male patient experienced two episodes of left parietal lobe hemorrhage ~4 weeks apart. **(A)** A noncontrast computerized tomography (CT) image after the second hemorrhage shows two intracerebral hematomas with different ages in the left parietal lobe. **(B)** An anteroposterior view of the left external carotid angiogram demonstrates left parasagittal dural arteriovenous fistulas (DAVFs) draining to a cortical vein which carries a venous aneurysm (arrow). Arrowhead indicates the fistula site. **(C)** An anteroposterior view left of the common carotid angiogram 6 months after embolization demonstrates complete obliteration of the DAVFs.

adjacent to the fistula site, which is usually curative and carries a low risk.[51,53] Indications for embolization are limited because of the risk to the vision by transarterial approach and inaccessibility by the transvenous approach.

■ Tentorial Incisural and Vein of Galen Dural Arteriovenous Fistulas

Tentorial incisural DAVFs are located along the margin of the tentorium and frequently present with

intraparenchymal or subarachnoid hemorrhage. These AVFs are supplied by tentorial branches of internal and external carotid arteries, and they can receive feeders from posterior cerebral and superior cerebellar arteries. The venous drainage is through the perimesencephalic veins and cerebellar veins and is frequently associated with focal dilatation and stenosis of outflow veins. Transarterial embolization with a liquid embolic agent is the first choice of treatment with a high cure rate (**Fig. 16–7**).[54] Some authors claim that surgical ligation of the origin of the draining vein is the first choice.[55] Although

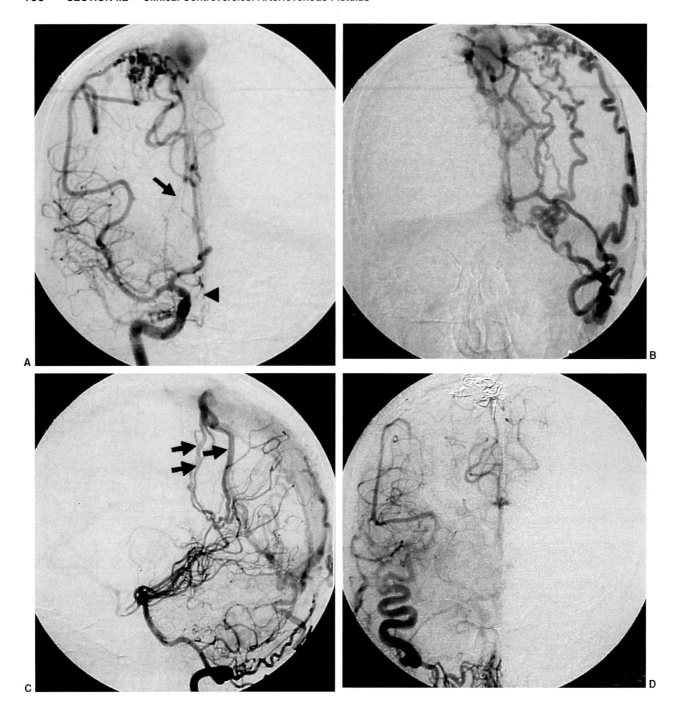

FIGURE 16–6 A 25-year-old woman presented with progressive headaches over the past 3 years. Prominent pulsation was noted over the scalp and large bruit was heard over the entire head. Neurological examination was normal without evidence of papilledema. **(A)** An anteroposterior view of the right internal carotid angiogram demonstrates parasagittal dural arteriovenous fistulas (DAVFs) supplied by the right anterior and middle cerebral artery branches. There is a small supply from the artery of free margin of the tentorium (arrow) from the cavernous internal carotid artery and faint opacification of the anterior falcine artery feeder (arrowhead), which is better seen from the left internal carotid artery injection. **(B)** An anteroposterior view of the left occipital artery angiogram shows multiple feeders to the right parasagittal DAVFs. There were additional feeders from the right occipital artery, bilateral superficial temporal arteries, and middle meningeal arteries (not shown). **(C)** A lateral view of the left vertebral artery angiogram shows supply to the parasagittal DAVFs by dural branches of the posterior cerebral artery along the falx (arrows). She underwent transarterial embolization through the external carotid artery branches. **(D)** An anteroposterior view of the right common carotid angiogram after embolization shows no residual arteriovenous fistulas.

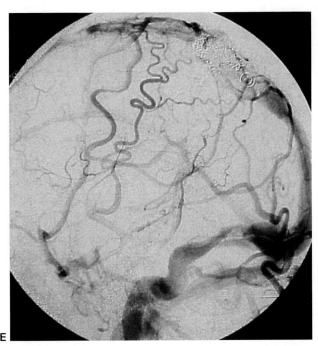

FIGURE 16–6 (*Continued*) **(E)** A lateral view of the late-venous phase of the left common carotid angiogram after embolization shows no remaining fistulas with preservation of the patency of the superior sagittal sinus. The patient's headaches disappeared after embolization and she refused follow-up angiography.

technically possible, transvenous embolization necessitates retrograde catheterization of a cortical vein that carries a higher risk of venous rupture than transvenous occlusion of the sinus.

Dural arteriovenous fistulas draining to the vein of Galen can be included in the same category in the sense that the lesion is close to the tentorial margin and supplied by the same feeders. However, AVFs in this location also receive feeders from the dural branches for the falx and falx cerebelli. Aneurysmal dilatation of the vein of Galen is a frequent finding as the result of anatomical or hemodynamic venous outflow restriction. If the outflow restriction is significant enough to cause cortical venous reflux, the patient can develop hemorrhage, focal neurological deficits, or dementia due to venous hypertension.[50] If the venous hypertension is not severe, the patient may present only with intracranial bruit. For treatment of the DAVFs in this location, transarterial embolization is the first choice of treatment. The treatment can result in cure,[56] but it may only be palliative to decrease the shunt and hence the degree of venous hypertension.

■ Pediatric Dural Arteriovenous Fistulas

Dural arteriovenous fistulas in the pediatric population are rare and should be considered as a distinct entity because they have specific clinical and angiographic features. They are classified into three categories by Lasjaunias[14]: dural sinus malformation, infantile-type DAVF, and adult-type DAVF.

Dural sinus malformations are congenital lesions and are present in the neonatal or infantile period with congestive heart failure, coagulation disorders, and symptoms of increased intracranial pressure such as macrocrania and seizures.[57,58] They can also be discovered by prenatal MRI study. Angiography shows a partially thrombosed large venous lake with relatively slow-flow DAVFs frequently involving the superior sagittal sinus and/or the transverse sinus. They are associated with occlusion, underdevelopment, or agenesis of the jugular bulb. Transarterial embolization is the only treatment option, and the prognosis after treatment depends on the extent of the malformation and brain injury already made in the developing brain. Only unilateral involvement of the sinus and well-developed collateral venous drainage through scalp veins indicate a better prognosis (**Fig. 16–8**). Extensive lesions involving the midline have a poor prognosis, because endovascular treatment frequently results in complete thrombosis of the involved sinus, unless the shunt is single or discreet.

Infantile DAVFs are also congenital lesions, are present in infants and children, and are characterized by high-flow shunting, which can persist or results in venous outlet occlusion. Patients who have persistent high-flow shunts present with relatively mild symptoms of venous congestion of the normal brain including focal neurological deficits, mental retardation, and seizures. Angiography may demonstrate multifocal AVFs and secondary development of pial AVFs remote from the original site of the DAVFs.[59] This pial AVF is a flow-related phenomenon and spontaneously disappears by occlusion of the original dural AVFs. Those that develop progressive venous outlet obstruction present with more severe symptoms of venous hypertension, and intracranial hemorrhage can occur if reflux to cortical veins develops. Transarterial embolization is the preferred approach, which usually can control the symptoms even for the extensive lesion. Complete obliteration of the lesion by only transarterial approach may be difficult for extensive lesions.

Adult type-DAVFs are acquired lesions similar to adult DAVFs. They are most common in the cavernous sinus followed by the sigmoid sinus. The symptoms and treatment are the same as adult DAVFs, but sacrificing the

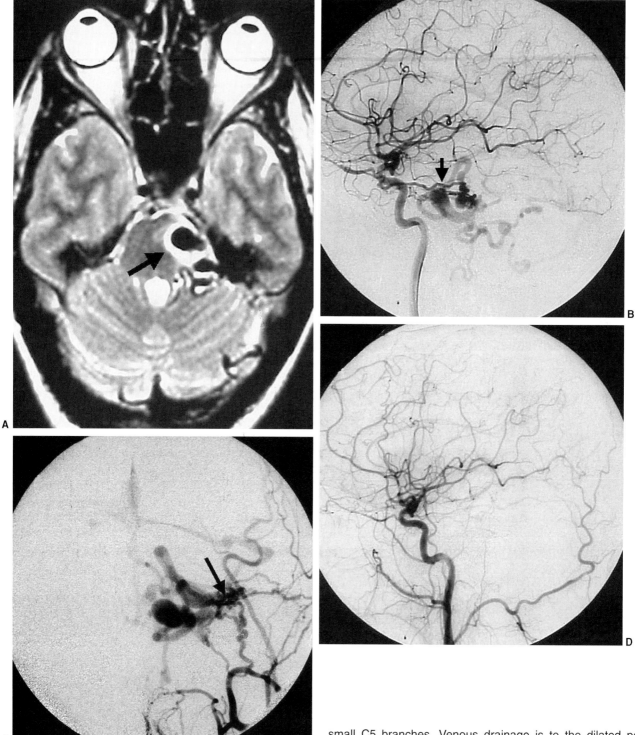

FIGURE 16–7 A 35-year-old woman presented with acute onset of right hemiparesis, numbness, and dysarthria. **(A)** A T2-weighted axial magnetic resonance image (MRI) demonstrates T2 high-signal abnormality in the upper pons (arrow) around a dilated signal void. There is no evidence of hemorrhage. **(B)** A lateral view of the internal carotid angiogram demonstrates dural arteriovenous fistulas (DAVFs) at the tentorial edge supplied by the artery of the free margin of the tentorium (arrow) originating from the ophthalmic artery as well as small C5 branches. Venous drainage is to the dilated perimesencephalic vein with reflux to cortical veins. **(C)** An anteroposterior view of the left distal external carotid angiogram shows DAVFs supplied by branches of the middle meningeal artery and drained by the dilated perimesencephalic vein with reflux to multiple cortical veins. The DAVFs were also supplied by left ascending pharyngeal artery and occipital artery branches (not shown). Arrow indicates the fistula site. **(D)** A lateral view of the left common carotid angiogram 4 months after embolization shows complete obliteration of the DAVFs.

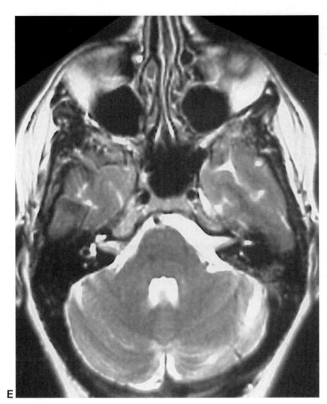

FIGURE 16–7 (*Continued*) **(E)** A follow-up T2-weighted axial MRI shows disappearance of T2 high-signal abnormality in the pons and flow voids of the draining vein.

sinus by transvenous embolization is generally not recommended in the pediatric population.

■ Dural Arteriovenous Fistulas with Spinal Perimedullary Venous Drainage

Some DAVFs located in the petrous ridge, posterior fossa, or skull base may drain to the brain stem and spinal cord perimedullary veins, causing venous hypertension of the brain stem or the spinal cord.[60] They tend to present with progressive brain stem dysfunction or myelopathy involving motor, sensory, and bladder/bowel/sexual functions, similar to spinal DAVFs. Congrad et al classified these DAVFs as type V. Abnormally dilated veins in the posterior fossa and in the cervical subarachnoid space can be detected by MRI. If the angiographic work-up is negative for spinal DAVF in a patient with typical clinical symptoms of spinal DAVFs, bilateral external carotid and vertebral artery angiogram should be performed to rule out this type of DAVFs. Transarterial embolization with a liquid agent is usually curative and is the first choice of treatment.

■ Spinal Dural Arteriovenous Fistulas

Spinal DAVFs are a distinct disease entity and should be separated from the spinal cord arteriovenous malformations (AVMs). They are an acquired disease that develops arteriovenous shunting within the dural layer covering the spinal nerve root. These AVFs are supplied by one or two radicular branches and drained by a single intradural radicular vein to the perimedullary veins, causing venous hypertension of the spinal cord. The lesion is usually located below the heart level and rarely occurs at the upper thoracic level. Nine to eighteen percent of cases occur in the territory supplied by the internal iliac artery. Angiographic study of the anterior spinal artery shows delayed circulation time without opacification of the venous drainage of the normal spinal cord, consistent with venous hypertension of the spinal cord.

The patients are usually over 40 years of age with a strong male predominance (85%) and present with progressive paraparesis, sensory disturbance, and bladder, bowel, and sexual dysfunction. Back pains are sometimes experienced and cause misdiagnosis as a herniated disk or a spinal stenosis. The functional prognosis is poor if untreated, due to progression of the disease resulting in the ascending necrotizing thrombosis of the spinal cord veins (Foix Alajouanine syndrome). Death can occur due to systemic complications of paraplegia, such as pulmonary infection and sepsis secondary to a decubitus ulcer or urinary tract infection, or pulmonary embolism.

Treatment can be performed by either transarterial liquid embolization[61,62] (**Fig. 16–9**) or surgery.[63–65] Good functional recovery can be expected if a patient is treated early before symptoms become severe.[66] Recovery occurs first in motor function, followed by sensory function. Bladder, bowel, and sexual dysfunctions recover last, if at all. Particle embolization has more than 50% recurrence rate[67,68] and should not be performed for this disease. For transarterial liquid embolization, careful analysis of angiography is important to rule out spinal cord arteries originating from the same pedicle as the feeder. If a spinal cord artery has the common trunk as the feeder to the AVF, transarterial embolization is usually contraindicated, unless the spinal cord artery is cleared by superselective catheterization. If those patients are excluded, successful obliteration of the lesion can be obtained in over 90% of cases.[61] For permanent occlusion of the lesion, the embolic material should be injected from a microcatheter wedged in the feeder to reach and occlude the proximal portion of the draining vein. Postembolization angiography sometimes demonstrates improved circulation of the anterior spinal artery, but it may not be noted until follow-up angiography. To confirm total obliteration and rule out recurrence of the lesion, a follow-up angiography is recommended in a few months.

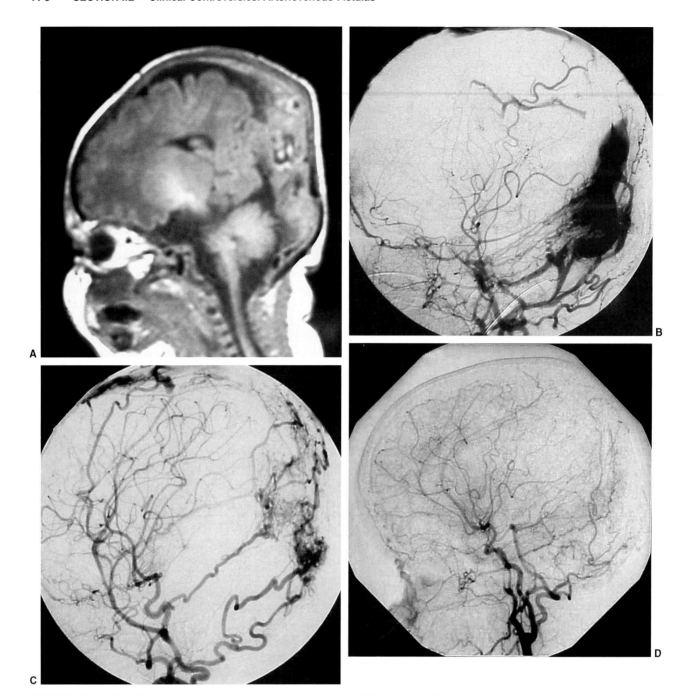

FIGURE 16–8 The diagnosis of dural arteriovenous fistulas (DAVFs) was made in uterus at 20 weeks of gestation on this female patient. She was born at 32 weeks of gestation with macrocephaly but was neurologically normal. At 3 weeks of age, she developed seizures. **(A)** A T1-weighted sagittal magnetic resonance image (MRI) at 11 days after birth demonstrates a partially thrombosed large sinus in the torcular area with multiple signal voids inside. **(B, C)** A lateral view of the left (B) and right (C) common carotid angiogram shows extensive DAVFs to the superior sagittal sinus and torcular area supplied by multiple dural branches of both internal and external carotid arteries. The patient underwent three transarterial embolization procedures. **(D)** A lateral view of the left common carotid angiogram 3 years after the last embolization shows no remaining DAVFs. The right common carotid artery and vertebral artery angiogram also showed no residual DAVFs (not shown).

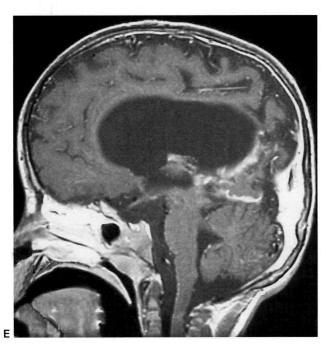

Embolization has several advantages over surgery, and we consider embolization as the primary route of treatment. Compared with surgery, embolization is less invasive without the necessity of skin incision and can be performed in the same setting as the diagnostic angiography. There is no risk of wound infection or postoperative cerebrospinal fluid leakage. The patient does not experience procedure-related pain and can start rehabilitation on the next day of the procedure. Also, if there is angiographic evidence of significant perimedullary venous thrombosis at the time of treatment, the patient can be fully heparinized immediately after occlusion of the fistula to prevent progressive venous thrombosis. If embolization is unsuccessful or contraindicated, surgery should be performed without delay. Surgery also has a high cure rate; it is considered as the first choice of treatment by some authors. Surgery is easily performed with intradural coagulation and disconnection of the draining vein. One point of caution for surgical treatment—there is a variation of spinal DAVFs in which venous drainage is directly to the epidural vein with reflux into the intradural perimedullary veins. Those cases should be recognized on presurgical angiographic evaluation, because intradural ligation of the draining vein for these cases may result in only partial obliteration of the fistula.

FIGURE 16–8 (*Continued*) **(E)** A T1-weighted sagittal MRI with contrast 3 years after the last embolization demonstrates shrinkage of torcular herophili. The ventricles and the subarachnoid space are enlarged. The patient is developing normally without focal neurological deficits. Her complex partial seizure is under control with Tegretol (Novartis, East Hanover, NJ).

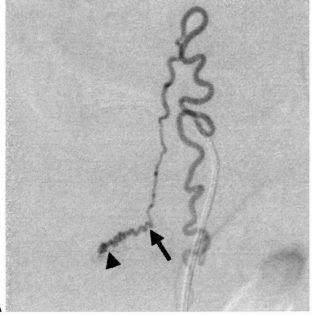

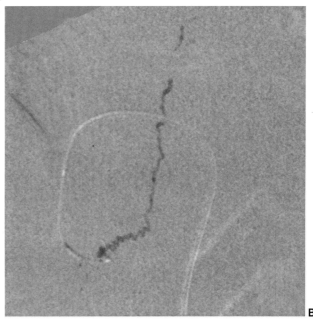

FIGURE 16–9 A 37-year-old male patient presented with progressive numbness and weakness of the lower extremities as well as difficulty in urination and constipation. He underwent laminectomy and biopsy of the spinal cord in an outside institution, which was nondiagnostic. The magnetic resonance image (MRI) study showed T2 high-signal abnormality in the lower spinal cord (not shown). **(A)** An anteroposterior view of the right T10 superselective angiogram shows the fistula site (arrow). The small feeding vessel is wedged by the tip of the microcatheter (arrowhead). The patient underwent embolization with *n*-butyl cyanoacrylate (NBCA) from this catheter position. **(B)** The cast of NBCA closes the venous side of the fistula. His neurological condition significantly improved and he was discharged to a rehabilitation facility. A follow-up MRI 5 months later showed improvement of T2 high-signal abnormality within the spinal cord (not shown).

■ Conclusion

Dural arteriovenous fistulas are a complex group of diseases with a wide range of radiological features and clinical symptoms and findings. Most symptoms are closely related to the pattern of venous drainage. Benign lesions with minor symptoms without cortical venous drainage can be conservatively observed. In contrast, malignant lesions with cortical venous drainage should be intensely treated. Treatment can be performed by transarterial embolization, transvenous embolization, surgery, or a combination of these. The indication and treatment strategy should be carefully determined based on the clinical symptoms, location, and angioarchitecture of the lesion. Careful analysis of pretherapeutic angiography including venous drainage of the lesion and normal brain is essential for adequate treatment planning.

■ References

1. Arnautovic K, Al-Mefty O, Angtuaco E, et al. Dural arteriovenous malformations of the transverse/sigmoid sinus acquired from dominant sinus occlusion by a tumor: report of two cases. Neurosurgery 1998;42:383–388

2. Houser O, Campbell J, Campbell R. Arteriovenous malformation affecting the transverse dural venous sinus: an acquired lesion. Mayo Clin Proc 1979;54:651–661

3. Lasjaunias P, Berenstein A. Dural Arteriovenous Malformations (DAVMs), Surgical Neuroangiography 2. Endovascular Treatment of Craniofacial Lesions. Berlin/Heidelberg/New York: Springer Verlag; 1987:273–315

4. Nishijima M, Takaku A, Endo S, et al. Etiological evaluation of dural arteriovenous malformations of the lateral and sigmoid sinuses based on histopathological examinations. J Neurosurg 1992;76:600–606

5. Uranishi R, Nakase H, Sakaki T. Expression of angiogenic growth factors in dural arteriovenous fistulas. J Neurosurg 1999;91:781–786

6. Lasjaunias P, Chiu M, TerBrugge K, et al. Neurological manifestations of intracranial dural arteriovenous malformations. J Neurosurg 1986;64:724–730

7. Borden J, Wu J, Shucart W. Proposed classification for spinal and cranial dural arteriovenous fistulous malformations and implications for treatment. J Neurosurg 1995;82:166–179

8. Cognard C, Gobin Y, Pierot L, et al. Cerebral dural arteriovenous fistulas: clinical and angiographic correlation with a revised classification of venous drainage. Radiology 1995;194:671–680

9. Davies M, TerBrugge K, Willinsky R, et al. The validity of classification for the clinical presentation of intracranial dural arteriovenous fistulas. J Neurosurg 1996;85:830–837

10. Barnwell S, Halbach V, Dowd C, et al. A variant of arteriovenous fistulas within the wall of dural sinuses. J Neurosurg 1991;74:199–204

11. Lalwani A, Dowd C, Halbach V. Grading venous restrictive disease in patients with dural arteriovenous fistulas of the transverse/sigmoid sinus. J Neurosurg 1993;79:11–15

12. Hurst R, LJB, Galetta S, et al: Dementia resulting from dural arteriovenous fistulas: the pathologic findings of venous hypertensive encephalopathy. AJNR Am J Neuroradiol 1998;19:1267–1273

13. Willinsky R, Terbrugge K, Montanera W, et al. Venous congestion: an MR finding in dural arteriovenous malformations with cortical venous drainage. AJNR Am J Neuroradiol 1994;15:1501–1507

14. Lasjaunias P. Dural Arteriovenous Shunts, Vascular Diseases in Neonates, Infants and Children. Berlin/Heidelberg/New York: Springer Verlag; 1997:321–371

15. Kupersmith M. Neuro-ophthalmic Manifestations of Intracranial Dural Venous Disorders, Neurovascular Neuro-ophthalmology. Berlin/Heidelberg/New York. Springer-Verlag, 1999:109–149

16. Davies M, Saleh K, Terbrugge K, et al. The natural history and management of intracranial dural arteriovenous fistulae. Part 1: benign lesions. Intervent Neuroradiol 1997;3:295–302

17. Davies M, Terbrugge K, Willinsky R, et al. The natural history and management of intracranial dural arteriovenous fistulae. Part 2: aggressive lesions. Intervent Neuroradiol 1997;3:303–311

18. Satomi J, van Dijk J, TerBrugge K, et al. Benign cranial dural arteriovenous fistulas: outcome of conservative management based on the natural history of the lesion. J Neurosurg 2002;97:767–770

19. Berenstein A, Lasjaunias P. Endovascular Treatment of Spine and Spinal Cord Lesions, Surgical Neuroangiography. Berlin: Springer-Verlag; 1992:1–109

20. Cognard C, Houdart E, Casasco A, et al. Long-term changes in intracranial dural arteriovenous fistulae leading to worsening in the type of venous drainage. Neuroradiology 1997;39:59–88

21. Nelson P, Russell S, Woo H, et al. Use of wedged microcatheter for curative transarterial embolization of complex intracranial dural arteriovenous fistulas: indications, endovascular technique, and outcome in 21 patients. J Neurosurg 2003;93:498–506

22. Lasjaunias P, Berenstein A. Technical Aspects of Surgical Neuroangiography, Surgical Neuroangiography 2. Endovascular Treatment of Craniofacial Lesions. Berlin/Heidelberg: Springer-Verlag; 1987:1–56

23. Houdart E, Saint-Maurice JP, Chapot R, et al. Transcranial approach for venous embolization of dural arteriovenous fistulas. J Neurosurg 2002; 97:280–286

24. Ohtakara K, Murano K, Kawaguchi K, et al. Selective transvenous liquid embolization of a Type I dural arteriovenous fistula at the junction of the transverse and sigmoid sinuses. J Neurosurg 2000; 92:1045–1049

25. Lewis A, Tomsick T Jr. Management of tentorial dural arteriovenous malformations: transarterial embolization combined with stereotactic radiation or surgery. J Neurosurg 1994;81:851–859

26. Friedman J, Pollock B, Nichols D, et al. Results of combined stereotactic radiosurgery and transarterial embolization for dural arteriovenous fistulas of the transverse and sigmoid sinuses. J Neurosurg 2001;94:886–891

27. Shin M, Kurita H, Tago M, et al. Stereotactic radiosurgery for tentorial dural arteriovenous fistulae draining into the vein of Galen: report of two cases. Neurosurgery 2000;46:730–734

28. Pan D, Chung W, Guo W, et al. Stereotactic radiosurgery for the treatment of dural arteriovenous fistulas involving the transverse-sigmoid sinus. J Neurosurg 2002;96:823–829

29. Satoh K, Satomi J, Nakajima N, et al. Cerebellar hemorrhage caused by dural arteriovenous fistula: a review of five cases. J Neurosurg 2001;94:422–426

30. Ishii K, Goto K, Ihara K, et al. High-risk dural arteriovenous fistulae of the transverse and sigmoid sinuses. AJNR Am J Neuroradiol 1987;8:1113–1120

31. Dawson RC 3rd, Joseph GJ, Owens DS, et al. Transvenous embolization as the primary therapy for arteriovenous fistulas of the lateral and sigmoid sinuses. AJNR Am J Neuroradiol 1998;19: 571–576

32. Halbach V, Higashida R, Hieshima G, et al. Transvenous embolization of dural fistulas involving the transverse and sigmoid sinuses. AJNR Am J Neuroradiol 1989;10:385–392

33. Gobin Y, Houdart E, Rogopoulos A, et al. Percutaneous transvenous embolization through the thrombosed sinus in transverse sinus dural fistula. AJNR Am J Neuroradiol 1993;14:1102–1105

34. Murphy K, Gailloud P, Venbrux A, et al. Endovascular treatment of a grade IV transverse sinus dural arteriovenous fistula by sinus

recanalization, angioplasty, and stent placement: technical case report. Neurosurgery 2000;46:497–501

35. Grove A Jr. The dural shunt syndrome. Pathophysiology and clinical course. Ophthalmology 1984;91:31–44

36. Kupersmith M, Berenstein A, Choi I, et al. Management of nontraumatic vascular shunts involving the cavernous sinus. Ophthalmology 1988;95:121–130

37. Sergott R, Grossman R, Savino P, et al. The syndrome of paradoxical worsening of dural-cavernous sinus arteriovenous malformations. Ophthalmology 1987;94:205–212

38. Golnik K, Newman S, Ferguson R. Angle-closure glaucoma consequent to embolization of dural cavernous sinus fistula. AJNR Am J Neuroradiol 1991;12:1074–1076

39. Miyachi S, Negoro M, Handa T, et al. Dural carotid cavernous sinus fistula presenting as isolated oculomotor nerve palsy. Surg Neurol 1993;39:105–109

40. Kurata A, Takano M, Tokiwa K, et al. Spontaneous carotid cavernous fistula presenting only with cranial nerve palsies. AJNR Am J Neuroradiol 1993;14:1097–1101

41. Halbach V, Higashida R, Hieshima G, et al. Dural fistulas involving the cavernous sinus: results of treatment in 30 patients. Radiology 1987;163:437–442

42. Lasjaunias P, Berenstein A, Ter Brugge K. The Skull Base and Extradural Arteries, Surgical Neuroangiography 1: Clinical Vascular Anatomy and Variations. Berlin/Heidelberg/New York: Springer-Verlag; 2001:387–478

43. Halbach VV, Higashida RT, Hieshima GB, et al. Transvenous embolization of dural fistulas involving the cavernous sinus. AJNR Am J Neuroradiol 1989;10:377–383

44. Teng M, Guo W, Huang C, et al. Occlusion of arteriovenous malformations of the cavernous sinus via the superior ophthalmic vein. AJNR Am J Neuroradiol 1987;9:539–546

45. Miller N, Monsein L, Debrun G, et al. Treatment of carotid-cavernous sinus fistulas using a superior ophthalmic vein approach. J Neurosurg 1995;83:838–842

46. Monsein L, Debrun G, Miller N, et al. Treatment of dural carotid cavernous fistulas via the superior ophthalmic vein. AJNR Am J Neuroradiol 1991;12:435–439

47. Kuwayama N, Endo S, Kitabayashi M, et al. Surgical transvenous embolization of a cortically draining carotid cavernous fistula via a vein of the Sylvian fissure. AJNR Am J Neuroradiol 1998;19:1329–1332

48. Hara T, Hamada J, Kai Y, et al. Surgical transvenous embolization of a carotid-cavernous dural fistula with cortical drainage via a petrosal vein: two technical case reports. Neurosurgery 2002;50:1380–1384

49. Chaloupka J, Goller D, Goldberg R, et al. True anatomical compartmentalization of the cavernous sinus in a patient with bilateral cavernous dural arteriovenos fistulae. Case report. J Neurosurg 1993;79:592–595

50. Halbach V, Higashida R, Hieshima G, et al. Treatment of dural arteriovenous malformations involving the superior sagittal sinus. AJNR Am J Neuroradiol 1988;9:337–343

51. Halbach V, Higashida R, Hieshima G, et al. Dural arteriovenous fistulas supplied by ethmoidal arteries. Neurosurgery 1990;26: 816–823

52. Reul J, Thron A, Laborde G, et al. Dural arteriovenous malformations at the base of the anterior cranial fossa: report of nine cases. Neuroradiology 1993;35:388–393

53. Lawton M, Chun J, Wilson C, et al. Ethmoidal dural arteriovenous fistulae: an assessment of surgical and endovascular management. Neurosurgery 1999;45:805–811

54. Tomak P, Cloft H, Kaga A, et al. Evolution of the management of tentorial dural arteriovenous malformations. Neurosurgery 2003;52:750–762

55. Awad I. Tentorial incisura and brain stem dural arteriovenous malformations. In: Awad IA, Barrow DL, eds. Dural Arteriovenous Malformations. Park Ridge, IL: American Association of Neurological Surgeons; 1993:131–146

56. Weigele J, Chaloupka J, Lesley W. Galenic dural arteriovenous fistula: unusual clinical presentation and successful endovascular therapy. J Neurosurg 2002;97:467–470

57. Ross D, Walker J, Edwards M. Unusual posterior fossa dural arteriovenous malformation in a neonate: case report. Neurosurgery 1986;19:1021–1024

58. Morita A, Meyer F, Nichols D, et al. Childhood dural arteriovenous fistulae of the posterior dural sinuses: Three case reports and literature review. Neurosurgery 1995;37:1193–1200

59. Garcia-Monaco R, Rodesch G, Terbrugge K, et al. Multifocal dural arteriovenous shunts in children. Childs Nerv Syst 1991;7:425–431

60. Gobin Y, Rogopoulos A, Aymard A, et al. Endovascular treatment of intracranial dural arteriovenous fistulas with spinal perimedullary venous drainage. J Neurosurg 1992;77:718–723

61. Niimi Y, Berenstein A, Setton A, et al. Embolization of spinal dural arteriovenous fistulae: results and follow-up. Neurosurgery 1997;40:675–683

62. Song J, Gobin Y, Duckwiler G, et al. N-butyl 2-cyanoacrylate embolization of spinal dural arteriovenous fistulae. AJNR Am J Neuroradiol 2001;22:40–47

63. Oldfield E, Di Chiro G, Quindlen E, et al. Successful treatment of a group of spinal cord arteriovenous malformations by interruption of dural fistula. J Neurosurg 1983;59:1019–1030

64. Symon L, Kuyama H, Kendall B. Dural arteriovenous malformation of the spine. Clinical features and surgical results in 55 cases. J Neurosurg 1984;60:238–247

65. Westphal M, Koch C. Management of spinal dural arteriovenous fistulae using an interdisciplinary neuroradiological/neurosurgical approach: experience with 47 cases. Neurosurgery 1999;45:451–458

66. Tacconi L, Lopez I, Symon L. Outcome and prognostic factors in the surgical treatment of spinal dural arteriovenous fistulas. A long-term study. Br J Neurosurg 1997;11:298–305

67. Morgan M, Marsh W. Management of spinal dural arteriovenous malformations. J Neurosurg 1989;70:832–836

68. Nichols D, Rufenacht D, Jack C Jr, et al. Embolization of spinal dural arteriovenous fistula with polyvinyl alcohol particles: experience in 14 patients. AJNR Am J Neuroradiol 1992;13:933–940

69. Komiyama M, Yamanaka K, Nagata Y, et al. Dural carotid-cavernous sinus fistula and central retinal vein occlusion: a case report and a review of the literature. Surg Neurol 1990;34:255–259

17

Surgical Treatment of Extracranial Vascular Occlusive Disease

BRIAN E. SNELL, ROBERT J. WIENECKE, AND CHRISTOPHER M. LOFTUS

Objectives: Upon completion of this chapter, the reader should be able to describe the surgical management of atherosclerotic disease and dissections involving the carotid and vertebral arteries, as well as the numerous clinical studies that have defined the indications for surgical therapy.

Accreditation: The AANS* is accredited by the Accreditation Council for Continuing Medical Education (ACCME) to sponsor continuing medical education for physicians.

Credit: The AANS designates this educational activity for a maximum of 15 credits in Category 1 credit toward the AMA Physician's Recognition Award. Each physician should claim only those hours of credit that he/she spent in the educational activity.

The Home Study Examination is online on the AANS Web site at: http://www.aans.org/education/books/controversy.asp

* The acronym AANS refers to both the American Association of Neurological Surgeons and the American Association of Neurosurgeons.

■ Carotid Artery Atherosclerotic Disease

Stroke resulting from atherosclerosis is a common cause of death in the United States. It results in ~150,000 deaths per year.[1,2] Approximately 400,000 to 500,000 new strokes are reported annually with a 20 to 50% recurrence rate within 5 years.[1,3] Stroke is also the leading cause of long-term physical and intellectual disability among adults.[4] Race, gender, and vascular risk factors may influence the distribution of atherosclerosis. Premenopausal women and Japanese, Chinese, Thai, and African-American populations are more likely to develop intracranial disease, whereas Caucasians and those with hypercholesterolemia are more likely to develop extracranial disease.[5] The most common extracranial sites for atherosclerotic disease are the carotid bifurcation, the subclavian arteries, and the proximal vertebral arteries[6,7]

The process of atherosclerosis is thought to occur at these sites secondary to the combined effects of turbulence, blood stagnation, hemodynamic sheer stress, and boundary separation.[8] The ratio of internal carotid artery area to common carotid artery area and the bifurcation angle result in a geometry at the bifurcation that produces vortex flow and increased contact of atherogenic substances and platelets with the site of maximal plaque development.[9] This current view of atherogenesis is referred to as the "response to injury" hypothesis.[10,11] According to this hypothesis, a variety of forces injures the endothelium, and the inflammatory response to this injury results in plaque development. Factors that may cause endothelial injury include hypercholesterolemia, cigarette smoking, hypertension, oxidative stress, advanced glycation end-products, and possibly infection.[12] Injury induces endothelial gene expression of platelet and leukocyte adhesion molecules and molecules involved in growth factor, cytokine, and coagulation protein synthesis.[13,14] Increased permeability secondary to endothelial injury allows monocytes and low-density lipoprotein to enter the intima. Monocyte-derived macrophages secrete mitogens that induce smooth muscle cell egress into the intima, with subsequent proliferation and extracellular collagen and proteoglycan synthesis. Oxidized lipoproteins fill macrophages turning them into foam cells that may rupture and release lipid and cytotoxic enzymes. This increases the fibroproliferative response of the smooth muscle cells.[15] Also, injured endothelium is more thrombogenic secondary to decreased expression of nitric oxide, prostacyclin, and fibrinolytic and antithrombotic glycoproteins.[14]

Stroke is defined as a sudden, nonconvulsive, focal neurological deficit. It is characterized by a specific temporal profile that includes abrupt onset of a neurological deficit, followed by subsequent arrest, and then regression in all but the most severe strokes. The type of neurological deficit is dependent upon the involved vascular territory but can include hemiplegia, mental confusion, varied sensory deficits, aphasia, visual field defects, diplopia, dizziness, or dysarthria.[16]

Atherosclerotic narrowing and ulceration at the carotid bifurcation is a major cause of thromboembolic stroke. The results of several prospective, randomized trials for symptomatic and asymptomatic carotid occlusive disease have provided evidence-based data for treatment. By 1990, seven trials were planned or in progress. Four of these trials addressed asymptomatic carotid occlusive disease (the Carotid Artery Stenosis Asymptomatic Narrowing Operation Versus Aspirin [CASANOVA] study, the Mayo Asymptomatic Carotid Endarterectomy [MACE] study, the Veterans Administration Asymptomatic Stenosis Trial [VAAST], and the Asymptomatic Carotid Atherosclerosis Study [ACAS]). Patients could not have symptoms from ipsilateral cerebral ischemia secondary to carotid occlusive disease, although contralateral symptoms were permitted in VAAST and ACAS. The four trials used similar exclusion criteria. Patients with neurological (e.g., seizures, dementia), cardiac (e.g., atrial fibrillation, severe valvular disease), or general medical conditions (e.g., diabetes, renal failure) that might affect stroke outcome were also excluded.[17] There is one asymptomatic carotid surgery randomized trial in the United Kingdom and Europe, the ACST trial.[18,18A]

The CASANOVA study randomized patients from the general population to immediate surgery versus antiplatelet therapy alone and best medical management. The stenosis criterion was 50 to 90% by noninvasive testing or angiography. Both arms received best medical management including aspirin (1000 mg/d) and dipyridamole (225 mg/d). The follow-up was 3 years and the study size was 410 patients. Endpoints were death and stroke. Two hundred six patients were randomized to immediate surgery, and 204 patients were randomized to antiplatelet therapy alone. One hundred eighteen of the 204 patients in the nonsurgical arm had delayed endarterectomy during the follow-up period secondary to transient ischemic attack (TIA), progressive severe stenosis (>90%), bilateral stenosis (>50%), or contralateral stenosis (>50%). The study found no statistically significant difference in outcome between the surgical and nonsurgical arms (10.7% and 11.3%, respectively).[19] The unusual study design of CASANOVA limits its statistical validity.

The MACE study enrolled 71 patients with >50% stenosis by noninvasive testing. The planned follow-up was 2 years. The nonsurgical arm received best medical management and aspirin (80 mg/d). The surgical arm did not receive aspirin. Only Mayo Clinic patients were randomized to the treatment arms. The study was terminated prematurely because of increased frequency of myocardial infarction in the surgical arm that did not receive aspirin. At termination, too few patients were enrolled to assess statistical significance. It was concluded that aspirin was appropriate for the perioperative and postoperative period unless contraindicated.[20]

The VAAST enrolled only men from VA centers and randomized them to surgical and nonsurgical arms, both of which received best medical management and aspirin (1300 mg/d). The stenosis criterion was >50% by angiography. The follow-up was 5 years and the study population was 444 patients (211 of 444 surgical and 233 of 444 nonsurgical patients). Participating centers were screened for perioperative morbidity and mortality of <3%. At 4-year follow-up, the combined incidence of ipsilateral TIA or stroke was 8% and 20.6% for the surgical and nonsurgical arms, respectively ($p < .001$). The sample size was not large enough to show statistical significance for stroke alone.[21]

The ACAS randomized 1662 patients with >60% stenosis (by angiography or Doppler ultrasound) to surgery versus best medical management. All patients received daily aspirin (325 mg). Nonwhite populations comprised only 5% of the study group. The projected risk of ipsilateral stroke at 5 years (mean follow-up of 2.7 years) was 5.1% for the surgical group and 11% for medical management. This represented an overall relative risk reduction of 53%. This risk reduction was more apparent for men and independent of degree of stenosis or contralateral disease. The calculated stroke risk for the medical management arm was 2.2% per year. The perioperative risk of stroke and death was 2.3% plus an additional risk of 1.2% for arteriography. Surgical benefit was noted at 10 months postrandomization and remained statistically significant at 3 years.[22] The European ACST also was a positive trial, confirming the benefit of surgery over medical therapy in a large number of asymptomatic patients.

Three trials focused on symptomatic carotid occlusive disease (the North American Symptomatic Carotid Endarterectomy Trial [NASCET], the Veterans Administration

Symptomatic Stenosis Trial [VASST], and the European Carotid Surgery Trial [ECST]). All three of these trials were terminated early. NASCET and VAAST maintained that participating centers must have surgical morbidity rates of <6%. Inclusion criteria were relatively similar among the trials and included transient retinal ischemia, transient cerebral ischemia, or minor completed stroke within 120 days of randomization in the distribution of the carotid lesion.[23]

The ECST stenosis criterion was 0 to 99%. The trial randomized 3018 patients, 1807 to surgery and 1211 to best medical management. The trial was terminated early at an interim analysis of 2200 patients. Follow-up was 5 years with a mean of 2.7 years for those with <30% stenosis and 3.0 years for those with >70% stenosis. Sample size was 374 for the <30% group and 395 for the >70% group. The primary endpoint was ipsilateral stroke. The mild stenosis group (<30%) revealed no statistically significant difference between surgical and nonsurgical arms with respect to stroke incidence. The severe stenosis group (>70%) revealed a benefit to the endarterectomy arm with a 10.3% total risk of stroke (i.e., 7.5% risk of stroke or death within 30 days plus an additional 2.8% risk of stroke) versus a 16.8% risk in the nonsurgical arm. The total 3-year risk of disabling or fatal stroke was 6.0% versus 11.0% in the surgical versus nonsurgical arms, respectively. Surgical benefit outweighed best medical management risk in patients with 70 to 80% stenosis. This benefit was realized 2- to 3-year status postrandomization.[24] The ECST data reanalysis using NASCET criteria revealed a significant surgical benefit for patients with 70% stenosis.

The NASCET was terminated early secondary to significant risk reduction in patients with >70% stenosis in the surgical arm. Six-hundred fifty-nine patients with symptomatic carotid stenosis between 70% and 99% were randomized to surgical (328 patients) and nonsurgical (331 patients) treatment arms. Ipsilateral stroke risk at 2-year follow-up was 9% for the surgical group versus 26% for the nonsurgical group. This represented a 71% relative risk reduction ($p < .001$), i.e., one stroke could be prevented for every 6 to 7 endarterectomies performed. A significant correlation was noted between severity of stenosis and surgical benefit. The protective effect of endarterectomy was durable over time and independent of age, gender, and stroke risk factors.[25] At 5-year follow-up for 2226 patients with 50 to 69% stenosis randomized to nonsurgical and surgical arms, the ipsilateral stroke rate was 22.2% versus 15.7% (nonsurgical vs. surgical, $p = .045$). Author estimates were that 15 endarterectomies would have to be performed to prevent one stroke in a 5-year period. Those individuals with <50% stenosis did not benefit from endarterectomy. Contralateral occlusion was a strong risk factor for stroke, though contralateral stenosis was not a

risk factor.[26] The timing of the surgery did not affect surgical risk.

The VASST was terminated early secondary to preliminary results from the two aforementioned trials. Though 5000 patients were screened at 16 participating VA centers, only 193 men were randomized to best medical management (98 men) and surgical (91 men) treatment arms.[27] Angiography was performed on all patients and greater than two-thirds of the population had >70% stenosis. There was a mean follow-up of 11.9 months. Risk of stroke or crescendo TIA was 7.7% versus 19.4% (surgical vs. nonsurgical, $p = .028$). Surgical benefit in patients with >70% stenosis was 7.9% versus 25.6% (surgical vs. nonsurgical). Sample size at 50 to 69% stenosis was too small to draw any statistically significant conclusions. Surgical benefit was appreciated as soon as 2-month status postrandomization and was maintained throughout follow-up. Total perioperative risk was 5.5% (perioperative morbidity of 2.2% plus perioperative mortality of 3.3%).

The above studies provide convincing evidence for the surgical treatment of carotid occlusive disease in asymptomatic patients with >60% stenosis and symptomatic patients with >50% stenosis. Note, however, that surgical benefit for women in ACAS was not apparent and that nonwhite patients comprised only 5% of the study population. Also, ACAS and VAAST surgeons and patients were specifically selected for low surgical risk. In the symptomatic carotid stenosis trials, the benefit of endarterectomy was observed in the setting of low surgical risk. Surgical benefit in nonselected populations may be less predictable.

Endovascular techniques including angioplasty and stenting are alternatives to carotid endarterectomy for the treatment of carotid occlusive disease. Presently, endovascular techniques are indicated for patients who are not candidates for conventional open reconstruction. This may include patients with extremely high lesions and patients with medical contraindications to general anesthesia (pulmonary or cardiac). Some experts feel that recurrent carotid stenosis and patients with contralateral carotid occlusion are better treated by endovascular techniques; the senior author (CML) feels that in most cases these patients remain excellent surgical candidates and can be operated on without undue risk in our experience.

Several studies have demonstrated acceptable morbidity and mortality data for the use of carotid angioplasty and stenting in carotid stenosis. Diethrich et al reported on 110 patients (117 vessels), 79 of whom were asymptomatic and 31 of whom were symptomatic with stenosis greater than or equal to 70%.[28] Two major and five minor neurological events resulted from the procedure, together representing 6.4% of the study population. Five patients had transient ischemic attacks, with 1.8% mortality. Asymptomatic occlusion occurred in 1.8%, and 2.7% ultimately required endarterectomy for failure or restenosis. Yadav et al reported on 107 patients, with

189 stents placed into 126 carotid arteries.[29] Mean stenosis was 78% preoperatively and 2% postoperatively. Eighty-two percent of these patients met NASCET criteria. There was a 10.8% complication rate for symptomatic patients and a 4% neurological event rate for asymptomatic patients. In follow-up, 4.9% experienced restenosis. The experience of Iyer[30] in 352 patients undergoing 384 procedures revealed a 0.7% major stroke rate, a 6% minor stroke rate, and 0.8% mortality. Nonneurological death occurred in 1.4%. Guterman and Hopkins[31] relayed their experience with 96 high–medical-risk patients with unstable angina or restenosis after endarterectomy. Patients with long stenotic segments or high carotid bifurcations were also included. Angioplasty and stent placement was undertaken in 62 patients, with the remainder receiving angioplasty alone. Two deaths of cardiac origin, two minor strokes, and no major complications were reported. The experience of Rosenwasser and Shanno[32] with 47 patients treated with angioplasty (45 of whom also had stents placed) revealed one major stroke 5 days postoperatively and one "cold foot" that resolved with heparin therapy. Sixty-three percent required temporary pacing during inflation (29 of 47 patients). Their indications for endovascular treatment of carotid occlusive disease were radiation-induced stenosis, recurrent stenosis, medically unstable patients (with cardiac or pulmonary risk factors), and lesions at C1–2 or long lesions extending into the petrous segment.

Complications of carotid endarterectomy include infection, bleeding, damage to local tissue structures (vessels, nerves, muscle), restenosis, myocardial infarction, stroke, and death. Complications applicable to endovascular techniques include pseudoaneurysm, arterial dissection or rupture, aberrant placement of prosthesis, infection, stroke, myocardial infarction, and death.

In conclusion, there is convincing evidence for the surgical treatment of carotid occlusive disease in asymptomatic patients with >60% stenosis and symptomatic patients with >50% stenosis. Though more studies need to be performed to define long-term benefit and durability of endovascular therapies for carotid occlusive disease, current studies are promising. For selected indications, e.g., radiation-induced stenosis, recurrent stenosis, medically unstable patients (with cardiac or pulmonary risk factors), and lesions at C1–2 or long lesions extending into the petrous segment, endovascular therapy is a viable alternative to surgical endarterectomy in selected centers with experienced teams.

■ Vertebral Artery Atherosclerotic Disease

Atherosclerosis of the vertebral artery may produce vertebrobasilar insufficiency (VBI) or stroke by way of embolism, hypoperfusion, or both. The diagnosis of VBI requires two or more of the following: bilateral sensory and/or motor symptoms occurring during the same event, diplopia, dysarthria, or homonymous hemianopsia. "Dizziness" not explained by orthostasis or inner ear pathology may be a symptom of VBI. Because the vertebral arteries exist as a pair, hypoperfusion typically results from bilateral vertebral atherosclerosis or unilateral atherosclerosis in combination with unilateral congenital hypoplasia or atresia.

The vertebral arteries arise from their respective subclavian arteries, with the left vertebral artery being dominant in ~50 to 60% of cases.[33] The vertebral arteries begin their ascent thru the transverse foramina at C6, and at the level of C2 break laterally to ascend thru the transverse foramina of C1. Once through the transverse foramina of C1 the vertebral arteries course posteriorly along the atlas before turning superiorly and medial to pierce the atlanto-occipital membrane and dura. The intracranial vertebral arteries give rise to the posterior inferior cerebellar arteries and the anterior spinal artery before joining as the basilar artery. The left vertebral artery has an aortic arch origin in ~5% of cases, and in some 40% of cases, the vertebral artery is hypoplastic.[34]

A commonly used system for naming the vertebral artery was developed by Krayenbuhl and Yasargil.[35] The vertebral artery is divided into four portions, V1 to V4. Portion V1 is the first portion of the vertebral artery extending from its origin to the C6 transverse foramen. The second portion, V2, is intraosseous, extending from the transverse foramen of C6 to that of C2. Postion V3 portends to that portion of the vertebral artery between the transverse foramen of C2 and the point of posterior fossa entry by way of the foramen magnum. The fourth portion, or intracranial portion of the vertebral artery (V4), travels a short distance before joining its homologue to become the basilar artery. The above-described system of vertebral artery nomenclature facilitates discussion regarding anatomy and pathology and, germane to this chapter, areas of atherosclerosis and surgical treatment.

In Western society, atherosclerosis is ubiquitous. The atherosclerotic lesion begins as an intimal fatty streak, which evolves over time to become a fibrous plaque. The fibrous plaque may grow to occlude or stenose the arterial lumen, or the plaque may rupture causing thrombosis or embolization. Risk factors for the development of atheromatous disease include hyperlipidemia, cigarette smoking, diabetes, hypertension, obesity, and a sedentary lifestyle. As noted by Fisher et al, atherosclerosis seems to affect the V1 segment primarily; however, distal V4 segment disease is more commonly symptomatic.[4] Subclavian steal of vertebral blood flow may occur if a flow-limiting atherosclerotic plaque extends into the proximal subclavian artery.

Very few published studies address the natural history of extracranial vertebral artery atherosclerotic occlusive disease. In 1984, Moufarrij et al published their data after following 96 patients with greater than 50% vertebral artery stenosis for approximately 4 years.[36] They concluded that proximal vertebral artery atherosclerotic stenosis was a relatively benign condition when not associated with basilar artery atherosclerosis.

Surgical treatment of extracranial vertebral artery atherosclerotic disease consists of endarterectomy, bypass grafting, or transposition. These surgical procedures are reserved typically for those individuals suffering from persistent vertebrobasilar insufficiency or transient ischemic attacks attributable to the vertebral artery. These procedures are made difficult by the relative inaccessibility and small size of the proximal vertebral artery, and as such are fraught with a relatively high morbidity and mortality. Published morbidity and mortality data for proximal vertebral artery reconstruction vary greatly, ranging between 1.9 and 20%.[37–39] Five-year patency rates vary between 75 and 80%.[37,38]

Balloon angioplasty and stent-supported angioplasty are now being used with increasing frequency to treat symptomatic extracranial vertebral artery disease. Stent-supported angioplasty utilizes the intraluminal rigidity of a stent to prevent elastic recoil and early restenosis. In 1996, a review of 268 vertebral balloon angioplasties performed by Kachel[40] reported an overall success rate of 95%, no mortality, and 0.7% morbidity. Although no long-term outcome studies exist for vertebral stent-supported angioplasty, the short-term results are promising.

Those patients with vertebrobasilar insufficiency or transient ischemic attacks attributable to the extracranial vertebral arteries are candidates for open surgical or endovascular revascularization procedures. Although no randomized prospective trial has compared the therapeutic efficacy of medical (platelet inhibitors and systemic anticoagulation) versus surgical versus endovascular treatment of symptomatic vertebral disease, the Warfarin-Aspirin Symptomatic Intracranial Disease Study[41] found that patients with a symptomatic stenosis of a major intracranial vessel had fewer strokes when taking Warfarin than when taking aspirin, and the results from this study are extrapolated to justify systemic anticoagulation in those with symptomatic extracranial atherosclerotic disease of the vertebral arteries. Certainly, surgical or endovascular procedures should be considered in those patients with a symptomatic stenosis of an extracranial vertebral artery who fail to respond to medical management.

Patients who are too medically ill to undergo general anesthesia may be better candidates for long-term systemic anticoagulation or endovascular revascularization. There are no absolute contraindications to endovascular treatment of a symptomatic vertebral artery stenosis; however, a recent posterior circulation stroke associated with a tight vertebral artery stenosis is a temporary contraindication to surgical or endovascular revascularization secondary to concern of reperfusion hyperemia and the potentially disastrous consequence of hemorrhagic stroke conversion.

The diagnosis of vertebral artery stenosis or occlusion is confirmed with conventional angiography. Contrast-enhanced magnetic resonance angiography is constantly improving with the use of new pulse-sequences and software[42]; however, conventional angiography remains the definitive test in those patients suspected to have stenotic vertebral arteries. Duplex ultrasound screening of the proximal vertebral arteries is relatively unreliable.[43]

As mentioned above, the therapeutic options for symptomatic stenosis of the vertebral artery include medical, surgical, and endovascular management. The modality of choice should be tailored to individual patient needs and expectations, and typically, even with endovascular and surgical revascularization procedures, antiplatelet drugs or anticoagulants are used in the short term. Obviously, long-term systemic anticoagulation with Warfarin is associated with significant morbidity and mortality, and the risks and benefits of any treatment modality must be discussed thoroughly with the patient. A long-term, multicenter, prospective, randomized trial is needed to establish reliable data and scientifically based recommendations regarding the treatment of extracranial vertebral artery atherosclerotic disease.

Potential complications of surgical revascularization include death, damage to soft tissues, infection, bleeding, stroke, and early restenosis or occlusion. Endovascular revascularization carries similar risks; however, complications related to arterial access (hematoma, infection, pseudoaneurysm) are included.

Iatrogenic dissection has been described with endovascular techniques; however, if evident at the time of treatment, placement of additional stents across the dissection is usually curative.[39]

■ Extracranial Vertebral and Carotid Artery Dissection

Carotid and vertebral artery dissection occurs spontaneously or following trauma; it is characterized by bleeding into the tunica media. Carotid dissection is more common than vertebral artery dissection.[44] Arterial dissection is a relatively common cause of stroke in the young, although dissections may occur at any age. Both vertebral and carotid dissection may be associated with headache (commonly ipsilateral), transient ischemic attack, stroke, or a palpable pulsatile mass in cases of pseudoaneurysm formation. Dissection may be asymptomatic and found incidentally on radiographic studies, or it may be symptomatic. Vessel stenosis and thromboembolism typically results from bleeding between the intima and media, or alternatively, pseudoaneurysm formation may follow bleeding between the media and adventitia.

Spontaneous dissection occurs more commonly in those predisposed by various disease states including fibromuscular dysplasia,[45] Marfan's syndrome, atherosclerosis, and various arteritides. Dissections may also follow relatively innocuous trauma such as sneezing, coughing, or shaving. Iatrogenic dissection following arterial catheterization is well described.[39]

The natural history of extracranial carotid and vertebral dissection is largely unknown because those with asymptomatic lesions rarely seek medical attention, and those with symptomatic dissections are treated via a medical, surgical, or endovascular route. It is generally held that thrombus within the tunica media resolves over several weeks and that the arterial lumen returns to its normal size spontaneously.

Dissection of the vertebral artery should be suspected in those complaining of severe spontaneous or posttraumatic neck pain associated with signs and symptoms of posterior circulation stroke or transient ischemia. A history of whiplash, a blow to the back of the neck, chiropractic manipulation, or cervical spine fracture should trigger suspicion of vertebral artery dissection. Vertebral artery dissection-induced pseudoaneurysms may produce a cervical radiculopathy, as described by Fournier et al. As mentioned above, carotid artery dissection may be associated with signs and symptoms of stroke or transient ischemia.[46] A patient with a Horner's syndrome complaining of headache should be considered to have carotid artery dissection until proven otherwise.

Arch and four-vessel cerebral angiography is the diagnostic modality of choice; however, duplex ultrasound, magnetic resonance imaging, and computed tomography are reasonable alternatives if contraindication exists to conventional angiography. Duplex ultrasonography should not be relied upon in cases of potential vertebral dissection, as the proximal vertebral artery is not well visualized with ultrasound.[43] Angiography classically reveals an area of severe narrowing or occlusion following a gradually tapered lumen. Extracranial carotid artery dissections usually begin distal to the carotid sinus and extend for a variable distance before ending proximal to the petrous carotid.[47] Vertebral artery dissections most commonly occur between the C2 vertebral body and the skull base (V3 segment).

In cases of vertebral or carotid artery dissection, medical management consisting of systemic anticoagulation should be started on an emergent basis. Typically, heparin provides immediate anticoagulation while oral anticoagulants are allowed to take effect. Systemic anticoagulation is contraindicated in those with stroke.

Three to six months of anticoagulation is usually sufficient prophylaxis against propagation of intramural thrombus and distal embolization.

Endovascular and surgical therapeutic modalities are reserved for those patients with dissection who remain symptomatic despite systemic anticoagulation. In cases of carotid dissection or pseudoaneurysm unresponsive or partially responsive to maximal medical therapy, attempts at open surgical bypass, external carotid to internal carotid bypass (EC-IC bypass) combined with internal carotid ligation, or internal carotid ligation alone may be made. Most of these surgical procedures are treacherous given the relative inaccessibility of the high cervical carotid artery and the friable nature of pseudoaneurysms. Muller et al reviewed 50 surgeries performed for symptomatic carotid artery dissection or pseudoaneurysm formation.[48] Forty-nine surgeries were performed for chronic symptomatology despite at least 6 months of anticoagulation, and one surgery was performed on a semi-emergent basis of fluctuating neurological symptoms. In their series one patient died of intracranial bleeding, five patients suffered the development of recurrent minor stokes, and 58% developed cranial nerve deficits, which, in most cases, were temporary.

Medically intractable vertebral dissections and pseudoaneurysms may also be treated surgically.[37,38] Ligation of the vertebral artery may be performed with or without bypass. Test balloon occlusion may help predict which patients have adequate collateral blood flow to withstand ligation of the carotid or vertebral arteries. Surgical ligation of the vertebral artery should take a common-sense approach with regard to the posterior inferior cerebellar artery (PICA). If the PICA takes off distal to the problematic area, then the dissection or pseudoaneurysm may be trapped between two ligatures. If the PICA originates within the area of dissection or pseudoaneurysm, one ligature may be placed just proximal to the PICA origin. In both of the above cases, the posterior inferior cerebellar artery will fill in a retrograde fashion from the contralateral vertebral artery.

Endovascular treatment of carotid and vertebral artery dissection and pseudoaneurysm has become feasible with the advent and optimization of coils and stents.[49–51] Saito et al described the endovascular treatment of a spontaneous carotid artery dissection with symptomatic pseudoaneurysm formation.[50] In their report, a self-expanding stent was used to cover the pseudoaneurysm neck while coils were passed through the stent into the pseudoaneurysm. Arteriography performed 4 months later confirmed thrombosis of the pseudoaneurysm with preservation of internal carotid artery blood flow. The patient reported symptomatic improvement. In 1999, Liu et al reported their 8-year experience of treating seven patients with symptomatic carotid artery dissections or pseudoaneurysms with stents.[49] Four patients received stents for large, nonhealing, pseudoaneurysms, and three patients received stents for severe preocclusive stenosis. In their series, no deaths or significant morbidity occurred; however, one patient developed asymptomatic occlusion of the treated carotid artery, and one patient required coil embolization of a persistent pseudoaneurysm. Use of stent-supported angioplasty is also well described in the treatment of noncarotid extracranial cerebrovascular disease[40,52] and dissection.[39]

Again, no long-term, prospective, randomized study has compared the efficacy and complication rates for the surgical and endovascular treatment of carotid and vertebral artery dissection and dissection-induced pseudoaneurysm; however, the seemingly good results and low complication rates associated with endovascular treatment modalities are impressive and should warrant the strong consideration for endovascular treatment to be the modality of choice.

■ Miscellaneous Lesions of the Extracranial Vertebral and Carotid Arteries

Fibromuscular dysplasia (FMD) is an idiopathic angiopathy that may affect the extracranial vertebral and carotid arteries. Pathologically, FMD is characterized by fibrous thickening of the arterial tunica media. Fibromuscular dysplasia affects the arterial wall intermittently giving an angiogram the classic "string-of-beads" appearance, and like carotid artery dissections, FMD typically affects the internal carotid artery at least 2 cm distal to the common carotid bifurcation. The carotid artery is affected in ~75% of cases, and the vertebral artery is affected in up to 25% of cases. Bilateral involvement occurs in 60 to 75% of all cases.[53] Fibromuscular dysplasia of the extracranial carotid and vertebral arteries predisposes to dissection, pseudoaneurysm formation, stenosis, and thromboembolic phenomena. Cases of symptomatic stenosis secondary to fibromuscular dysplasia have traditionally been treated surgically with the graduated internal dilation technique[54]; however, in recent times endovascular stent-supported angioplasty has proven to be effective in cases of simple stenosis and in cases of FMD-induced pseudoaneurysms.[55]

Carotid artery injury secondary to penetrating neck wounds is a significant cause for morbidity and mortality in the urban young. Carotid artery laceration or transection may be accompanied by exsanguination, or lesser injury may cause thrombosis, dissection, or pseudoaneurysm formation. Those patients who are hemodynamically unstable from a carotid artery injury should be taken immediately to the operative suite for repair, reconstruction, or ligation of the damaged artery.

Patients with no neurological deficit, or with a noncoma deficit, should preferentially undergo carotid repair or reconstruction instead of ligation.[56] Comatose individuals may have the carotid artery ligated, and hemodynamically stable patients suspected to have a carotid injury should undergo angiography prior to neck exploration.

Head and neck neoplasms that affect the extracranial carotid or vertebral arteries should be removed if possible, by dissecting the tumor off the vessel. If tumor invasion of the arterial wall has occurred, then various reconstructions may be employed. Preoperative test balloon occlusion of the extracranial vessels coupled with intraoperative monitoring may provide invaluable information in difficult cases when sacrifice of an artery is considered. Carotid body tumors arise from paraganglion cells; they are typically benign and slow growing. Surgical resection of these tumors classically is associated with a relatively high morbidity and mortality.

■ References

1. American Heart Association. Heartfacts: 1994 Cardiovascular Statistics. Dallas: American Heart Association; 1994
2. Blatter DD, Bahr AL, Parker DL, et al. Cervical carotid MR angiography with multiple overlapping thin-stab acquisition: comparison with conventional angiography. AJR Am J Roentgenol 1993;161: 1269–1277
3. Zwiebel WJ. Duplex sonography of the cerebral arteries: efficacy, limitations, and indications [comments]. AJR Am J Roentgenol 1992;158:29–36
4. Fleck JD, Biller J, Loftus CM. Medical and surgical management of stroke and extracranial carotid artery disease. In: Grossman RG, Loftus CM, eds. Principles of Neurosurgery, ed 2. New York: Lippincott-Raven; 1999:271
5. Caplan LR, Gorelick PB, Hier DB. Race, sex, and occlusive cerebrovascular disease: a review. Stroke 1986;17:648–655
6. Fisher CM, Gore I, Okabe N, et al. Atherosclerosis of the carotid and vertebral arteries—extracranial and intracranial. J Neuropathol Exp Neurol 1965;24:455–476
7. Hutchinson HC, Yates PO. Carotico-vertebral stenosis. Lancet 1957;1:2–8
8. Warlow C. Disorders of the cerebral circulation. In: Walton J, ed. Brain's Diseases of the Nervous System, ed 10. Oxford: Oxford University Press; 1993:217
9. Fisher M, Fieman S. Geometric factors of the bifurcation in carotid atherogenesis. Stroke 1990;21:267–271
10. Fuster V, Badimon L, Badimon JJ, et al. The pathogenesis of coronary artery disease and the acute coronary syndromes. N Engl J Med 1992;326:242–250
11. Ross R. The pathogenesis of atherosclerosis: a perspective for the 1990s. Nature 1993;362:801–809
12. Drexler H. Endothelial dysfunction: clinical implications. Prog Cardiovasc Dis 1997;39:287–324
13. Cybulsky MI, Gimbrone MA. Endothelial expression of a mononuclear leukocyte adhesion molecule during atherogenesis. Science 1991;251:788–791
14. O'Brien KD, McDonald TO, Chait A, et al. Neovascular expression of E-selectin, intracellular adhesion molecule-1, and vascular cell adhesion molecule-1 in human atherosclerosis and their relation to intimal leukocyte content. Circulation 1996;93:672–682

15. Schussheim AE, Fuster V. Antibiotics for myocardial infarction? A possible role of infection in atherogenesis and acute coronary syndromes. Drugs 1999;57:283–291

16. Adams RD, Victor M, Ropper AH. Principles of Neurology, ed 6. New York: McGraw-Hill; 1997:779–780

17. Harrison GS, Mayberg MR. Prospective randomized studies for carotid endarterectomy. Neurosurg Clin N Am 2000;11:225–227

18. Halliday AW. The asymptomatic carotid surgery trial (ACST) rationale and design. Eur J Vasc Surg 1994;8:703–710

18A. MRC Asymptomatic Carotid Artery Surgery Trial. Prevention of disabling and fatal strokes by successful carotid endarterectomy in patients without recent neurological symptoms: randomized clinical trial. Lancet 2004;363:1491–1502

19. CASANOVA Study Group. Carotid surgery versus medical therapy in asymptomatic carotid stenosis. Stroke 1991;22:1229–1235

20. Mayo Asymptomatic Carotid Endarterectomy Study Group. Effectiveness of carotid endarterectomy for asymptomatic carotid stenosis: Design of a clinical trial. Mayo Clin Proc 1989;64:897–904

21. Hobson RW, Weiss DG, Fields WS, et al. Efficacy of carotid endarterectomy for asymptomatic carotid stenosis. N Engl J Med 1993;328:221–227

22. Asymptomatic Carotid Atherosclerosis Study Group. Endarterectomy for asymptomatic carotid artery stenosis. JAMA 1995;273:1421–1428

23. Harrison GS, Mayberg MR. Prospective randomized studies for carotid endarterectomy. Neurosurg Clin N Am 2000;11:227–232

24. European Carotid Surgery Trialists' Collaborative Group. Randomised trial of endarterectomy for recently symptomatic carotid stenosis: final results of the MRC European Carotid Surgery Trial (ECST). Lancet 1998;351:1379–1387

25. North American Symptomatic Carotid Endarterectomy Trial Collaborators. Beneficial effect of carotid endarterectomy in symptomatic patients with high-grade carotid stenosis. N Engl J Med 1991;325:445–453

26. Barnett HJ. Status report on the North American Symptomatic Carotid Surgery Trial. J Mal Vasc 1993;18:202–208

27. Mayberg MR, Wilson SE, Yatsu F, et al. Carotid endarterectomy and prevention of cerebral ischemia in symptomatic carotid stenosis. JAMA 1991;266:3289–3294

28. Diethrich EB, Ndiaye M, Reid DB. Stenting in the carotid artery: Initial experience in 110 patients. J Endovasc Surg 1996;3:42–62

29. Yadav JS, Roubin GS, Iyer S, et al. Elective stenting of the extracranial carotid arteries [see comments]. Circulation 1997;95:376–381

30. Iyer S. Carotid angioplasty. Paper presented at: The New York University Cerebrovascular Conference; 1999; New York, NY.

31. Guterman L, Hopkins N. Carotid Angioplasty and Stenting. Philadelphia: American Association of Neurological Surgeons; 1998

32. Rosenwasser RH, Shanno GB. Angioplasty and stenting for carotid atherosclerotic disease. Neurosurg Clin N Am 2000;11:323–330

33. Osborn AG. Diagnostic Neuroradiology. St. Louis: Mosby-Year Book; 1994:142–143

34. Arnold V, Lehrmann R, Kursawe HK, et al. Hypoplasia of the vertebrobasilar arteries. Neuroradiology 1991;33(suppl):426–447

35. Krayenbuhl H, Yasargil MG. Die Vaskularen Erkrankungen im Giebert der Arteria Vertebralis und Arteria Basilaris. Stuttgart: Thieme; 1957:1–170

36. Moufarrij NA, Little JR, Furlan AJ, et al. Vertebral artery stenosis: long-term follow-up. Stroke 1984;15:260–263

37. Berguer R, Flynn LM, Kline Ra, et al. Surgical reconstruction of the vertebral artery: management and outcome. J Vasc Surg 2000;31:9–18

38. Berguer R, Morasch MD, Kline RA. A Review of 100 consecutive reconstructions of the distal vertebral artery for embolic and hemodynamic disease. J Vasc Surg 1998;27:852–859

39. Fessler RD, Wakhloo AK, Lanzino G, et al. Stent placement for vertebral artery occlusive disease: preliminary clinical experience. Neurosurg Focus 1998;5:41–45

40. Kachel R. Results of balloon angioplasty in the carotid arteries [see comments]. J Endovasc Surg 1996;3:22–30

41. Chimowitz MI, Kokkinos J, Strong J, et al. The Warfarin-Aspirin Symptomatic Intracranial Disease Study. Neurology 1995;45:1488–1493

42. Leclerc X, Gauvrit JY, Nicol L, et al. Contrast-enhanced MR angiography of the craniocervical vessels: a review. Neuroradiology 1999;41:867–874

43. Ackerstaff RG, Grosveld WJ, Eikelboom BC, et al. Ultrasonic duplex scanning of the prevertebral segment of the vertebral artery in patients with cerebral atherosclerosis. Eur J Vasc Surg 1988;2:387–393

44. Leys D, Lesoin F, Pruvo JP, et al. Bilateral spontaneous dissection of extracranial vertebral arteries. J Neurol 1987;234:237–240

45. Anson J, Crowell RM. Craniocervical arterial dissection. Neurosurgery 1991;29:89–96

46. Fournier JY, Amsler U, Weder B. Extracranial vertebral artery dissection causing cervical root lesion. J Neuroimaging 2000;10:125–128

47. Anson J, Crowell RM. Craniocervical arterial dissection. Neurosurgery 1991;29:89–96

48. Muller BT, Luther B, Hort W, et al. Surgical treatment of 50 carotid dissections: indications and results. J Vasc Surg 2000;31:980–988

49. Liu AY, Paulsen RD, Marcellus ML, et al. Long-term outcomes after carotid stent placement for treatment of carotid artery dissection. Neurosurgery 1999;45:1368–1373

50. Saito R, Ezura M, Takahashi A, et al. Combined neuroendovascular stenting and coil embolization for cervical carotid artery dissection causing symptomatic mass effect. Surg Neurol 2000;53:318–322

51. Simionato F, Righi C, Scotti G. Post-traumatic dissecting aneurysm of extracranial internal carotid artery: endovascular treatment with stenting. Neuroradiology 1999;41:543–547

52. Phatouros CC, Higashida RT, Malek AM, et al. Endovascular treatment of noncarotid extracranial cerebrovascular disease. Neurosurg Clin N Am 2000;11:331–350

53. Goldberg HI. Angiography of extra- and intracranial occlusive cerebrovascular disease. Neuroimaging Clin N Am 1992;2:487–507

54. Starr DS, Lawrie GM, Morris GC. Fibromuscular disease of the carotid arteries: long-term results of graduated internal dilation. Stroke 1981;12:196–199

55. Manninen HI, Koivisto T, Saari T, et al. Dissecting aneurysms of all four cervicocranial arteries in fibromuscular dysplasia: treatment with self-expanding stents, coil embolization, and surgical ligation. AJNR Am J Neuroradiol 1997;18:1216–1220

56. Weaver F, Yellin A, Wagner W, et al. The role of arterial reconstruction in penetrating carotid injuries. Arch Surg 1988;123:1106–1109

18

Endovascular Revascularization of Carotid Artery Disease

PHILIP M. MEYERS, SEAN D. LAVINE, AND RANDALL T. HIGASHIDA

Objectives: Upon completion of this chapter, the reader should be able to describe balloon angioplasty and stenting of atherosclerotic disease involving the carotid artery, as well as the numerous clinical studies that have defined the indications for endovascular therapy.

Accreditation: The AANS* is accredited by the Accreditation Council for Continuing Medical Education (ACCME) to sponsor continuing medical education for physicians.

Credit: The AANS designates this educational activity for a maximum of 15 credits in Category 1 credit toward the AMA Physician's Recognition Award. Each physician should claim only those hours of credit that he/she spent in the educational activity.

The Home Study Examination is online on the AANS Web site at: http://www.aans.org/education/books/controversy.asp

* The acronym AANS refers to both the American Association of Neurological Surgeons and the American Association of Neurosurgeons.

More than 750,000 people suffer a stroke annually in the United States costing an estimated $52 billion in treatment and lost productivity. This makes cerebrovascular disease the third leading cause of death in the United States. While there are many causes of stroke, carotid occlusive disease accounts for 25% of all strokes. Carotid stenosis affects 0.5% of Americans after age 60 and increases to 10% in persons >80 years of age, yet most cases remain asymptomatic. In this chapter, we will evaluate the evolution in the treatment of carotid stenosis using stent-supported angioplasty.

Surgical carotid endarterectomy has historically enjoyed an unchallenged role in the treatment of carotid stenosis and remains the accepted standard of care for revascularization of extracranial carotid occlusive disease. Such a pre-eminent position is relatively rare in medical practice and has been validated by multiple, randomized, controlled trials demonstrating its efficacy over medical therapy. Any challenger will have to prove efficacy over and above this well-characterized methodology.

During the past 24 years, endovascular techniques for the treatment of cerebrovascular atherosclerotic disease have undergone technical advancement and increasing clinical application. Starting with balloon angioplasty alone, percutaneous revascularization procedures have progressed to the use of metallic stents for improved immediate and long-term results. Stent-supported angioplasty now offers a therapeutic alternative to traditional methods of surgical revascularization and treatment for those individuals without surgical options who have failed maximal medical therapy. Additionally, endovascular techniques offer treatment for a variety of non-atherosclerotic diseases affecting the craniocervical arteries including inflammatory, radiation-induced, and postsurgical strictures; acute intimal dissection; traumatic and spontaneous arteriovenous fistulas; aneurysms; and pseudoaneurysms.

For patients at high risk for surgical complications, endovascular procedures have gained clinical, if not scientific, preference as the therapeutic modality of choice. Continued innovation and refinement of endovascular technology and techniques will further improve technical success, reduce procedural morbidity, and broaden the endovascular therapeutic spectrum for extracranial and intracranial cerebrovascular disease. The first NIH-sponsored trial to compare carotid endarterectomy with stent-angioplasty (CREST) has now begun enrollment. In time, stent-angioplasty may supersede endarterectomy as the procedure of choice to treat carotid stenosis.

■ Endovascular Treatment of Carotid Occlusive Disease

Carotid Balloon Angioplasty

Kerber is often credited with the first reported case, in 1980, of percutaneous transluminal balloon angioplasty for carotid artery stenosis.[1] Seven years later, Theron published a study of 48 patients treated for de novo atherosclerosis or postsurgical restenosis using carotid angioplasty. Technical success was achieved in 94% of cases, with a 4.1% rate of serious morbidity.[2] By 1995, 96.2% technical success had been demonstrated in 523 carotid angioplasty procedures with 2.1% permanent morbidity, 6.3% transient minor complications, and no deaths.[3] In 1996, Gil-Peralta described 85 balloon-angioplasty procedures in 82 patients with symptomatic carotid stenoses greater than 70%. The results showed a 92% technical success, 0% 30-day mortality, and 4.9% major morbidity, which compare very favorably to the European Carotid Surgery Trial (ECST) and the North American Symptomatic Carotid Endarterectomy Trial (NASCET.)[4] Restenosis at 18.7 months follow-up occurred in 6.7%, predominantly between 3 to 6 months post treatment, and was entirely asymptomatic. Restenosis within 2 years of treatment has been reported in other large angioplasty series and ranges between 0 to 16%.[5,6] Meanwhile, carotid endarterectomy series report 10% early restenosis.[7]

Limitations to balloon angioplasty include vessel wall recoil, intimal dissection, and plaque disruption with particulate embolization. Angioplasty of atherosclerotic lesions generates emboli composed of atheroma, cholesterol crystals, thrombus, and platelet aggregates.[8,9] Similarly, embolization of microparticles has also been shown during and after carotid endarterectomy correlating with complex plaque morphology[10] and with clinical postoperative cerebral ischemia.[11]

Studies examining the frequency of emboli during carotid balloon angioplasty using transcranial Doppler (TCD) have failed to show a clear-cut correlation between number of insonated emboli and neurological sequelae.[9] By using transcranial Doppler ultrasound in 28 patients evenly divided between carotid angioplasty and endarterectomy, Crawley reported an average of 202

embolic signals during carotid balloon angioplasty compared with 52 during carotid endarterectomy. During a 20-minute postoperative recovery period, the tables turned and the average number of embolic signals was 5 for balloon angioplasty versus 19 for endarterectomy. However, no correlation was found between the number of high-intensity transient signals (HITS) and the rate of periprocedural stroke.[8]

The risk of stroke from embolic debris is thought to depend upon size and composition as well as the extent and location of brain involvement. It is difficult to accurately distinguish between air and particulate emboli using TCD[12]; therefore, the lack of correlation between emboli and clinical sequelae has led to the suggestion that the large majority of emboli detected during balloon angioplasty are either gaseous or small platelet aggregates <200 μm in diameter, both of which correlate with a more benign outcome.[8] Premedication with antiplatelet agents to prevent larger platelet aggregates is now commonly endorsed.[13]

Endovascular revascularization of carotid occlusive disease may result in cerebral hypoperfusion from luminal compromise by catheters and guidewires crossing the stenotic lesion and/or during balloon inflation. This is of even greater relevance in the presence of contralateral carotid artery occlusion or stenosis. Eckert monitored 22 patients undergoing carotid balloon angioplasty using TCD, noting that a >50% reduction of middle cerebral artery mean blood flow velocity compared with baseline values represented a critical threshold for the development of ischemic symptoms in conscious patients, even with short occlusion times of 10 to 40 seconds.[14] By contrast, Crawley reported significantly greater hemodynamic ischemia during endarterectomy than balloon angioplasty.[8] Consequently, balloon inflation and occlusion times are commonly brief (less than 30 seconds) in these circumstances to avoid the risk of potential cerebral ischemia. If there is attendant compromise of the contralateral carotid artery, assessment of the cerebral collateral circulation becomes even more important, and the procedure should be performed with minimal sedation to facilitate neurological monitoring.

Stent-Supported Angioplasty

The impetus for carotid stenting has arisen principally from the descriptions of the efficacy of stent-supported angioplasty in the coronary circulation that has consistently demonstrated persistent benefit in event-free survival at 1 year and a reduced need for repeat angioplasty.[15] The theoretical advantages of stent-supported angioplasty over angioplasty alone include reduction in symptomatic plaque embolization, intimal dissection, elastic vessel recoil, and early and late restenosis. Although it remains unknown whether or not these benefits apply to the carotid circulation, endovascular carotid revascularization is now most commonly performed with stents.

Since 1996, there have been 11 large carotid stent series published in which the total number of patients is 1311.[6,16–26] Comparative analysis of these reports is difficult due to inconsistencies in the sample populations, lesion characteristics, endovascular techniques, and outcome data. Overall, technical success is >95%; procedural mortality rates including cardiac deaths are 0.6 to 4.5%; major stroke rates are 0 to 4.5%; minor stroke rates are 0 to 6.5%; and the 6-month restenosis rate is <5%. This excludes other studies on high-risk patient populations.[27–30] Similarly, favorable results were reported by Al-Mubarak on 51 patients undergoing simultaneous or staged carotid artery stenting and percutaneous coronary intervention. Technical success was achieved in all carotid arteries with 4% minor stroke and no major strokes, myocardial infarctions, or deaths.[31] In NASCET, the perioperative stroke and death rate was 5.8%, with 0.6% mortality predominantly due to myocardial infarction.[32]

Vitek reviewed a series of 404 patients treated for carotid stenosis using stent-angioplasty with 98% technical success, 1.9% 30-day morbidity–mortality, 0.7% major stroke rate, 5.8% minor stroke, and 5% restenosis.[33] Lower complication rates were noted in the last 122 patients, presumably due to increased operator experience with 2.5% minor stroke and no major strokes or deaths. Finally, Wholey published the results of a worldwide stent survey in which 3047 carotid stent procedures from 24 centers in America, Europe, and Asia, with 0.98% 30-day procedural mortality, 1.35% major stroke, 2.53% minor stroke, 2.23% restenosis at 6 months, and 2.48% restenosis at 12 months.[34] Centers performing fewer than 50 cases experienced 6.4% major stroke and death, compared with 2.3% for centers performing between 50 to 100 cases. Consequently, Wholey suggests a 50-case learning curve for carotid stent angioplasty.

Operator experience appears to have an important role in treatment outcome.[35] It is evident that some threshold for excellent outcomes exists but the exact training and experience the treating physician must have remains to be determined. Furthermore, the impact of case performance on complication rates must be clarified. For centers that performed fewer than 50 cases, there was a 5.9% rate of major stroke and death. By comparison, in those centers with a throughput of 50 to 100 cases, the complication rate fell to 2.6%, while a complication rate of 1.7% was found at centers contributing 100 to 200 cases. Interestingly, participating centers with 200 to 300 and 300 to 400 cases reported increasing periprocedural complications.[35]

Treatment outcomes for NASCET-ineligible patients (ie, those considered higher risk for surgery) undergoing stent angioplasty have been studied. In NASCET, the perioperative stroke and death rate was 5.8%.[32] NASCET criteria were applied to patients enrolled in five carotid

stent series demonstrating that 79% of these 574 patients would have failed NASCET eligibility because of medical comorbidities.[16,20,24,36] (**Fig. 18–1**). Nevertheless, 2.0 to

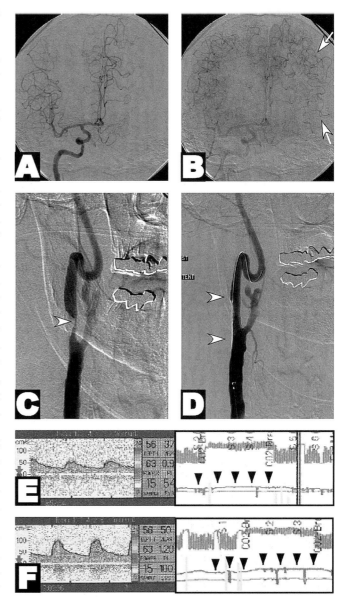

FIGURE 18–1 A 70-year-old man presented with known left carotid occlusion developed episodic right hemiparesis and expressive aphasia. **(A, B)** Right common carotid arteriography in the frontal projection during early and late arterial phases demonstrates that the left middle cerebral artery distribution depends predominantly upon leptomeningeal collaterals (arrows) from the anterior cerebral artery circulation. **(C, D)** Right common carotid arteriography demonstrates 95% eccentric stenosis (arrowhead) of the right internal carotid artery origin treated with an 8 × 30 mm nitinol stent. **(E, F)** Transcranial Doppler sonography before **(E)** and after **(F)** inhalation of 5% carbon dioxide demonstrates dramatic improvement in cerebral vascular reactivity (arrowheads) associated with improved cerebral blood flow. This method has been shown to be a strong predictor of cerebral hemodynamic failure and stroke.[109]

7.9% morbidity and 0.6 to 2.0% mortality in these early stent series compare favorably both with NASCET and ECST. Still, 41% of these patients had asymptomatic carotid stenosis for which lower endarterectomy morbidity and mortality rates might be expected. For another group of NASCET ineligible patients, Yadav reported 22 patients treated for postendarterectomy carotid stenosis, with stent angioplasty resulting in no major and only one (4.5%) minor stroke.[37] Lanzino reported favorable results in 18 patients undergoing stent angioplasty for recurrent stenosis following endarterectomy with no periprocedural strokes and one transient ischemic attack.[38] Mericle described 23 patients with high-grade carotid stenosis and contralateral carotid occlusion treated electively using stent angioplasty with no 30-day perioperative stroke or deaths.[39] In NASCET, the perioperative stroke and death rate in the presence of contralateral carotid occlusion was 14.3%.[32]

Mathur retrospectively analyzed stroke risk factors in 231 patients undergoing elective stenting of the extracranial carotid arteries in which only 14% of patients were NASCET eligible.[40] The overall 30-day stroke rate was 6.9%, while the comparable stroke rate was only 2.7% in the NASCET-eligible group. Advanced age beyond 80 years, long or multiple stenoses were found to be independent predictors of periprocedural stroke. Contralateral carotid occlusion, prior carotid endarterectomy, and combined carotid and coronary procedures, all of which are associated with a higher incidence of complications in carotid endarterectomy, did not result in an increased rate of adverse outcome in stent patients.[40,41] Chastain also found that age was a risk factor for carotid stent angioplasty. One hundred eighty-two patients treated with carotid stent angioplasty were stratified into three age groups: >80 years; 75 to 79 years; ≤74 years. Neurological complications were significantly more frequent in

patients >80 years (25%) than in patients ≤74 years (8.6%). Major stroke and death occurred in 1.6%, with a 0.5% rate of myocardial infarction.[42]

There are few published studies directly comparing carotid endarterectomy with carotid stenting. Jordan retrospectively compared 107 endarterectomy patients with 166 prospectively treated stent angioplasty patients and found a higher early minor stroke rate in the stent group (6.6% vs. 0.6%) but a greater risk of major stroke and death in the surgical cohort (4.2% vs. 2.8%).[43] Jordan compared outcomes from a subset of 109 endarterectomy patients treated under regional anesthesia with 268 stent angioplasty patients at the same institution. The early stroke and death rate was greater in the stent-angioplasty group: 9.7% versus 0.9%. Yet, most strokes were minor. The major stroke rates between the two groups were more similar: 1.5% stent versus 0% endarterectomy. Naylor reported an early prospective, randomized study in 17 patients treated for symptomatic stenoses of >70% with no complications in 10 endarterectomy patients, while five of seven stent patients suffered strokes, three of which remained disabling at 30 days.[44] This trial was prematurely terminated in favor of endarterectomy; methodological problems may explain the unusually disappointing results associated with stent angioplasty.

In general, review of the current literature on carotid stent angioplasty reveals technical success rates, procedure-related morbidity and mortality, and restenosis rates comparable with the results of endarterectomy.[45–47] Unfortunately, inconsistencies in trial design, reporting criteria, and follow-up render direct comparison of endarterectomy with endovascular revascularization difficult (**Table 18–1**). The validity of comparisons between such disparate clinical data are unsound. In the case of carotid endarterectomy, there is Class I evidence of efficacy,

TABLE 18–1 Carotid Stent versus Endarterectomy Series Data

Study	Stenosis %	Symptomatic	No. Points (CEA)	High-Risk Excluded	Minor Stroke %	Major Stroke	Myocardial Infarction	Death	Ipsilateral Stroke %	Ipsilateral Disabling stroke %	Any stroke %	Death %	Duration
					Perioperative				**Annual**				
CAVATAS[51]	>30*	90	253 CEA		4[†]	4	NA	2	4.1	2	NA	2.7[‡]	3
			251 Stent	Yes	4	4	NA	2	3.2	1.1	NA	3.7	3
Wallstent[52]	>60	Yes	112 CEA			4.5[§]				0.9[ǁ]	3.6		1
			107 Stent	NA		12.1				3.7	12.1[¶]		1
Brooks et al[53]	>70%	Yes	51 CEA		0	2	1	1					
			53 Stent	No	2	0	0	0					
SAPPHIRE[54]	≥50%[#]	Yes, >48 hour	151 CEA		3.3	2	7.3	2					
			156 Stent	No	3.2	0.6	2.6	0.6					

* Minimum stenosis not specified.
[†] Defined as modified Rankin Scale less than 3 at 30 days.
[‡] Estimated from figures presented for death and disabling stroke.
[§] Defined as any stroke or death.
[ǁ] Includes any major stroke.
[¶] Includes any major stroke, vascular death, or procedural death.
[#] ≥50% symptomatic stenosis, ≥80% asymptomatic stenosis.
Abbreviation: NA, not available; CEA, Carotid endarterectomy.

whereas the bulk of the endovascular data are derived from nonrandomized, uncontrolled single institution data.[48] For a more direct comparison, five prospective, randomized multicenter trials comparing carotid endarterectomy with stent angioplasty have been undertaken thus far.

The Carotid and Vertebral Transluminal Angioplasty Study (CAVATAS) was a prospective, randomized, multicenter trial including 504 patients randomized to endarterectomy, stent angioplasty, or medical therapy.[49] Patients with symptomatic stenoses (at least 30% luminal diameter reduction) suitable for surgery were randomized between endarterectomy and stent angioplasty over 5 years. Patients unsuitable for endarterectomy were randomized to stent angioplasty or medical treatment alone. The findings are remarkable: There was no significant difference in procedural risk of stroke or death between endarterectomy and stent angioplasty. The rate of any stroke lasting more than 7 days or death within 30 days of first treatment was nearly 10%, while the rate of disabling stroke or death within 30 days of first treatment was 6% in both surgical and endovascular groups. Preliminary analysis of long-term survival showed no difference in the rate of ipsilateral stroke or any disabling stroke in patients up to 3 years after randomization.[49] In CAVATAS, the 30-day stroke or death rates are higher than those in many prior studies but are not significantly different from the 7% stroke and death rate in ECST.[50] Cranial nerve injury and myocardial ischemia were only reported at the time of treatment in the endarterectomy group but not thereafter. Long-term follow up beyond 3 years is not yet available.[51]

The Carotid Artery Stenting versus the Carotid Endarterectomy trial (the Wallstent Trial) was an industry supported prospective, randomized trial comparing endarterectomy and stent angioplasty for treatment of symptomatic stenosis ≥60%. The results were disappointing and were only published as an abstract.[52] In this study, 219 patients with symptomatic 60 to 90% carotid stenosis were randomized to endarterectomy or stent angioplasty. The perioperative risk of stroke or death was 4.5% for surgery but 12.1% for stent angioplasty. At 1 year, the major stroke rates were widely disparate at 0.9% for surgery versus 3.7% for stent angioplasty. Consequently, this trial was prematurely halted due to poor results from stent angioplasty.

Brooks reported a single community hospital's experience randomizing 104 symptomatic patients to either carotid endarterectomy or stent angioplasty without distal protection.[53] Perioperative stroke or death was 2% for endarterectomy and 0% for stent angioplasty. Other endarterectomy complications totaled 16% including hematoma requiring treatment, cranial nerve injury, and hypotension requiring treatment. Stent angioplasty complications totaled 45% including transient cerebral

ischemia, leg amputation, retroperitoneal hemorrhage, bradycardia requiring temporary pacing, and symptomatic hypotension.

The Stenting and Angioplasty with Protection in Patients at High Risk for Endarterectomy (SAPPHIRE) trial randomized 307 high-risk patients to endarterectomy or stent angioplasty using distal protection. High risk was defined as congestive heart failure (class III/IV) or ejection fraction <30%, open-heart surgery needed within 6 weeks, recent myocardial infarction (24 hours to 4 weeks), or unstable angina (CCS class III/IV). Among randomized patients, the cumulative risk for stroke, death, or myocardial infarction at 30 days was 39% lower with stenting than endarterectomy. The combined risk for the two primary endpoints at 1 year was 7.9% lower with stenting. The authors concluded that stenting with embolic protection is not inferior to endarterectomy ($p = 0.004$). The data narrowly missed the mark for statistical superiority with stenting ($p = 0.053$). Moreover, fewer patients with stents required reoperation than those who underwent endarterectomy.[54]

However, the SAPPHIRE trial remains controversial. Of enrolled patients, 55% were excluded from randomization as poor surgical candidates, a number that appears high and may introduce bias. More than 20% of randomized patients were being treated for restenosis following prior endarterectomy, likely favoring the endovascular approach. Finally, myocardial infarction was included in the composite endpoint; hence, the effects of less-frequent strokes and deaths were obscured, which were the primary endpoints in previous large endarterectomy trials. The SAPPHIRE trial was not powered to evaluate stroke and death alone.

The Carotid Revascularization Endarterectomy versus Stent Trial (CREST) is the National Institute of Health–funded North American, multicenter, randomized, controlled trial comparing the efficacy of surgical endarterectomy with carotid stenting.[55] In CREST, patients with symptomatic extracranial carotid stenosis of ≥50% are randomized to stent angioplasty or endarterectomy. To demonstrate a clinically significant difference between the two treatments, CREST will require at least 2500 patients. To evaluate for differences among clinical subgroups, such as groups affected by recurrent stenosis, an even greater number will be required. Predominantly because of political and contractual issues, the trial has been slow to enlist centers ready to enroll patients, thus risking withdrawal of government funding for this endeavor.

Additional multicenter trials will help to provide supporting evidence for the role of stent angioplasty. Currently, there are three other major trials in progress. EVA-3S is a French trial randomizing 900 patients with ≥70% (by NASCET criteria) symptomatic atherosclerotic carotid stenosis to surgery or stentangioplasty.[32] The Stent-Protected Percutaneous Angioplasty of the Carotid versus Endarterctomy (SPACE) trial is a German study comparing 950 patients in both endarterectomy and stent-angioplasty groups with symptomatic carotid stenosis measuring ≥50%.[56] The International Carotid Stenting Study (ICSS) is a multinational study undertaken on four continents that will randomize 2000 patients with symptomatic carotid stenosis measuring ≥70% by common carotid measurement method to endarterectomy or stent angioplasty as a randomized follow-on trial of CAVATAS.[57]

Procedural Technique

Depending on existence of comorbidities, medical therapy may need to be adjusted before arteriography and intervention. Patients on long-term oral anticoagulation should be converted to heparin. Patients with pre-existing renal disease may be admitted on the prior day for intravenous hydration or monitored vasodilator therapy. Oral enteric-coated aspirin and clopidogrel (Plavix Bristol-Meyers Squibb, New York, New York) have been recommended at least 3 days before the procedure to reduce periprocedural platelet emboli. Experimental data suggest aspirin and clopidogrel have a synergistic effect on platelet aggregation, thrombotic activity, and prevention of restenosis due to fibromyointimal proliferation.[58] Following the procedure, oral antiplatelet agents are usually continued. We usually will continue Plavix for 6 weeks and aspirin indefinitely.

Although the procedure may be performed under general anesthesia, stent angioplasty of the cervical carotid artery is most commonly performed under local anesthesia at the puncture site with or without light conscious sedation which allows continuous monitoring of the patient's neurological status.[59] While the decision to proceed with treatment may have been made based on prior noninvasive imaging or arteriography, the final determination of stenosis severity is made based upon the arteriogram at the time of intervention. Carotid stenosis may be eccentric; therefore, the optimal projection to demonstrate the stenosis should be found, which may require multiple projections or even rotational angiography.[60] In the case of presumed ICA occlusion, prolonged filming is necessary, as otherwise delayed, faint, antegrade opacification due to an angiographic "string sign" of critical ICA stenosis may be missed.[61] Standard anteroposterior (AP) and lateral intracranial views should be obtained in all cases to establish the adequacy of the intracranial collateral circulation via the external carotid and anterior communicating arteries, and also to document any distal intracranial stenotic lesions. Many experienced operators also advocate routine vertebral angiography to assess collateral flow via the posterior communicating arteries and to document any extracranial or intracranial vertebrobasilar stenoses. Certainly, in cases of contralateral carotid occlusion, bilateral severe stenosis, or deficient anterior collateral pathways, evaluation of the adequacy of collateral flow via the posterior circulation becomes even more important.

The use of systemic heparin is standard. Angiomax (bivalirudin, The Medicines Company, Parsippany, New Jersey), a newer alternative to heparin, may have some preferable properties.[62] Glycoprotein IIb/IIIa inhibitors such as abciximab have been shown to decrease mortality and morbidity in several coronary stent studies and also potentially improve long-term patency rates, but their role remains undefined in carotid artery stenting.[63] These agents may have a potential role in the uncommon event of acute stent thrombosis because white thrombus (platelet aggregates) represents the primary mechanism of thrombosis.[64]

The decision to pre-dilate the lesion using balloon angioplasty depends upon the type and size of stent being used, the narrowest lumen diameter, and the morphological configuration of the stenotic segment. Many operators perform routine pre-dilatation to ~2.5 to 4.0 mm diameter. However, others suggest that the risk of embolism is high during this part of the procedure and if atraumatic crossing of the lesion with a filtration device or the stent-delivery-catheter is possible without pre-dilatation, then this may be preferable.

The currently used stents are either balloon-expandable or self-expanding, with the self-expanding stents made of either stainless steel or Nitinol (nickel-titanium alloy). Early reports of carotid stenting mainly utilized balloon-expandable stents such as the Palmaz, or the newer Genesis stent (Johnson & Johnson Interventional Systems Co., Warren, New Jersey), which allow greater precision than self-expanding types. Balloon-expandable stents are not optimal for cervical carotid revascularization because of reports documenting a 2 to 16% rate of Palmaz stent collapse on follow-up imaging, which has led to increased use of self-expanding types.[65] Furthermore, carotid Doppler ultrasound performed retrospectively was only 29% sensitive at identifying seven patients with stent compression.[65] In Wholey's global survey of 3047 carotid stenting procedures including 3033 endovascular carotid stents, balloon-expandable Palmaz stents were used in 47% of cases, and all 28 stent deformations occurred exclusively with the Palmaz stent.[65] However, Bergeron reported no instances of compression at a mean 13-month follow-up among 96 patients with carotid stenosis all treated with Palmaz stents.[25] Similarly, compression of balloon-expandable stents has been found to be a significant cause of restenosis in the superficial femoral arteries and hemodialysis grafts.[66] Thus, the balloon-expandable stent may not be an ideal choice for superficially exposed arteries such as the internal carotid. For nonexposed locations such as the vertebral artery or great vessel origins, the superior positional deployment accuracy of balloon-expandable stents may be advantageous. Self-expanding Nitinol stents offer the purported advantage of crush recoverability due to their "spring-like" behavior. If an external force compresses or deforms a Nitinol stent, it will resume its expanded shape upon removal of the external stress.

In terms of stent sizing, the stent margins should optimally extend 1 cm beyond the proximal and distal margins of the stenotic plaque. This may necessitate "caging" or "jailing" of the external carotid artery origin by the stent mesh, which does not usually result in vessel occlusion or significant clinical sequelae. The stent diameter should be at least 1 to 2 mm larger than the largest vessel diameter the stent will need to appose. Stent oversizing leads to a greater metallic coverage of the lesion per unit area, which is theoretically advantageous in preventing distal embolism and reducing tissue prolapse through the stent and does not appear to be associated with a higher rate of restenosis.[67]

Postdeployment angioplasty using a high-pressure (12 to 20 atm), semi-compliant balloon may then be performed to closely appose the stent and intima, and moreover, to expand regions of residual stent narrowing. This may require the use of varying diameter balloons, particularly if the stent extends into the common carotid artery. Obvious gaps between the stent circumference and endoluminal surface potentially increase the risk of acute or delayed thromboembolism.[68] Angioplasty beyond the stent margins is not recommended because this may cause acute vessel dissection, symptomatic vasospasm, or subsequent restenosis beyond the stent margins. Some operators do not advocate routine postdeployment angioplasty of the stent other than for obvious gaps between the stent and vessel wall and regions of residual stenosis, suggesting this reduces the risk of embolic complications and improves restenosis rates because of reduced intimal injury.

What defines technical success remains controversial. There is insufficient information to define technical success scientifically. For extremity and renal angioplasty, technical success requires <30% diameter residual stenosis by angiography and may require improvement in transstenotic pressure gradient.[69] In the coronary literature, technical success for balloon angioplasty and stenting had originally been defined as at least 20% relative improvement with a decrease in stenosis to less than 50%, but it has recently been revised to a decrease in stenosis to less than 20% diameter.[70] However, unlike extremity, renal, or coronary stenoses, carotid stenoses are very rarely symptomatic due to hemodynamic compromise. Rather, symptoms usually arise first from thromboembolism formation on carotid plaque with distal embolism.

It is unknown what degree of correction of carotid stenosis is necessary to reduce the risk of embolization, but removal of the embolic source is fundamental to procedural success. During stent angioplasty, it is possible that an attempt to eliminate residual stenosis more completely by complete balloon dilation can liberate additional emboli during the procedure that could cause a higher risk of procedural complications. Alternatively, severe residual stenosis may lead to a higher risk of late restenosis, which remains of uncertain clinical significance. Some carotid stenting trials have defined technical success as residual stenosis <30%.[54] Others have used a definition of residual stenosis <50%.[71] By recent consensus, technical success is arbitrarily defined as stent placement resulting in improvement of the stenosis by >20% with a final residual stenosis <50% using NASCET measurement criteria.[72]

Iatrogenic vasospasm may occur during the procedure, but it usually resolves shortly after removal of the guidewire from the internal carotid artery. Some investigators describe the use of injectable nimodipine (200 μg diluted in 10 ml injected slowly as a 2 to 3 ml bolus)[68] or nitroglycerin (100 μg),[36] and verapamil (5 mg diluted in 5 cc saline injected as a 1 to 2 mg bolus)[73] into the carotid artery to treat mechanically induced vasospasm. Recalcitrant iatrogenic vasospasm usually responds well to low-pressure balloon angioplasty (<3 atm).

Anteroposterior and lateral cerebral angiograms are obtained following stent angioplasty to exclude any embolic branch occlusion and document changes in cerebral blood flow. Heparin anticoagulation is generally allowed to taper physiologically rather than be reversed using protamine sulfate. The arteriotomy may be closed immediately after the procedure with one of several percutaneous closure devices. Some operators have experimented with "outpatient" stent angioplasty of the extracranial carotid artery; however, patients are usually monitored in an intensive care setting for 12 to 24 hours post treatment. Antiplatelet agents are usually continued post procedure, currently including clopidogrel for 4 to 6 weeks and enteric-coated aspirin indefinitely.

The patient should be carefully examined neurologically following the procedure. Neurological deficits may be due to intracranial embolism, hemorrhage, or reperfusion injury.[74] Following successful revascularization, reduction in mean arterial pressure 10 to 20% below baseline may be desirable to prevent cerebral hyperperfusion injury.[74] Intravenous diltiazem (Cardizem, Bioval Pharmaceuticals, Mississauga, Ontario) may be used post procedurally to control elevated blood pressure, particularly if associated with headache or neurological sequelae, as it has minimal cerebral vasodilatory effects.[75] Clonidine (Catapres, Boehringer-Ingelheim, Ingelheim, Germany) has been used in an effort to control the sympathetic autonomic neuronal pathways thought responsible for the hypertensive response following carotid baroreceptor injury.[76] Metoprolol (Lopressor, Novartis Pharmaceuticals, Basel, Switzerland), or another β-blocker, may be useful to control the carotid pulsatility index following stent angioplasty.[77] Prolonged postprocedural bradycardia or hypotension may occur as a result of carotid sinus dysfunction necessitating the use of intravenous vasopressors or inotropic agents,[78] possibly even cardiac pacing.[79]

Posttreatment Evaluation

Posttreatment evaluation should include periodic evaluation for recurrent carotid stenosis. Recurrent carotid stenosis following endarterectomy is usually asymptomatic, but repeat revascularization is necessary in ~5% of patients who undergo carotid endarterectomy.[80] Similarly, repeat endovascular revascularization for restenosis has been reported in 8% of patients undergoing carotid stenting,[81] although the rate may be higher in patients for whom the original carotid stent was placed to treat a recurrent stenosis due to endarterectomy.[82] Follow-up evaluation is easily performed with carotid duplex ultrasound and should be obtained at least 2 to 4 weeks post procedure, 10 to 12 months post procedure, and if ischemic symptoms recur. More frequent surveillance intervals may be useful in certain circumstances.[83]

■ Complications

Stroke is both a complication of carotid revascularization and an outcome measure of the effectiveness of the revascularization. The stroke may be ipsilateral or contralateral to the treated vessel. Neurological deficits as a complication of the procedure may be due to intracranial embolism, hemorrhage, or reperfusion injury.[84] The phenomenon of reperfusion hemorrhage following surgical endarterectomy is well described. Ouriel in a review of 1471 patients undergoing surgical endarterectomy reported a 0.75% incidence of intracerebral hemorrhage. Hemorrhage occurred at a median of 3 days postoperatively and accounted for 35% of the total perioperative neurological events. Death from massive hemorrhage and herniation occurred in 36% of cases. Factors correlating with an increased hemorrhage risk were hypertension, high-grade ipsilateral stenosis, high-grade contralateral stenosis or occlusion, and younger age.[85] This complication has been reported with carotid angioplasty as well. Schoser reported two patients with reperfusion hemorrhage—one intraparenchymal hemorrhage and one subarachnoid hemorrhage following balloon angioplasty for carotid and vertebral artery stenosis.[84] In a high-risk patient cohort, we found an unusually high 5% incidence of cerebral hyperperfusion phenomenon poststent angioplasty requiring intensive medical management to prevent sequelae such as seizure, stroke, and hemorrhage.[74]

Minor, major, and disabling stroke have not been uniformly defined in previous studies of endarterectomy or carotid stenting (**Table 18–2**). Other major complications include myocardial infarction and death, which in combination with stroke, are the major adverse events used to compare carotid stenting and endarterectomy. Some complications are unique to endovascular as compared with surgical revascularization. Carotid stent angioplasty may cause severe bradycardia and hypotension because of carotid sinus dysfunction requiring treatment.[78] Endovascular revascularization may produce vascular injuries such as dissection, perforation, hematoma, pseudoaneurysm, and groin infection. By contrast, complications unique to surgical revascularization include cranial nerve injuries, local wound hematomas, and infections.

■ Costs

Retrospective studies examining the cost of endarterectomy versus stenting have indicated lower costs for their respective procedures.[86–88] Surgical procedures include the costs of anesthesia and operating room time, while endovascular procedures include costs for catheters, stents, and angiographic room time. Cost-effectiveness analysis includes costs with respect to outcomes and may favor endarterectomy or stent angioplasty depending on major and minor complication rates.[89] Randomized, prospective data are needed to accurately estimate this cost differential based on patient outcomes.

■ Future Developments: Making Stent Angioplasty Safer

Potential areas of innovation include cerebral protection using intravascular filters or temporary occlusion balloons; smaller diameter, more flexible, and hence, less-traumatic stent delivery systems; reduction of restenosis from fibromyointimal hyperplasia by using catheter brachytherapy, radiation-emitting stents,[90] or biologically active coatings,[91] and improved adjuvant pharmacological regimes utilizing antiplatelet agents such as the glycoprotein IIb/IIIa inhibitors, which could reduce the risk of acute thromboembolism and improve long-term patency.[92] The potential for future technical and pharmacological improvement has prompted some investigators to suggest that a direct comparison of stent angioplasty with endarterectomy may be premature.

Distal embolization during carotid angioplasty and stenting has generated tremendous interest and financial speculation in methods of cerebral protection (**Fig. 18–2**). A triple-coaxial catheter system, designed to provide cerebral protection, has been described by Theron,[93]

TABLE 18–2 Carotid Stent Series Data

		Roubin[26]	Theron[6]	Diethrich[17]	Yadav[20]	Vozzi[19]	Criado[18]	Wholey[36]	Henry[94]	Teitelbaum[23]	Waigand[24]	Bergeron[25]
Patient Data	No. patients	528	69	110	107	22	33	108	163	22	50	99
	No. stents	604	69	129	189	19	33	108	178	31	56	99
	Asymptomatic stenosis, %	48	NS	72	36	55	27	44	35	32	72	42
Technical Success Rate		98	100	99.1	100	96	100	95	99.4	96.2	100	97
Complications	30-day morbidity	7.4	NS, 3% embolic complications, no deaths	7.3	7.9	NS	NS	NS	NS	27.3	2	7.1
	Mortality	1.6		1.8	0.9	4.5	0	1.9	0	4.5	2	0
	Minor stroke	4.8		4.5	6.5	4.5	0	1.8	1.2	13.6	2	1
	Major stroke	1.0		2.0	1.9	4.5	0	1.8	1.8	18.2	2	0
Restenosis Rate	6-month					4.9	3 (mean 8 months.)	1 (mean 6 months.)	2.3	14.3	8.7 (mean 8 months.)	4.2 (mean 13 months.)
	12-month	3	4	NS	NS	NS			NS	NS		
	Remarks			1 cardiac death				1 cardiac death	distal protection in 32 cases	high-risk cohort, 1 cardiac death	high-risk cohort	

Abbreviations: NS, not specified.

who reported distal embolic complications in 3 of 38 patients (8%) undergoing internal carotid artery balloon angioplasty without distal protection versus 0 of 43 patients (0%) undergoing the same procedure using distal balloon protection.[68] However, Henry used Theron's distal occlusion balloon technique in 32 of 163 carotid stenting cases in which 2 of the 3 major strokes occurred in conjunction with use of this device. Henry cited prolonged procedure time and increased embolic risk when traversing ulcerated lesions as potential problems associated with use of this particular system.[94] Albuquerque employed a similar technique using distal balloon protection for the angioplasty portion of the stent-angioplasty procedure during 17 procedures on 16 patients with 94% technical success, 1 (6%) transient neurological complication, and no major strokes.[95]

Numerous commercial devices aimed at reducing the microembolic burden associated with stent angioplasty of the carotid bifurcation, using filters or guidewire attached balloons, are currently under development. These include low-profile embolic filters deployed and retrieved on 0.014- or 0.018-inch guidewires that subsequently guide balloon and stent delivery. Ex vivo models have demonstrated near complete capture of particles >200 μ and 100% capture of particles >500 μ in size.[96]

An early progenitor device similar with that described by Theron involves a temporary occlusion balloon mounted on a 0.014-inch guidewire. Following angioplasty and stenting with the protection balloon inflated, an over-the-wire aspiration catheter is passed through the dilated area to clear debris.[97] This balloon-protection method has the disadvantage of temporary occlusion of carotid flow, whereas filter devices allow uninterrupted cerebral perfusion.

It remains unclear whether endovascular carotid revascularization with stent angioplasty reduces the number of particulate emboli by trapping them beneath the metallic meshwork. Current stent designs may trap larger fragments but not efficiently prevent microemboli because the interstice's size is too large.[68] As mentioned previously, a study using transcranial Doppler ultrasound demonstrated a greater number of embolic signals or HITS during stent angioplasty than endarterectomy, but a greater number of HITS were recorded after endarterectomy than stent angioplasty. A recent prospective study examined patients before and after stent angioplasty with magnetic resonance imaging (MRI) and failed to demonstrate evidence of brain signal abnormality referable to embolic ischemia. However, a similar prospective study examining 17 patients with

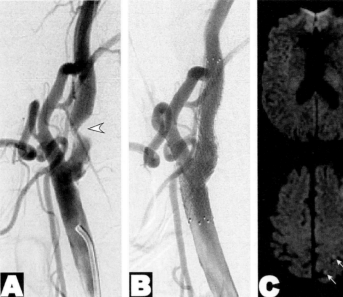

FIGURE 18–2 A 62-year-old man presented with transient confusion and aphasia. **(A, B)** Left common carotid arteriography demonstrates severe stenosis of the left internal carotid artery behind the angle of the mandible. Because of the relatively high cervical location of the plaque (arrowhead), the patient was referred for stent angioplasty. The stenosis was treated with a 9 × 40-mm nitinol stent subsequently dilated with a 5-mm diameter balloon without availability of a distal protection device. Several hours after the procedure, the patient developed recurrent episodes of expressive aphasia. **(C)** Diffusion-weighted magnetic resonance image scan demonstrates punctate infarcts (arrows) in the left middle cerebral artery distribution compatible with procedure-related thromboembolism.

diffusion-weighted MRI showed new but clinically silent ischemic foci in three cases.[98]

The equipment and techniques for endovascular revascularization of the carotid artery are evolving rapidly. Currently, stents used for carotid revascularization are adaptations of peripheral vascular or biliary stent designs. Dedicated carotid stent designs accommodating the size discrepancy between the common and internal carotid artery may better conform to vessel anatomy and improve patency rates. Other potential areas of innovation under present investigational focus include methods of providing cerebral protection using intravascular filters or balloons.[99–101] Early evidence from the SAPPHIRE trial indicates that stent angioplasty with distal protection has half the neurological risk of carotid endartectomy.[54] Smaller diameter, more flexible and less traumatic delivery systems; lowering rates of restenosis secondary to intimal hyperplasia and prevention of in-stent restenosis by using local catheter brachytherapy, radiation-emitting stents[102]; drug-eluting stents with antiproliferative chemicals such as paclitaxel or sirolimus[91,103–105]; and improved adjuvant pharmacological agents[63] have been observed in a small case series to improve short- and long-term outcomes.[106]

Several commercial devices aimed at reducing the microembolic burden associated with carotid angioplasty and/or stenting, using filters or balloons attached to guidewire, are currently under investigation. Studies in in vitro models have shown 88% capture of particles released during angioplasty and stenting of the carotid plaque lesion.[96] Alternatively, a protection balloon incorporated into the guidewire tip has been utilized. Following angioplasty and stenting with the protection balloon inflated, an over-the-wire aspiration catheter is passed through the dilated area to clear debris. This balloon-protection method has the disadvantage of temporary occlusion of carotid flow, whereas filter devices allow constant cerebral perfusion. A nonrandomized study comparing carotid stenting with and without a distal protection balloon device showed a significant reduction in microembolic signals (MES) during the procedure in the former group, leading us to find support for clinical efficacy.[96] The observed reduction in MES during critical procedural stages (pre- and postdilation, stent deployment) coincides with particularly misleading phases of transcranial Doppler monitoring with showers of "microemboli" that are only unreliably differentiated from gaseous signals. Furthermore, another surrogate marker frequently utilized to reinforce the notion of microembolizations, diffusion-weighted imaging, was not reported, and no cliniconeurological differences were found.

Long-term results on the effectiveness of distal protection devices are not yet available, but preliminary data

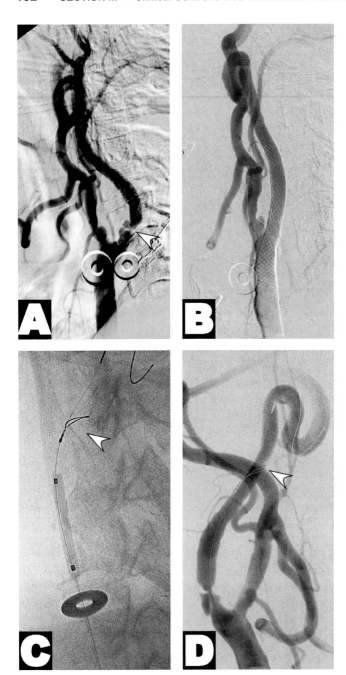

FIGURE 18–3 A 70-year-old man presented with multifocal atherosclerotic cardiovascular disease, prior stroke, and progressive bilateral carotid stenosis. **(A)** Right common carotid arteriography in the lateral projection demonstrates severe, focal stenosis in the bulbar segment of the right internal carotid artery (arrowhead). **(B)** Shown is a right common carotid arteriography following stent-supported angioplasty with an 8 × 29 mm self-expanding stainless steel stent under distal protection using a proprietary filtration device. **(C, D)** This fluoroadiograph and digital subtraction arteriogram of the right carotid artery shows the filtration device (arrows) in position. The filtration membrane permits near-normal blood flow but is highly effective at capturing emboli to 150 μm in size.

comparing carotid stenting assisted by a basket-like protection device (AngioGuard, Cordis, Miami, Florida) with endarterectomy in surgically high-risk patients were reported in June 2002[54] (**Fig. 18–3**). Among the 307 randomized patients (156 stenting, 151 endarterectomy), the combined endpoint of death, stroke, or myocardial infarction within the first 30 days after procedure was significantly lower in the stenting group (5.8 vs. 12.6%); however, stratification in symptomatic and asymptomatic patients led to statistically nonsignificant differences. The rates of TIAs and major bleedings within 30 days did not differ between the two groups.

Further research progress and technical improvement may also be expected from biocompatibility issues of the stent material. Although very little is known about the histopathological changes following stent angioplasty in the human carotid artery, a recent case report on a patient who died 8 months after placement of a self-expanding stent described the autopsy findings. Stent placement for asymptomatic left internal carotid artery stenosis in this individual revealed good neointimal coverage of the stent struts within the internal carotid artery segment compatible with healing. However, there was very poor neointimal coverage of the stent within the common carotid artery segment in association with scattered inflammatory cellular reaction and thrombotic material adherent to the struts indicative of poor incorporation of the stent into the vessel wall.[108]

▪ Conclusion

The early results of carotid angioplasty and stent-supported angioplasty vary. Certain case series show results comparable to endarterectomy, particularly in NASCET ineligible patients. The prospective, randomized trials offer encouraging results: CAVATAS and SAPPHIRE demonstrated favorable results with stent angioplasty compared with endarterectomy, while the WALLSTENT trial was prematurely discontinued due to inferior results from stent angioplasty compared with surgery. Given these discordant results, inconsistencies in patient selection, and definitions used to report outcomes, uniform reporting standards are needed, along with guidance for study design. A uniform set of reporting standards has recently been published to guide data collection, interpretation, and reporting to allow broader comparability across study designs.[72] This will allow creation of reliable trials to study the safety and effectiveness of carotid endovascular revascularization using current and future technology.

■ References

1. Kerber CW, Cromwell LD, Loehden OL. Catheter dilatation of proximal carotid stenosis during distal bifurcation endarterectomy. AJNR Am J Neuroradiol 1980;1(4):348–349
2. Theron J, Raymond J, Casasco A, Courtheoux F. Percutaneous angioplasty of atherosclerotic and postsurgical stenosis of carotid arteries. AJNR Am J Neuroradiol 1987;8(3):495–500
3. Kachel R. Results of balloon angioplasty in the carotid arteries. J Endovasc Surg 1996;3(1):22–30
4. Gil-Peralta A, Mayol A, Marcos JR, et al. Percutaneous transluminal angioplasty of the symptomatic atherosclerotic carotid arteries. Results, complications, and follow-up. Stroke 1996;27(12):2271–2273
5. Higashida RT, Meyers PM, Phatouros CC, et al. Reporting standards for carotid artery angioplasty and stent placement. Stroke 2004;35:112–133
6. Theron JG, Payelle GG, Coskun O, Huet HF, Guimaraens L. Carotid artery stenosis: treatment with protected balloon angioplasty and stent placement. Radiology 1996;201(3):627–636
7. Moore W, Kempczinski R, Nelson J, Toole J. Recurrent carotid stenosis: results of the asymptomatic carotid atherosclerosis study. Stroke 1998;29:2018–2025
8. Crawley F, Clifton A, Buckenham T, Loosemore T, Taylor RS, Brown MM. Comparison of hemodynamic cerebral ischemia and microembolic signals detected during carotid endarterectomy and carotid angioplasty. Stroke 1997;28(12):2460–2464
9. McCleary AJ, Nelson M, Dearden NM, Calvey TA, Gough MJ. Cerebral haemodynamics and embolization during carotid angioplasty in high-risk patients. Br J Surg 1998;85(6):771–774
10. Gaunt ME, Brown L, Hartshorne T, Bell PR, Naylor AR. Unstable carotid plaques: preoperative identification and association with intraoperative embolisation detected by transcranial Doppler. Eur J Vasc Endovasc Surg 1996;11(1):78–82
11. Gaunt ME, Martin PJ, Smith JL, et al. Clinical relevance of intraoperative embolization detected by transcranial Doppler ultrasonography during carotid endarterectomy: a prospective study of 100 patients. Br J Surg 1994;81(10):1435–1439
12. Ringelstein EB, Droste DW, Babikian VL, et al. Consensus on microembolus detection by TCD. International Consensus Group on Microembolus Detection. Stroke 1998;29(3):725–729
13. Goertler M, Baeumer M, Kross R, et al. Rapid decline of cerebral microemboli of arterial origin after intravenous acetylsalicylic acid. Stroke 1999;30(1):66–69
14. Eckert B, Thie A, Valdueza J, Zanella F, Zeumer H. Transcranial Doppler sonographic monitoring during percutaneous transluminal angioplasty of the internal carotid artery. Neuroradiology 1997;39(3):229–234
15. Serruys PW, van Hout B, Bonnier H, et al. Randomised comparison of implantation of heparin-coated stents with balloon angioplasty in selected patients with coronary artery disease (Benestent II). Lancet 1998;352(9129):673–681
16. Roubin G, Yadav S, Iyer S, Vitek J. Carotid stent-supported angioplasty: a neurovascular intervention to prevent stroke. Am J Cardiol 1996;78(3A):8–12
17. Diethrich EB, Ndiaye M, Reid DB. Stenting in the carotid artery: initial experience in 110 patients. J Endovasc Surg 1996;3(1):42–62
18. Criado FJ, Wellons E, Clark NS. Evolving indications for and early results of carotid artery stenting. Am J Surg 1997;174(2):111–114
19. Vozzi CR, Rodriguez AO, Paolantonio D, Smith JA, Wholey MH. Extracranial carotid angioplasty and stenting. Initial results and short-term follow-up. Tex Heart Inst J 1997;24(3):167–172
20. Yadav JS, Roubin GS, Iyer S, et al. Elective stenting of the extracranial carotid arteries. Circulation 1997;95(2):376–381
21. Wholey MH, Jarmolowski CR, Eles G, Levy D, Buecthel J. Endovascular stents for carotid artery occlusive disease. J Endovasc Surg 1997;4(4):326–338
22. Henry M, Amor M, Klonaris C, et al. Angioplasty and stenting of the extracranial carotid arteries. Tex Heart Inst J 2000;27(2):150–158
23. Teitelbaum GP, Lefkowitz MA, Giannotta SL. Carotid angioplasty and stenting in high-risk patients. Surg Neurol 1998;50(4):300–311 discussion 311–2
24. Waigand J, Gross CM, Uhlich F, et al. Elective stenting of carotid artery stenosis in patients with severe coronary artery disease. Eur Heart J 1998;19(9):1365–1370
25. Bergeron P, Becquemin JP, Jausseran JM, et al. Percutaneous stenting of the internal carotid artery: the European CAST I Study. Carotid Artery Stent Trial. J Endovasc Surg 1999;6(2):155–159
26. Roubin GS, New G, Iyer SS, et al. Immediate and late clinical outcomes of carotid artery stenting in patients with symptomatic and asymptomatic carotid artery stenosis: a 5-year prospective analysis. Circulation 2001;103(4):532–537
27. Phatouros CC, Higashida RT, Malek AM, et al. Clinical use of stents for carotid artery disease. Neurol Med Chir (Tokyo) 1999;39(12):809–827
28. Malek AM, Higashida RT, Phatouros CC, et al. Stent angioplasty for cervical carotid artery stenosis in high-risk symptomatic NASCET-ineligible patients. Stroke 2000;31(12):3029–3033
29. Malek AM, Higashida RT, Phatouros CC, et al. Treatment of posterior circulation ischemia with extracranial percutaneous balloon angioplasty and stent placement. Stroke 1999;30(10):2073–2085
30. Malek AM, Higashida RT, Phatouros CC, et al. Endovascular management of extracranial carotid artery dissection achieved using stent angioplasty. AJNR Am J Neuroradiol 2000;21(7):1280–1292
31. Al-Mubarak N, Roubin GS, Liu MW, et al. Early results of percutaneous intervention for severe coexisting carotid and coronary artery disease. Am J Cardiol 1999;84(5):600–602
32. The North American Symptomatic Carotid Endarterectomy Trial Collaborators. Beneficial effect of carotid endarterectomy in symptomatic patients with high-grade cartod stenosis. N Engl J Med 1991;325:445–453
33. Vitek J, Roubin G, Iyer S. Immediate and Late Outcome of Carotid Angioplasty with Stenting. Vol. 43. Nashville, Tennessee: AANS/CNS/ASITN;1999:41
34. Wholey M, Wholey MH, Eles G. Cervical carotid artery stent placement. Semin Interv Cardiol 1998;3(2):105–115
35. Wholey MH, Wholey M, Mathias K, et al. Global experience in cervical carotid artery stent placement. Catheter Cardiovasc Interv 2000;50(2):160–167
36. Wholey M, Wholey MH, Jarmolowski CR, et al. Endovascular stents for carotid artery occlusive disease. J Endovasc Surg 1997;(4):326–338
37. Yadav JS, Roubin GS, King P, Iyer S, Vitek J. Angioplasty and stenting for restenosis after carotid endarterectomy. Initial experience. Stroke 1996;27(11):2075–2079
38. Lanzino G, Mericle RA, Lopes DK, Wakhloo AK, Guterman LR, Hopkins LN. Percutaneous transluminal angioplasty and stent placement for recurrent carotid artery stenosis. J Neurosurg 1999;90(4):688–694
39. Mericle RA, Kim SH, Lanzino G, et al. Carotid artery angioplasty and use of stents in high-risk patients with contralateral occlusions. J Neurosurg 1999;90(6):1031–1036
40. Mathur A, Roubin GS, Iyer SS, et al. Predictors of stroke complicating carotid artery stenting. Circulation 1998;97(13):1239–1245
41. Meyer FB, Piepgras DG, Fode NC. Surgical treatment of recurrent carotid artery stenosis. J Neurosurg 1994;80(5):781–787
42. Chastain HD II, Gomez CR, Iyer S, et al. Influence of age upon complications of carotid artery stenting. UAB Neurovascular Angioplasty Team. J Endovasc Surg 1999;6(3):217–222
43. Jordan Jr WD, Schroeder PT, Fisher WS, McDowell HA. A comparison of angioplasty with stenting versus endarterectomy for the treatment of carotid artery stenosis. Ann Vasc Surg 1997;11(1):2–8

44. Naylor AR, Bolia A, Abbott RJ, et al. Randomized study of carotid angioplasty and stenting versus carotid endarterectomy: a stopped trial. J Vasc Surg 1998;28(2):326–334

45. Higashida RT, Malek AM, Phatouros CC, et al. Stenting and angioplasty for cerebrovascular disease. In: Fisher M, Fieschi C, eds. Prevention of Ischemic Stroke. London: Martin Dunitz Publishers; 1999:231–252

46. Phatouros CC, Higashida RT, Lefler JE, et al. Angioplasty and stent placement in the extracranial circulation. In: Marks, MP, Do, HM, eds. Endovascular and Percutaneous Therapy of the Brain and Spine. Philadelphia: Lippincott Williams and Wilkins; 2002:43–47

47. Phatouros CC, Higashida RT, Malek AM, et al. Carotid artery stent placement for atherosclerotic disease: rationale, technique, and current status. Radiology 2000;217(1):26–41

48. Beebe HG. Scientific evidence demonstrating the safety of carotid angioplasty and stenting: do we have enough to draw conclusions yet? J Vasc Surg 1998;27(4):788–790

49. Endovascular versus surgical treatment in patients with carotid stenosis in the Carotid and Vertebral Artery Transluminal Angioplasty Study (CAVATAS): a randomised trial. Lancet 2001; 357(9270):1729–1737

50. The European Carotid Surgery Trialists' Collaborative Group. Randomised trial of endarterectomy for recently symptomatic carotid stenosis: final results of the MRC European Carotid Surgery Trial (ECST). Lancet 1998;351(9113):1379–1387

51. Brown MM. Vascular surgical society of Great Britain and Ireland: results of the carotid and vertebral artery transluminal angioplasty study. Br J Surg 1999;86(5):710–711

52. Alberts MJ. Results of a Multicenter Prospective Randomized Trial of Carotid Artery Stenting vs. Carotid Endarterectomy. Stroke 2001;32:325 -d.

53. Brooks WH, McClure RR, Jones MR, Coleman TC, Breathitt L. Carotid angioplasty and stenting versus carotid endarterectomy: randomized trial in a community hospital. J Am Coll Cardiol 2001;38(6):1589–1595

54. Yadav J, Wholey M, Kuntz KM, et al. Protected carotid-artery stenting versus endarterectomy in high-risk patients. N Engl J Med 2004;351(15):1493–1501

55. Hobson RW II. CREST (Carotid Revascularization Endarterectomy versus Stent Trial): background, design, and current status. Semin Vasc Surg 2000;13(2):139–143

56. Stent-protected percutaneous angioplasty of the carotid vs. endarterectomy. Available at: http://www.strokecenter.org/trials/TrialDetail.aspx?tid=214&search_string=stent. Accessed November 16, 2005

57. International Carotid Artery Study (CAVATAS-2) http://www.strokecenter.org/trials/TrialDetail.asp?ref = 86. Accessed November 16, 2005

58. Herbert JM, Dol F, Bernat A, Falotico R, Lale A, Savi P. The anti-aggregating and antithrombotic activity of clopidogrel is potentiated by aspirin in several experimental models in the rabbit. Thromb Haemost 1998;80(3):512–518

59. Luginbuhl M, Remonda L. Interventional neuroradiology. Recent developments and anaesthesiologic aspects. Minerva Anestesiol 1999;65(6):445–454

60. Elgersma OE, Buijs PC, Wust AF, van der Graaf Y, Eikelboom BC, Mali WP. Maximum internal carotid arterial stenosis: assessment with rotational angiography versus conventional intraarterial digital subtraction angiography. Radiology 1999;213(3):777–783

61. Mehigan JT, Olcott C IV. The carotid "string" sign. Differential diagnosis and management. Am J Surg 1980;140(1):137–143

62. Cho L, Chew DP, Moliterno DJ, et al. Safe and efficacious use of bivalirudin for percutaneous coronary intervention with adjunctive platelet glycoprotein IIb/IIIa receptor inhibition. Am J Cardiol 2003;91(6):742–743

63. Investigators TE. Platelet glycoprotein IIb/IIIa receptor blockade and low-dose heparin during percutaneous coronary revascularization. N Engl J Med 1997;336(24):1689–1696

64. Jeong MH, Owen WG, Staab ME, et al. Porcine model of stent thrombosis: platelets are the primary component of acute stent closure. Cathet Cardiovasc Diagn 1996;38(1):38–43

65. Mathur A, Dorros G, Iyer SS, Vitek JJ, Yadav SS, Roubin GS. Palmaz stent compression in patients following carotid artery stenting. Cathet Cardiovasc Diagn 1997;41(2):137–140

66. Rosenfield K, Schainfeld R, Pieczek A, Haley L, Isner JM. Restenosis of endovascular stents from stent compression. J Am Coll Cardiol 1997;29(2):328–338

67. Piamsomboon C, Roubin GS, Liu MW, et al. Relationship between oversizing of self-expanding stents and late loss index in carotid stenting. Cathet Cardiovasc Diagn 1998;45(2):139–143

68. Theron J, Guimaraens O, Coskun L, Sola J, Martin T, Rufenacht D. Complications of carotid angioplasty and stenting. Neurosurgical Focus 1998;5(6):1–19

69. Martin LG, Rundback JH, Sacks D, et al. Quality improvement guidelines for angiography, angioplasty, and stent placement in the diagnosis and treatment of renal artery stenosis in adults. J Vasc Interv Radiol 2002;13(11):1069–1083

70. Smith SC Jr, Dove JT, Jacobs AK, et al. ACC/AHA guidelines of percutaneous coronary interventions (revision of the 1993 PTCA guidelines)–executive summary. A report of the American College of Cardiology/American Heart Association Task Force on Practice Guidelines (committee to revise the 1993 guidelines for percutaneous transluminal coronary angioplasty). J Am Coll Cardiol 2001;37(8):2215–2239

71. Illig KA, Zhang R, Tanski W, Benesch C, Sternbach Y, Green RM. Is the rationale for carotid angioplasty and stenting in patients excluded from NASCET/ACAS or eligible for ARCHeR justified? J Vasc Surg 2003;37(3):575–581

72. Higashida RT, Meyers PM, Phatouros CC, Connors JJ III, Barr J, Sacks D. Reporting standards for carotid artery angioplasty and stent placement. Stroke 2003; In press

73. Feng L, Fitzsimmons BF, Young WL, et al. Intraarterially administered verapamil as adjunct therapy for cerebral vasospasm: safety and 2-year experience. AJNR Am J Neuroradiol 2002;23(8):1284–1290

74. Meyers PM, Higashida RT, Phatouros CC, et al. Cerebral hyperperfusion syndrome after percutaneous transluminal stenting of the craniocervical arteries. Neurosurgery 2000;47(2):335–343 discussion 343–345

75. Hirayama T, Katayama Y, Kano T, Tsubokawa T. Control of systemic hypertension with diltiazem, a calcium-antagonist, in patients with a mildly elevated intracranial pressure: a comparative study. Neurol Res 1994;16:97–99

76. Ille O, Woimant F, Pruna A, Corabianu O, Idatte JM, Haguenau M. Hypertensive encephalopathy after bilateral carotid endarterectomy. Stroke 1995;26(3):488–491

77. Felding M, Jakobsen CJ, Cold GE, Davidsen B, Jensen K. The effect of metoprolol upon blood pressure, cerebral blood flow and oxygen consumption in patients subjected to craniotomy for cerebral tumours. Acta Anaesthesiol Scand 1994;38(3):271–275

78. Qureshi AI, Luft AR, Lopes DK, et al. Postoperative hypotension after carotid angioplasty and stenting: report of three cases. Neurosurgery 1999;44(6):1320–1323 discussion 1324

79. Harrop JS, Sharan AD, Benitez RP, Armonda R, Thomas J, Rosenwasser RH. Prevention of carotid angioplasty-induced bradycardia and hypotension with temporary venous pacemakers. Neurosurgery 2001;49(4):814–820 discussion 820–822

80. O'Hara PJ, Hertzer NR, Karafa MT, Mascha EJ, Krajewski LP, Beven EG. Reoperation for recurrent carotid stenosis: early results and late outcome in 199 patients. J Vasc Surg 2001;34(1):5–12

81. Chakhtoura EY, Hobson RW II, Goldstein J, et al. In-stent restenosis after carotid angioplasty-stenting: incidence and management. J Vasc Surg 2001;33(2):220–225 discussion 225–226

82. Leger AR, Neale M, Harris JP. Poor durability of carotid angioplasty and stenting for treatment of recurrent artery stenosis after

carotid endarterectomy: an institutional experience. J Vasc Surg 2001;33(5):1008–1014

83. Hobson RW II, Goldstein JE, Jamil Z, et al. Carotid restenosis: operative and endovascular management. J Vasc Surg 1999;29(2): 228–235 discussion 235–238

84. Schoser BG, Heesen C, Eckert B, Thie A. Cerebral hyperperfusion injury after percutaneous transluminal angioplasty of extracranial arteries. J Neurol 1997;244(2):101–104

85. Ouriel K, Shortell CK, Illig KA, Greenberg RK, Green RM. Intracerebral hemorrhage after carotid endarterectomy: incidence, contribution to neurologic morbidity, and predictive factors. J Vasc Surg 1999;29(1):82–87 discussion 87–89

86. Jordan WD Jr, Roye GD, Fisher WS III, Redden D, McDowell HA. A cost comparison of balloon angioplasty and stenting versus endarterectomy for the treatment of carotid artery stenosis. J Vasc Surg 1998;27(1):16–22 discussion 22–24

87. Ricotta JJ, Hargadon T, O'Brien-Irr M. Cost management strategies for carotid endarterectomy. Am J Surg 1998;176(2):188–192

88. Fisher WS III, Jordan WD. Carotid angioplasty. Surg Neurol 1998;50(4):295–298 discussion 298–299

89. Kilaru S, Korn P, Kasirajan K, et al. Is carotid angioplasty and stenting more cost effective than carotid endarterectomy? J Vasc Surg 2003;37(2):331–339

90. Teirstein PS, Massullo V, Jani S, et al. Catheter-based radiotherapy to inhibit restenosis after coronary stenting. N Engl J Med 1997;336(24):1697–1703

91. Morice MC, Serruys PW, Sousa JE, et al. A randomized comparison of a sirolimus-eluting stent with a standard stent for coronary revascularization. N Engl J Med 2002;346(23):1773–1780

92. Oesterle SN, Whitbourn R, Fitzgerald PJ, et al. The stent decade: 1987 to 1997. Stanford Stent Summit faculty. Am Heart J 1998;136(4 Pt 1):578–599

93. Theron J, Courtheoux P, Alachkar F, Bouvard G, Maiza D. New triple coaxial catheter system for carotid angioplasty with cerebral protection. AJNR Am J Neuroradiol 1990;11(5):869–874 discussion 875–877

94. Henry M, Amor M, Masson I, et al. Angioplasty and stenting of the extracranial carotid arteries. J Endovasc Surg 1998;5(4):293–304

95. Albuquerque FC, Teitelbaum GP, Lavine SD, Larsen DW, Giannotta SL. Balloon-protected carotid angioplasty. Neurosurgery 2000;46(4):918–921 discussion 922–923

96. Ohki T, Roubin GS, Veith FJ, et al. Efficacy of a filter device in the prevention of embolic events during carotid angioplasty and stenting: an ex vivo analysis. J Vasc Surg 1999;30(6):1034–1044

97. Henry M, Amor M, Henry I, et al. Carotid stenting with cerebral protection: first clinical experience using the PercuSurge Guard Wire System. J Endovasc Surg 1999;6(4):321–331

98. Van Heeswijk HP, Vos JA, Louwerse ES, et al. New brain lesions at MR imaging after carotid angioplasty and stent placement. Radiology 2002;224(2):361–365

99. Al-Mubarak N, Roubin GS, Vitek JJ, Iyer SS. Microembolization during carotid stenting with the distal-balloon antiemboli system. Int Angiol 2002;21(4):344–348

100. Ohki T, Veith FJ, Grenell S, et al. Initial experience with cerebral protection devices to prevent embolization during carotid artery stenting. J Vasc Surg 2002;36(6):1175–1185

101. Whitlow PL, Lylyk P, Londero H, et al. Carotid artery stenting protected with an emboli containment system. Stroke 2002;33(5): 1308–1314

102. Chan AW, Roffi M, Mukherjee D, et al. Carotid brachytherapy for in-stent restenosis. Catheter Cardiovasc Interv 2003;58(1): 86–92

103. Liistro F, Stankovic G, Di Mario C, et al. First clinical experience with a paclitaxel derivate-eluting polymer stent system implantation for in-stent restenosis: immediate and long-term clinical and angiographic outcome. Circulation 2002;105(16):1883–1886

104. Virmani R, Liistro F, Stankovic G, et al. Mechanism of late in-stent restenosis after implantation of a paclitaxel derivate-eluting polymer stent system in humans. Circulation 2002;106(21): 2649–2651

105. Degertekin M, Serruys PW, Foley DP, et al. Persistent inhibition of neointimal hyperplasia after sirolimus-eluting stent implantation: long-term (up to 2 years) clinical, angiographic, and intravascular ultrasound follow-up. Circulation 2002;106(13):1610–1613

106. Topol EJ, Lincoff AM, Kereiakes DJ, et al. Multi-year follow-up of abciximab therapy in three randomized, placebo-controlled trials of percutaneous coronary revascularization. Am J Med 2002; 113(1):1–6

107. Al-Mubarak N, Roubin GS, Vitek JJ, Iyer SS, New G, Leon MB. Effect of the distal-balloon protection system on microembolization during carotid stenting. Circulation 2001;104(17):1999–2002

108. Toma N, Matsushima S, Murao K, et al. Histopathological findings in a human carotid artery after stent implantation. Case report. J Neurosurg 2003;98(1):199–204

109. Marshall RS, Rundek T, Sproule DM, Fitzsimmons BF, Schwartz S, Lazar RM. Monitoring of cerebral vasodilatory capacity with transcranial Doppler carbon dioxide inhalation in patients with severe carotid artery disease. Stroke 2003;34(4):945–949

19

Diagnosis and Medical and Endovascular Treatment of Intracranial Atherosclerotic Disease

HUNALDO VILLALOBOS, ALAN S. BOULOS, AND LEE R. GUTERMAN

Objectives: Upon completion of this chapter, the reader should be able to identify the indications for and technical steps involved in treating intracranial atherosclerotic disease with angioplasty, stenting, or some combination.

Accreditation: The AANS* is accredited by the Accreditation Council for Continuing Medical Education (ACCME) to sponsor continuing medical education for physicians.

Credit: The AANS designates this educational activity for a maximum of 15 credits in Category 1 credit toward the AMA Physician's Recognition Award. Each physician should claim only those hours of credit that he/she spent in the educational activity.

The Home Study Examination is online on the AANS Web site at: http://www.aans.org/education/books/controversy.asp

* The acronym AANS refers to both the American Association of Neurological Surgeons and the American Association of Neurosurgeons.

The treatment of intracranial atherosclerotic disease has centered on a symptomatic patient population. Patients presenting with transient ischemic attack (TIA) or stroke without cervical carotid disease have increasingly been studied by means of magnetic resonance (MR) angiography. This new trend has been responsible for uncovering an increasing number of patients with intracranial stenosis. When the stenosis correlates with the neurological signs and symptoms, treatment should be initiated. Antiplatelet (aspirin) and anticoagulant (sodium warfarin) therapies have been the focus of medical management. A prospective randomized trial (Warfarin-Aspirin Symptomatic Intracranial Disease [WASID]) to determine whether aspirin or warfarin is more effective for the treatment of symptomatic intracranial atherosclerotic lesions has recently been completed, and the results demonstrated a significantly increased hemorrhage and death rate in the warfarin group (compared with the aspirin group) without any benefit with warfarin for stroke prevention in patients with symptomatic intracranial stenosis.[1,2] Technological advancements in angioplasty catheters and stents have driven the application of these devices for revascularization of the intracranial circulation. To date, only small patient series have been reported in the literature.

In this chapter, we will review the current literature concerning the natural history of intracranial atherosclerotic disease and primary angioplasty, primary stenting, and provisional stenting procedures for the treatment of symptomatic intracranial atherosclerotic lesions. Methods of diagnosis and patient selection for endoluminal revascularization will be reviewed. Selected case presentations will be made. Finally, complication avoidance and management will be discussed.

■ Natural History and Medical Management of Intracranial Stenosis

The management of intracranial atherosclerosis remains perplexing. Unlike for atherosclerosis of the extracranial vasculature, only one prospective randomized trial has influenced therapeutic approaches for intracranial disease. The Extracranial-to-Intracranial (EC-IC) Cooperative Bypass Study demonstrated the inefficacy of bypass surgery to prevent stroke recurrence.[3] This study and other smaller prospective studies have allowed us to define the natural history of intracranial arterial stenosis.

There are several studies, including the EC-IC bypass study, in which a subgroup of patients was treated with aspirin alone. In the bypass study, 714 patients with intracranial internal carotid artery or middle cerebral artery (MCA) stenosis who received 1300 mg of aspirin on a daily basis were observed. The ipsilateral annual stroke rate was 7%, with an overall stroke rate of 10%. In prospective nonrandomized studies conducted by Craig et al (58 patients) and Marzewski et al (66 patients), distal ICA stenosis carried a 3.2 to 7.6% annual stroke rate ipsilateral to the stenosis, with an overall stroke rate of 4 to 11.6%.[4,5]

The retrospective arm of the WASID study examined the efficacy of warfarin compared with aspirin for the prevention of major vascular events (stroke, myocardial infarction, or sudden death).[1] Among 63 patients treated with aspirin, the rate of a major vascular event was 18.1 per 100 patient-years. The associated stroke rate of 10.4 per 100 patient-years corroborates well with that of other studies. Among patients receiving warfarin, however, the major vascular event rate decreased to 8.4 per 100 patient-years in 88 patients. The stroke rate was 3.6 per 100 patient years. Three patients (3%) had major hemorrhagic complications, with two being fatal. The rate of hemorrhagic complications for the warfarin-treatment group was 7.8 per 100 patient-years, compared with 1.4 per 100 patient-years for the aspirin-treatment group.[1] In addition, a European trial, Stroke Prevention in Reversible Ischemia Trial (SPIRIT), has demonstrated a high hemorrhagic complication rate associated with warfarin therapy in patients who have experienced previous cerebral ischemic events, adding to the complexity of medication choices.[6]

The mechanism by which warfarin eliminates strokes is unclear. In the WASID trial, warfarin treatment resulted in near-elimination of strokes in territories outside the significant stenosis.[1] Among six patients who had strokes, five strokes were in the territory of the compromised vessel. With aspirin, 15 strokes occurred, of which 9 were in the territory of the stenotic artery. This suggests that warfarin may affect other pathophysiological mechanisms of stroke besides large artery occlusive disease (e.g., mechanisms such as small vessel arteriopathy or cardioembolic events). Cardioembolic sources of stroke may well be prevalent in this population, and warfarin may be a more effective treatment for these embolic sources than aspirin.

The WASID study also provides interesting data on posterior circulation events, with respect to daily aspirin use.[1] For posterior circulation stenosis, stroke rates approached those for symptomatic extracranial carotid stenosis exceeding 70%. For intracranial vertebral artery stenosis, a 7.8% annual stroke rate was found, whereas basilar artery stenosis was associated with a 10.7% annual stroke rate.

Further studies have implicated a very high recurrence of neurological symptoms once antithrombotic therapy has failed.[7] Recurrent ischemic events typically occur within 1 month after failure of therapy.[7] There is, therefore, some urgency to change the form of treatment once failure has occurred. In addition, most patients with intracranial disease are more likely to present with a major event (such as a catastrophic stroke) than with TIAs or minor stroke.[3] This further complicates medical decision-making, as the question arises whether medical management should even be attempted initially.

■ Pathophysiology of Cerebral Infarction from Arterial Stenosis

There is considerable debate about the mechanism responsible for large vessel intracranial stenosis that results in stroke. Unlike the extracranial carotid where artery-to-artery embolism is the predominant mechanism, increasing evidence in the literature supports a hemodynamic cause for large vessel infarctions. Certainly, a subset of patients has demonstrated a higher rate of stroke recurrence associated with hemodynamic failure.[8–10] More likely, there is an ongoing interaction between the stenosis providing an embolic source and reduced blood flow resulting in diminished ability to clear the emboli. The ischemic events are thus a shift in the balance between embolic load and blood flow.[11]

Another medical concern regarding stroke prevention is hypertension. Blood pressure control is the most important factor in preventing recurrent stroke even in patients with evidence of impaired cerebrovascular reserve.[12] Hypertension is the most important risk factor for small vessel disease in penetrating arteries and large vessel atherosclerosis, yet aggressive control of blood pressure may precipitate ischemia in a territory with diminished cerebrovascular reserve. Therefore, a difficult medical decision must be made as to the optimal blood pressure for patients with stenosis and functional tests that suggest relative hemodynamic insufficiency.

Bypass surgery limitations probably relate to the reasons mentioned above. Bypass surgery can improve cerebral blood flow and reduce hemodynamic risk of future strokes, but it has little ability to reduce artery-to-artery embolism. The EC-IC bypass study failed to demonstrate a reduction in stroke frequency, partly because the patient population could not be selected to a hemodynamic failure arm.[3] In addition, the EC-IC bypass procedure would occasionally precipitate MCA occlusion at the site of the stenotic segment (usually the M1 segment).[13,14] This thrombosis likely causes perforator occlusion, resulting in deep brain infarction. The Carotid Occlusion Surgery Study (COSS) is evaluating the rate of stroke reduction after the performance of EC-IC bypass procedure in patients with symptomatic carotid occlusion and an increased oxygen extraction fraction, as measured by positron emission tomography.[15]

In summary, aspirin has demonstrated only mild efficacy for stroke prevention. Warfarin was associated with significantly higher rates of intracranial hemorrhage and provided no benefit over aspirin in the WASID prospective trial.[2] Endoluminal revascularization, therefore, may have a role in the treatment of both embolic and hemodynamic sources of infarction from the stenotic vessel.

■ Angiographic Progression of Intracranial Atherosclerosis

A brief explanation of the angiographic appearance of intracranial atherosclerosis is a necessary prelude to a discussion of endovascular techniques for the treatment of this condition. Intracranial stenosis is a dynamic process whereby repeat imaging can reveal sometimes dramatically different degrees of arterial blockage. In a retrospective series of serial angiographic studies obtained to determine the natural history of intracranial stenosis, 40% of stenoses progressed and 20% regressed.[16] The distal internal carotid artery did not seem as predisposed to disease progression as did the more distal branches (MCA, anterior cerebral artery, posterior cerebral artery). In three patients, regression of the intracranial stenosis was impressive, suggesting that a thrombus was present within the already diseased vessel. More recently, significant angiographic improvement of a stenotic vertebrobasilar artery segment was seen after the administration of high-dose atorvastatin, a potent HMG-CoA reductase inhibitor, for a 2-week period.[17] This improvement may have been from resolution of thrombus as statins promote endogenous fibrinolysis and plaque remodeling.

■ Endoluminal Revascularization

The three methods for achievement of endoluminal revascularization are primary angioplasty, primary stenting, or provisional stenting. Primary angioplasty means that the physician is placing an angioplasty balloon to expand the stenotic segment and does not intend to place a stent. Primary stenting means that the physician intends to place a stent and may or may not dilate the lesion with an angioplasty balloon before stent placement. If no previous dilation is required, the procedure

is referred to as direct stenting. Initial patient series presented the feasibility and demonstrated the limitations of primary angioplasty alone.[13,18–20] More recent series have documented the decreased incidence of complications, demonstrating a considerable learning curve for these techniques.[21–24] The periprocedural neurological event rate in these four series, which comprise more than 10 patients each, is less than 10%,[21–24] whereas the event rate in the four initial studies, comprising more than 10 patients each, ranged from 8 to 33%.[18–20,25]

The results of these numerous reports are mirrored in the angioplasty series presented by Connors and Wojak.[21] These authors divided their experience from 1989 to 1998 into three periods. A higher rate of complications was encountered in 17 patients treated during the early and middle periods from 1989 to 1993, including dissection, 82%; neurological events, 6%; and death, 6%. Subsequent to 1993, the rates among 41 patients were dissection, 14%; neurological events, 8% (of which 4% were TIAs); and death, 2%. Connors and Wojak attribute the improvements to decreasing the balloon diameter to restore the vessel lumen, very slow inflation of the balloon (over 2 to 5 minutes), and the routine use of glycoprotein IIb/IIIa receptor inhibitors, such as abciximab, during angioplasty. Two hemorrhages (included in the neurological events rate) occurred during this period. They also avoid crossing a lesion more than once with the angioplasty balloon because that maneuver is likely to raise an intimal flap and cause the vessel to become occluded. One intrinsic advantage that endovascular approaches have over surgery is the ability to re-angioplasty. A stenotic vessel that has been suboptimally dilated initially can be further dilated on subsequent interventions. Another "pearl" discovered by these authors is the use of shorter angioplasty balloons to prevent straightening of the intracranial vessels after balloon inflation, making an injury or dissection less likely.

Mori et al demonstrated in several published case series the effectiveness of angioplasty in patients with short (≤5 mm), mildly eccentric or concentric (type A) lesions.[23] In their hands, these lesions had a periprocedural complication rate of 8% (1 stroke in 12). During the 2-year follow-up period, no ipsilateral stroke, neurological event, or angiographic stenosis occurred, and no bypass surgery or repeat angioplasty was needed. In angiographic lesions that were longer and more eccentric or chronically occluded, the procedure yielded less effective results. For lesions that were 5 to 10 mm in length or totally occluded and were less than 3 months from initial angioplasty (type B), the success rate was 86%. Angiographic restenosis occurred in 33% of the lesions within the 2-year follow-up period. Angioplasty attempts were unsuccessful in 2 of 21 patients. Patients with chronically occluded lesions that were 3 months or older or highly angular or long (>10 mm in length; type C) fared the worst. Angioplasty was associated with an initial success rate of 33% (3 of 9 patients) and a restenosis rate of 100% at 1 year. These results suggest that angiographic characteristics may help determine feasibility and periprocedural risks. One of nine patients with type C lesions experienced a stroke from abrupt closure of the stenotic vessel, suggesting that vessels harboring these lesions are extremely tenuous. The cumulative risk of ipsilateral stroke was 12% for type B lesions and 56% for type C lesions. Of note, the natural history of these lesions was not delineated according to lesion type in either the WASID study or the EC-IC bypass study. The studies by Mori et al[26,27] suggest that type C and possibly type B lesions as well should not be treated by angioplasty alone but rather may benefit from another endovascular technique or surgery.

In another series, 20 patients with intracranial vertebrobasilar stenosis were treated with angioplasty alone.[24] One dissection resulting in a stroke and one TIA occurred, for a 10% complication rate. Restenosis occurred in 14% during an average follow-up period of 8 months. The two cases of restenosis were in patients in whom residual stenosis of 20 to 30% remained at the end of the revascularization procedure.

Marks et al report a low periprocedural risk of 5% in their intracranial angioplasty series.[22] These authors also undersize the balloon and allow for residual stenosis. They frequently include anticoagulation (warfarin) therapy in their postprocedural regimen (prescribed for 18 of 23 patients), particularly if there was significant (>50%) residual stenosis or dissection. Two complications occurred in the immediate postprocedural period among this group of 23 patients. A vessel ruptured, which resulted in death, and an angioplasty site became occluded by a thrombus. The clot was successfully lysed with intraarterial tissue plasminogen activator. Two strokes occurred during the respective follow-up periods of 37 and 32 months. Only one of the strokes involved the territory supplied by the treated vessel. This stroke occurred in a vessel with 50% residual stenosis. Including the vessel rupture, the annual rate of stroke in the territory of the previously treated vessel was 3.2%, and the overall rate of stroke during the average 35.4 months of follow-up was 4.8%. This dramatically low frequency of strokes should be acknowledged because it occurred while warfarin therapy was often used in conjunction with revascularization therapy. This combination of therapies may best reduce the risk of strokes from hemodynamic, embolic, and small vessel arteriopathy sources.

In summary, angioplasty remains a new modality of therapy for intracranial atherosclerotic disease. Although no prospective randomized trials are available for review, numerous retrospective series suggest that this approach has promise. In all of the series, numerous dissections occurred, and mortality was usually a result of vessel

rupture or wire perforation. Strokes occurred rarely during the procedure, but on occasion, emboli were generated; and the vessels at greatest risk for restenosis or further strokes were those with residual stenosis. Furthermore, angioplasty eliminates one of the factors confounding optimal blood pressure management. With aggressive blood pressure control, no ischemia should be precipitated.

Procedural improvements are ongoing. New developments in wire technology and the introduction of catheters with soft hydrophilic coatings have made perforations rare. Undersizing the balloon makes rupture unlikely. Embolic phenomena can now be treated with medications such as glycoprotein IIb/IIIa receptor inhibitors. A caveat is that the use of IIb/IIIa inhibitors may increase the hemorrhagic risk of these procedures. In the future, protection devices may be available to collect plaque debris during angioplasty. This technology, whether it involves a filter or a balloon aspiration device placed distal to the angioplasty site, is on the horizon and is currently being used in the extracranial carotid distribution. Dissections can be prevented by use of either slower inflation techniques or shorter balloons (of note, the balloon length still must span the entire stenotic segment). If dissection does occur, intracranial stents can be placed to tack the intimal layer down. Stents have been used to improve the results of coronary angioplasty by restoring vessel luminal diameter and preventing restenosis. This strategy should apply to the intracranial circulation. Self-expanding stent characteristics of less radial force and enhanced navigational flexibility represent the technology that is advancing to become the appropriate tool for the treatment of intracranial stenosis. Unfortunately, stent navigation in tortuous anatomy can be hazardous, sometimes leading to complications.

There are two series of at least 10 patients each who underwent intracranial primary stenting for atherosclerotic lesions.[28,29] Both report excellent results with minimal residual stenosis and no neurological complications. Mori et al were unable to deliver a stent in two of 12 lesions.[29] They were able to successfully angioplasty these lesions. Improvements in trackability and flexibility will make stents easier to deliver. In the series reported by Mori et al, two lesions were type C, and eight lesions were type B lesions.[29] One type C lesion could not be accessed for stent delivery, which again demonstrates the difficulty in treating this kind of lesion. No restenosis or neurological events have been reported in the early postprocedural (<4 months) period. Gomez et al reported that three of their 12 patients had headaches and two had cranial nerve deficits, all of which resolved in 8 to 12 weeks.[28] The cranial nerve deficits were likely related to nerve injury resulting from basilar artery movement during stent placement.

Ramee et al proposed a combined approach.[30] They used primary angioplasty for revascularization. If the lesion was complex or long, primary stenting was attempted. If the results of primary angioplasty were sub-optimal because of either dissection or vessel recoil with residual stenosis, stenting was used. The combined approach yielded an excellent short-term outcome with a 93% success rate and a 53% "unexpected benefit" rate in that 8 of 15 patients had reversal of what was initially thought to be a permanent deficit from a prior stroke. This method is described in the coronary literature as provisional stenting; it has become popular for coronary revascularization.

Levy et al presented a series of 10 patients who underwent stent placement for medically refractory, symptomatic atherosclerotic disease of the basilar artery at our center.[31] Four patients were treated with direct stent placement, three with a staged procedure (angioplasty followed ≥1 month later by stent placement with or without repeated angioplasty), and three with conventional stent placement. In the group treated with direct stent placement, a dense quadriparesis developed in two patients after the procedure, with infarction of the ventral pons in these patients. In the staged stent placement group, no permanent neurological complications occurred after the procedure, and in the conventional stent placement group, one of three patients experienced a neurological complication involving homonymous hemianopsia. Based on these data, direct stent placement in the basilar artery is associated with a relatively high complication rate, compared with a staged procedure. Complications may result from an embolic shower following disruption of atheromatous plaque debris by high-profile devices such as stents, as demonstrated by the postprocedural imaging appearance of acute pontine infarctions. Additionally, displacement of debris by the stent into the ostia (snowplowing) of small brainstem perforating vessels may be responsible for the complications noted.

■ Patient Selection and Preparation

We use endoluminal revascularization for only symptomatic patients with high-grade intracranial stenosis because of the intrinsic risks of these procedures. A screening MR angiogram is performed that documents the target lesion. Direct correlation between the neurological deficit and the lesion location must be made prior to treatment. Dizziness alone, without a corresponding neurological deficit, is not adequate motivation for revascularization of the anterior circulation.

Initially, we treat all patients with antiplatelet therapy using aspirin and clopidogrel before consideration of the patient for revascularization. Patients in whom pharmacologic treatment has failed are scheduled for revascularization. We recently modified our treatment regimen after a few patients, each with posterior circulation atherosclerosis,

suffered devastating strokes while receiving pharmacologic therapy. At present, patients with severe stenotic symptomatic lesions are considered for revascularization primarily.

Cerebral blood flow measurements have played an increasingly important role in the treatment of symptomatic atherosclerotic lesions. Single-photon emission CT (SPECT) scans are used to study vascular perfusion and reserve.[8,12] Patients with symptomatic high-grade lesions and evidence of severe hypoperfusion ipsilateral to the stenosis are good candidates for revascularization. Patients with poor vascular reserve, as evidenced by acetazolamide-challenge SPECT, are also good candidates for revascularization. Computerized tomography (CT) perfusion techniques are being evaluated and analyzed to determine their correlation with actual vascular perfusion.[32–34] At our center, perfusion CT scans have gained acceptance as a means of studying vascular perfusion and reserve.

Patients with recent infarctions are considered for treatment within 2 to 4 weeks of the ictus. The volume of the infarction governs the timing from ictus until treatment. Large infarctions are permitted to stabilize as a means of reducing the risk of reperfusion injury. In addition, neurological signs and symptoms fluctuate in the immediate period after the onset of stroke, which makes interpretation of the periprocedural examination difficult. It is crucial that outcomes be monitored carefully during our early experience with device-based intracranial revascularization.

Before patients are considered for intracranial revascularization, it is essential that the cervical carotid artery, carotid artery origin, vertebral artery, and vertebral artery origin be free of significant atherosclerotic disease. Cervical carotid disease can be easily imaged by use of duplex ultrasonography. Vertebral artery or carotid origin disease cannot be adequately imaged by use of this technology. MR angiography can provide adequate images of the aortic arch and vertebral artery, especially if gadolinium bolus techniques are used. We have found that digital subtraction angiography is the "gold standard" for uncovering lesions in these locations.

If significant stenosis within the proximal vasculature is discovered, consideration should be given to a staged revascularization. The proximal lesion can be treated first. The intracranial lesion can be treated within 6 to 8 weeks after the proximal lesion has healed. Sometimes, the flow limitation created by the proximal lesion will make the distal lesion appear more severe on the angiographic image.

■ Pre- and Perioperative Procedure

Patients undergo routine preprocedural testing that includes blood cell count, electrolytes, EKG, chest X-ray, and coagulation profile. They are maintained on aspirin and clopidogrel for 72 hours before the procedure. Preprocedural inspection of lower-extremity pulses and distal perfusion are helpful as a means of avoiding periprocedural lower extremity ischemia.

The procedure is performed after midazolam and fentanyl have been administered to induce mild neuroleptic analgesia. Oxygen saturation, heart rate, blood pressure, urine output, and neurological status are monitored throughout the procedure. A 6-French sheath is placed into the femoral artery. This sheath is perfused with heparin saline flush (4 U heparin per cc of normal saline solution). A 5-French Sim II catheter (Terumo Medical, Somerset, New Jersey) is used for access to the brachiocephalic vessel. A three- or four-vessel, diagnostic contrast X-ray angiogram is performed to facilitate lesion characterization and to assess collateral circulation. Measurements are made of the target lesion. Proximal and distal vessel diameters and lesion length are measured. The tortuosity of the intracranial vascular pathway should be carefully assessed. In some cases, tight curves or bends in the artery that are proximal and distal to the lesion may prevent delivery of devices to the target vessel.

Anticoagulation

Anticoagulation is initiated by use of an intravenous or intraarterial bolus of heparin in the range of 70 U/kg. All saline flush bags are infused with heparin as previously mentioned. Activated coagulation time (ACT) is measured and maintained within the range of 250 to 300 seconds. Numerous practitioners have suggested the use of intravenous IIb/IIIa inhibitors as a means of preventing acute or subacute thrombosis in instrumented plaque. Although this has been widely accepted in cardiology, judicious application of this pharmacologic therapy in neurointerventional procedures is warranted. Revascularization of a chronically ischemic vascular bed can result in reperfusion hemorrhage. Bleeding in the face of platelet-receptor blockade can result in uncontrolled intracranial hemorrhage and death. Careful blood pressure monitoring and aggressive blood pressure control are tantamount to safe use of IIb/IIIa inhibitors in this patient population. If IIb/IIIa inhibitors are to be used, a smaller bolus of heparin (40 or 50 U/kg) is given with an ACT objective of 225 seconds.

Surgical Technique

The procedure is performed by use of a biplane digital subtraction angiography (DSA) fluoroscopy unit (Toshiba Medical Systems, Tustin, California). After the diagnostic catheter is positioned in the target vessel and the ACT has been adequately adjusted with heparin, an exchange-length *glidewire* (Terumo Medical, Somerset, New Jersey) is placed through the diagnostic catheter into the target vessel. The diagnostic catheter is then removed. A 6-French straight Envoy catheter (Cordis Neurovascular, Miami Lakes, Florida) is placed over the wire and into the internal carotid or vertebral artery. The position of the catheter

is critical. If a stent is to be used, the catheter tip should be placed as distal in the target vessel as possible. Positioning of the guide catheter can lead to spasm, vessel telescoping, and dissection. Roadmap fluoroscopy can be very useful to avoid vessel injury.

Once the guide catheter is in position, a micro-catheter (Prowler14, Cordis Neurovascular) and microwire (Transcend Wire; Boston Scientific Scimed, Natick, Massachusetts) are used to cross the lesion. The microcatheter is advanced through the lesion into the distal target vessel. The microwire is removed, and a 300-cm exchange length 0.014-inch wire (light- or medium-weight balance, Guidant/ACS, Temecula, California) is placed through the microcatheter. The microcatheter is then removed. Great care must be taken to ensure that the position of the distal wire does not change during device exchange.

Revascularization Strategies

The strategy governing the choice of devices for revascularization is fueled with controversy. Initially, the use of intracranial stents was reserved for patients who had failed previous angioplasty because of significant vessel recoil or dissection. This strategy is supported by the work of Connors and Wojak, who advocate angioplasty with a low-profile coronary balloon.[21] They routinely avoid oversizing the balloon relative to the vessel diameter. They perform slow inflation and deflation of the balloon at low pressures, typically below 6 atm. In this way, the plaque is stretched and not cracked. They postulate that this prevents dissections and limits vessel recoil. Connors and Wojak have not seen a need for intracranial stent placement. Their angioplasty series includes more than 50 patients.

In Buffalo, we advocate the use of staged angioplasty and stent placement.[35] We stent vessels after angioplasty whenever the anatomy of the vessels permits safe delivery of the device. Preliminary results, albeit without long-term angiographic follow-up, indicate a reduced rate of restenosis.

To facilitate balloon delivery, the shortest balloon length that covers the lesion should be chosen. We routinely undersize the balloon relative to the vessel diameter; for example, for an MCA lesion, a balloon diameter of 1.5 or 2 mm would be chosen. For short lesions, a 10-mm length balloon would be used. For longer lesions, a 15 or 20 mm balloon can be used. Longer balloons may be more difficult to deliver and may require distal wire purchase. Inflations are kept below 8 atm, and the balloon is slowly inflated and deflated.

Stent delivery, placement, and deployment involve a steep learning curve. Our experience with intracranial stents was preceded by a robust animal experience.[36] We would suggest practice in models prior to clinical application. As mentioned previously, the decision to perform stent placement should be based on postangioplasty results. Excessive vessel recoil or dissection may mandate stent placement. The stent diameter should be larger than the vessel diameter by ~10 to 20%. The stent length should be chosen so that the entire lesion will be covered with an additional 1 to 2 mm overlap onto the healthy vessel on each side.

Stent delivery can be difficult, especially when the radius of curvature of the carotid siphon or vertebral artery near the C1 vertebra is low. It is critical that the wire has a firm purchase in the distal vessel. For a stent to be positioned in the supraclinoid carotid artery, the wire should be positioned in the M2 or M3 segment of the ipsilateral MCA. For a midbasilar stenosis, the wire should be positioned in the P2 or P3 segment of the posterior cerebral artery. During delivery, the position of the distal end of the guide catheter should be carefully monitored. As the stent impacts tight turns in the vasculature, the guide catheter may back out. This movement can result in loss of guide catheter position and distal wire purchase. Great care must be taken to advance the guide catheter distally to ensure adequate support for stent delivery. On occasion, a second wire (V18 Control; Boston Scientific Scimed, Natick, Massachusetts) is placed in the guide catheter for improved stability.

Once the stent has crossed the lesion, careful attention must be paid to positioning. Prior to deployment, we routinely perform numerous DSA studies to ensure that the lesion is adequately covered by the stent. Rarely will patients become symptomatic due to flow obstruction caused by the stent before deployment. It is advisable to take time to ensure that the stent is positioned properly prior to deployment. Deployment should be performed slowly and evenly. The balloon should be expanded fully, and the stent should be imbedded into normal vessel proximal and distal to the lesion. A DSA study performed after the procedure should confirm placement, patency, and apposition of the stent to the wall of the vessel. Poststent angioplasty can be performed with a slightly larger balloon if needed. If the stent does not adequately cover the lesion, another stent should be placed. Sluggish flow or evidence of thrombus in the stent may require the administration of IIb/IIIa inhibitors to prevent acute or subacute thrombosis. Runoff in the distal vasculature must be carefully examined to ensure that distal embolization has not occurred.

At the conclusion of the procedure, the effect of the heparin is allowed to reverse on its own. The groin sheath can be left in place and removed when the coagulation cascade has normalized, after which pressure can be applied to the groin region to ensure hemostasis. Alternatively, a femoral artery closure device can be used while the patient is receiving anticoagulant or antiplatelet therapy.

In the perioperative period, blood pressure is closely monitored and controlled. Clopidogrel is continued for 30 days. Aspirin is continued for the life of the patient.

■ Case Study

This 73-year-old man presented with unstable angina and prior coronary angiography demonstrating three-vessel coronary disease. He was being prepared for coronary artery bypass grafting and had a 1-year history of right hemisphere TIAs. Diagnostic cerebral angiography revealed a 90% petrous carotid stenosis (**Fig. 19–1**). A brain SPECT scan using 99 m Tc-bicisate (Neurolite; DuPont Pharmaceutical Co., Wilmington, DE) demonstrated hypoperfusion of the right internal carotid distribution—particularly of the watershed areas in the dorsolateral MCA and between the anterior cerebral and middle cerebral arteries. Petrous carotid revascularization was indicated to reduce his perioperative stroke risk, particularly in the setting of hypotension during bypass (**Fig. 19–1B–D**).

■ Conclusion

The natural history of intracranial atherosclerosis must be well understood to better make decisions regarding who should undergo endovascular revascularization and when treatment should be performed. Our techniques have evolved such that we perform revascularization in symptomatic patients with high-grade intracranial stenosis and blood-flow assessment revealing hypoperfusion in the threatened territory. We are increasingly using stent-assisted angioplasty for complex plaques as well as when initial angioplasty results are suboptimal.

The decision to perform revascularization becomes more difficult when hypoperfusion on SPECT imaging is not demonstrated or the patient has not failed a course of treatment with antiplatelet agents. This group of patients could be candidates for endovascular revascularization. Another challenging group includes asymptomatic patients with magnetic resonance angiography evidence of intracranial stenosis. We do not treat these patients unless SPECT imaging reveals moderate or severe hypoperfusion or lack of reserve in a patient who is to undergo a coronary bypass procedure.

Our techniques for endoluminal revascularization of intracranial stenosis have evolved in accordance with the literature. We use short, undersized angioplasty balloons with slower inflations. We continue to administer two different antiplatelet agents for 72 hours before the procedure and may use IIb/IIIa inhibitors during revascularization of longer, ulcerated lesions. We use stent-assisted angioplasty to rescue prior angioplasty dissections or occlusions.[21] We use staged angioplasty and stent secondarily to reduce residual stenosis.

Given the constant evolution of microcatheters, microwires, and angioplasty balloons and stents, our ability to treat these lesions continues to improve. There

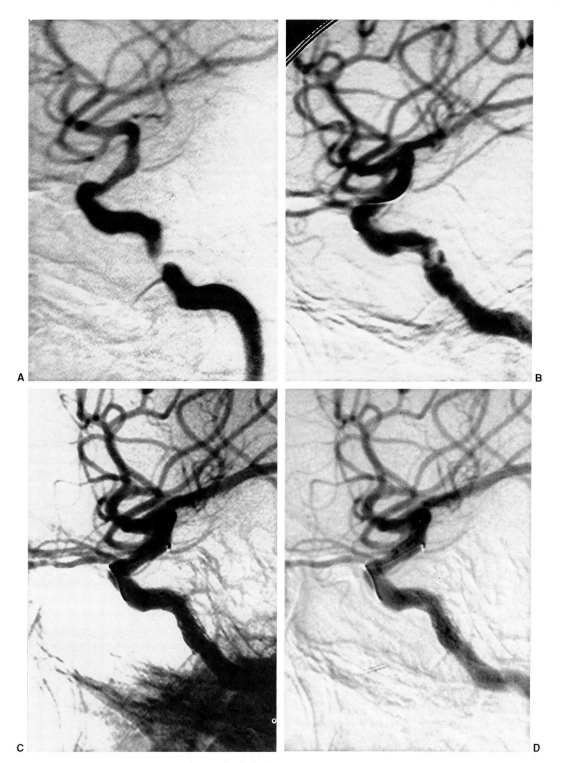

FIGURE 19–1 (A) Preoperative right internal carotid arteriography in reverse oblique orientation demonstrates high-grade petrous carotid artery stenosis. **(B)** A microcatheter (Rapid Transit, Cordis Neurovascular, Miami Lakes, FL) was advanced with an AllStar microguidewire (ACS; Guidant, Santa Clara, CA). After being placed across the lesion, the microcatheter was exchanged for a 2 × 11-mm coronary artery balloon catheter (Chubby; Boston Scientific Schneider, Plymouth, MN). These devices were exchanged after two balloon angioplasty inflations were completed. Improvement in the lumen is seen, but significant stenosis of the vessel and irregularity within the plaque remain. **(C)** The Chubby balloon catheter is exchanged for a 4 × 12-mm AVE GFX coronary artery stent (Medtronic AVE, Santa Rosa, CA). This is after initial deployment of the stent. There is considerable improvement in the lesion. No significant stenosis remains. **(D)** Oblique view demonstrates improvement in luminal diameter and a marked improvement in flow through the middle cerebral artery.

appears to be a role for revascularization, particularly in the concentric, short stenosis.

■ Acknowledgment

We thank Paul H. Dressel for preparation of the figure.

■ References

1. Chimowitz MI, Kokkinos J, Strong J, et al. The Warfarin-Aspirin Symptomatic Intracranial Disease Study. Neurology 1995;45(8):1488–1493

2. Chimowitz MI, Lynn MJ, Howlett Smith H, et al. Comparison of warfarin and aspirin for symptomatic intracranial arterial stenosis. N Engl J Med 2005;352:1305–1316

3. The EC-IC bypass study. N Engl J Med 1987;317(16):1030–1032

4. Craig DR, Meguro K, Watridge C, Robertson JT, Barnett HJ, Fox AJ. Intracranial internal carotid artery stenosis. Stroke 1982;13(6):825–828

5. Marzewski DJ, Furlan AJ, St Louis P, Little JR, Modic MT, Williams G. Intracranial internal carotid artery stenosis: longterm prognosis. Stroke 1982;13(6):821–824

6. Gorter JW. Major bleeding during anticoagulation after cerebral ischemia: patterns and risk factors. Stroke Prevention in Reversible Ischemia Trial (SPIRIT). European Atrial Fibrillation Trial (EAFT) study groups. Neurology 1999;53(6):1319–1327

7. Thijs VN, Albers GW. Symptomatic intracranial atherosclerosis: outcome of patients who fail antithrombotic therapy. Neurology 2000;55(4):490–497

8. Ozgur HT, Kent Walsh T, Masaryk A, et al. Correlation of cerebrovascular reserve as measured by acetazolamide-challenged SPECT with angiographic flow patterns and intra- or extracranial arterial stenosis. AJNR Am J Neuroradiol 2001;22(5):928–936

9. Webster MW, Makaroun MS, Steed DL, Smith HA, Johnson DW, Yonas H. Compromised cerebral blood flow reactivity is a predictor of stroke in patients with symptomatic carotid artery occlusive disease. J Vasc Surg 1995;21(2):338–345

10. Yonas H, Pindzola RR, Meltzer CC, Sasser H. Qualitative versus quantitative assessment of cerebrovascular reserves. Neurosurgery 1998;42(5):1005–1012

11. Caplan LR, Hennerici M. Impaired clearance of emboli (washout) is an important link between hypoperfusion, embolism, and ischemic stroke. Arch Neurol 1998;55(11):1475–1482

12. Yokota C, Hasegawa Y, Minematsu K, Yamaguchi T. Effect of acetazolamide reactivity on [corrected] long-term outcome in patients with major cerebral artery occlusive diseases. Stroke 1998;29(3):640–644

13. Awad I, Furlan AJ, Little JR. Changes in intracranial stenotic lesions after extracranial- intracranial bypass surgery. J Neurosurg 1984;60(4):771–776

14. Awad IA, Little JR, Furlan AJ. Conversion of an intracranial arterial stenosis to a symptomatic occlusion after EC/IC bypass surgery. Neurosurgery 1983;13(6):734

15. Grubb RL Jr, Powers WJ, Derdeyn CP, Adams HP Jr, Clarke WR. The carotid occlusion surgery study. Neurosurg Focus 2003 Mar 15;14(3):e9

16. Akins PT, Pilgram TK, Cross DT III, Moran CJ. Natural history of stenosis from intracranial atherosclerosis by serial angiography. Stroke 1998;29(2):433–438

17. Callahan AS III, Berger BL, Beuter MJ, Devlin TG. Possible short-term amelioration of basilar plaque by high-dose atorvastatin: use of reductase inhibitors for intracranial plaque stabilization. J Neuroimaging 2001;11(2):202–204

18. Clark WM, Barnwell SL, Nesbit G, O'Neill OR, Wynn ML, Coull BM. Safety and efficacy of percutaneous transluminal angioplasty for intracranial atherosclerotic stenosis. Stroke 1995;26(7):1200–1204

19. Higashida RT, Tsai FY, Halbach VV, Barnwell SL, Dowd CF, Hieshima GB. Interventional neurovascular techniques in the treatment of stroke—state-of-the-art therapy. J Intern Med 1995;237(1):105–115

20. Takis C, Kwan ES, Pessin MS, Jacobs DH, Caplan LR. Intracranial angioplasty: experience and complications. AJNR Am J Neuroradiol 1997;18(9):1661–1668

21. Connors JJ III, Wojak JC. Percutaneous transluminal angioplasty for intracranial atherosclerotic lesions: evolution of technique and short-term results. J Neurosurg 1999;91(3):415–423

22. Marks MP, Marcellus M, Norbash AM, Steinberg GK, Tong D, Albers GW. Outcome of angioplasty for atherosclerotic intracranial stenosis. Stroke 1999;30(5):1065–1069

23. Mori T, Fukuoka M, Kazita K, Mori K. Follow-up study after intracranial percutaneous transluminal cerebral balloon angioplasty. AJNR Am J Neuroradiol 1998;19(8):1525–1533

24. Nahser HC, Henkes H, Weber W, Berg-Dammer E, Yousry TA, Kuhne D. Intracranial vertebrobasilar stenosis: angioplasty and follow-up. AJNR Am J Neuroradiol 2000;21(7):1293–1301

25. Terada T, Higashida RT, Halbach VV, et al. Transluminal angioplasty for arteriosclerotic disease of the distal vertebral and basilar arteries. J Neurol Neurosurg Psychiatry 1996;60(4):377–381

26. Mori T, Kazita K, Mori K. Cerebral angioplasty and stenting for intracranial vertebral atherosclerotic stenosis. AJNR Am J Neuroradiol 1999;20(5):787–789

27. Mori T, Mori K, Fukuoka M, Arisawa M, Honda S. Percutaneous transluminal cerebral angioplasty: serial angiographic follow-up after successful dilatation. Neuroradiology 1997;39(2):111–116

28. Gomez CR, Misra VK, Liu MW, et al. Elective stenting of symptomatic basilar artery stenosis. Stroke 2000;31(1):95–99

29. Mori T, Kazita K, Chokyu K, Mima T, Mori K. Short-term arteriographic and clinical outcome after cerebral angioplasty and stenting for intracranial vertebrobasilar and carotid atherosclerotic occlusive disease. AJNR Am J Neuroradiol 2000;21(2):249–254

30. Ramee SR, Dawson R, McKinley KL, et al. Provisional stenting for symptomatic intracranial stenosis using a multidisciplinary approach: acute results, unexpected benefit, and one- year outcome. Catheter Cardiovasc Interv 2001;52(4):457–467

31. Levy EI, Hanel RA, Boulos AS, et al. Comparison of periprocedure complications resulting from direct stent placement compared with those due to conventional and staged stent placement in the basilar artery. J Neurosurg 2003;99(4):653–660

32. Latchaw RE, Yonas H, Hunter GJ, et al. Guidelines and recommendations for perfusion imaging in cerebral ischemia: a scientific statement for healthcare professionals by the writing group on perfusion imaging, from the Council on Cardiovascular Radiology of the American Heart Association. Stroke 2003;34(4):1084–1104

33. Hamberg LM, Hunter GJ, Maynard KI, et al. Functional CT perfusion imaging in predicting the extent of cerebral infarction from a 3-hour middle cerebral arterial occlusion in a primate stroke model. AJNR Am J Neuroradiol 2002;23(6):1013–1021

34. Hunter GJ, Silvennoinen HM, Hamberg LM, et al. Whole-brain CT perfusion measurement of perfused cerebral blood volume in acute ischemic stroke: probability curve for regional infarction. Radiology 2003;227(3):725–730

35. Levy EI, Hanel RA, Bendok BR, et al. Staged stent-assisted angioplasty for symptomatic intracranial vertebrobasilar artery stenosis. J Neurosurg 2002;97(6):1294–1301

36. Levy EI, Boulos AS, Hanel RA, et al. In vivo model of intracranial stent implantation: a pilot study to examine the histological response of cerebral vessels after randomized implantation of heparin-coated and uncoated endoluminal stents in a blinded fashion. J Neurosurg 2003;98(3):544–553

20

Microsurgical Treatment of Cavernous Malformations

MUSTAFA K. BAŞKAYA, ANDREW JEA, AND JACQUES J. MORCOS

Objectives: After completing this chapter, the reader should be able to report options for managing a cavernous malformation patient, and the appropriate indications and approaches for surgical resection.

Accreditation: The AANS* is accredited by the Accreditation Council for Continuing Medical Education (ACCME) to sponsor continuing medical education for physicians.

Credit: The AANS designates this educational activity for a maximum of 15 credits in Category 1 credit toward the AMA Physician's Recognition Award. Each physician should claim only those hours of credit that he/she spent in the educational activity.

The Home Study Examination is online on the AANS Web site at: http://www.aans.org/education/books/controversy.asp

* The acronym AANS refers to both the American Association of Neurological Surgeons and the American Association of Neurosurgeons.

Cavernous malformations (CMs), also known as cavernous angiomas or cavernomas, are compact lesions comprised of sinusoidal vascular channels lined by a single layer of endothelium and lacking the full complement of mature vessel wall components. Between the vascular channels in the core of the lesion, there is loose connective tissue stroma without intervening brain parenchyma. Varying degrees of gliotic neural tissue may be found in the periphery of the lesion. The channels are often filled with stagnated blood in varying degrees of thrombosis and degradation.[1]

The spectrum of cerebrovascular malformations includes arteriovenous malformations, cavernous malformations, venous angiomas, and capillary telangiectasias. In a representative autopsy series, almost 5% of the general population harbored one of these malformations.[1,2] Although there is no reliable study which reflects the true incidence and prevalence of CMs in the population at present, the prevalence of CMs has been estimated to be between 0.4 and 0.9% of the population and 8 to 15% of all vascular malformations.[1–3]

The majority of CMs are located supratentorially. Of the supratentorial CMs, most are located in the white matter of the cerebral hemispheres. The infratentorial CMs are located in the cerebellum, pons, midbrain, and medulla. Less-frequent locations of CMs are the lateral and third ventricles, cranial nerves, and optic chiasm. Acute hemorrhage from a chiasmal CM is a rare cause of permanent visual loss.[4] Of the extracerebral locations the cavernous sinus, the orbits, and the spinal cord are the most common.

Because CMs are low-flow lesions without arterialized veins or large feeding arteries, they are poorly visualized by angiography and thus labeled "occult." Computerized tomography (CT) is more sensitive at detecting CMs, but its specificity is low because most appear simply as high-density lesions with little or no contrast enhancement. This is in contrast to the high sensitivity and specificity of magnetic resonance imaging (MRI) for CMs. The MRI appearance of CMs has been categorized into four types: a hyperintense core on T1- and T2-weighted images representing subacute hemorrhage (type I); a "classic" picture of mixed-signal, reticulated core surrounded by a low-signal rim (type II); a iso- or hypointense lesion on T1 and markedly hypointense lesion with hypointense rim on T2, which corresponds to chronic hemorrhage (type III); and punctate, poorly visualized hypointense foci, which can be visualized only on gradient echo MRI, representing tiny CM or telangiectasia (type IV).[5,25]

With most asymptomatic CMs, particularly when the diagnosis is relatively clear by MRI characteristics, the right approach for the patient is conservative management with close follow-up, with a few exceptions. In contrast to a bleeding episode from an arteriovenous malformation (AVM), a bleeding episode from a CM is rarely life threatening.[6] However, there is more controversy with symptomatic cavernous malformations which hemorrhage in deep, difficult-to-access surgical locations. Here, there are arguments for and against treatment, as well as regarding the type of treatment—open surgery versus stereotactic radiosurgery. The key to making the proper recommendation to the patient is an understanding of the natural history of cavernous malformations. The available data, however, is not as solid as with cerebral AVMs.

■ Natural History and Clinicopathological Features

The rate of hemorrhage for CMs is not as well defined as for AVMs. Several reasons explain this discrepancy. First, some of the published studies dealing with natural history of CMs calculated the *retrospective* hemorrhage rate, whereas others calculated the *prospective* hemorrhage rate by using newer databases. The latter studies seem to be more likely to reflect the true risk of hemorrhage from a CM, but their period of follow-up is understandably shorter.

The second reason is the definition of hemorrhage in published series in the literature. Hemorrhage from a CM may not always be identifiable clinically or radiologically in contrast to hemorrhage from an AVM. This is because there is no uniform pattern of bleeding from CMs, nor is there homogenous terminology to define hemorrhagic episodes. A report suggested that radiologically defined hemorrhage might miss clinically significant events. It therefore proposed the use of "event rates"—defining neurological deterioration that is experienced by the patient as a subjective worsening, and associated with objective worsening of clinical status, independent of the radiological findings.[7] A study described the three patterns of hemorrhage from CMs: "slow ooze" producing the hemosiderin ring seen on MRI, "intralesional hemorrhage" producing an expansion of the lesion on MRI with or without subtle increase in symptomatology, and "gross hemorrhage" producing acute severe symptoms and intra- or extralesional acute hemorrhage on MRI.[8]

Third, the clinical importance of hemorrhage from a CM is dependent not only on the severity of hemorrhage but also on the location of the CM in the brain. For example, a moderate-size intracerebral hemorrhage (ICH) in the nondominant anterior frontal lobe may not cause any neurological symptoms that may warrant radiological work-up, while even a small intralesional hemorrhage from a CM in the brainstem or optic chiasm may produce significant disability.

Epilepsy and focal neurological deficits were found to be the most common symptoms in a series of 30 children with an average age of 9.4 years.[9] A study of 36 children demonstrated higher hemorrhage risk and lower incidence of epilepsy—which may be related to chronic or recurrent microbleeding—when compared with adults.[10]

A retrospective study calculated an annual hemorrhage rate of 1.3% per patient-year[11]; a second study[12] calculated a rate of 0.25% per patient-year[12]; and still a third study reported a rate of 2.3% per patient-year.[13] A prospective study reported a 0.7% hemorrhage rate per lesion-year.[15] Another prospective study of 11 patients with CMs reported an overall hemorrhage rate of 2.6% per patient-year.[11] Rebleeding rate in patients with previous hemorrhage from their CMs was 4.5% per year, in contrast to a bleeding rate of 0.6% in patients without prior evidence of hemorrhage. In a retrospective review of 141 patients with CM and previous hemorrhage, the cumulative incidence of a second hemorrhage was 14% after 1 year and 56% after 5 years; during the first 2.5 years after a hemorrhage, the monthly rehemorrhage rate was 2%, and the risk then decreased spontaneously to less than 1% per month, a 2.4-fold decline.[14] Rehemorrhage rates were higher in younger patients. **Table 20–1** summarizes the overall hemorrhage rates found in published case series.

The actual population hemorrhage rates likely lie between the lowest retrospective and the highest prospective rates. Patients with asymptomatic lesions have traditionally included those presenting with mild headache and nonspecific symptoms. Although there is insufficient data to precisely identify which patients progress to develop symptoms or the risk factors associated with symptomatic transformation, several authors have implicated the following putative "predisposing" factors.[6] A report mentioned that the hemorrhage risk may be higher in females and in CMs located in the brainstem.[15] Others also found that females have a higher risk of hemorrhage. In one study, estrogen receptors were demonstrated in a few CMs in females.[16]

Immunohistochemical studies demonstrated the presence of proliferating cell nuclear antigen and angiogenic growth factors (vascular endothelial growth factor, basic fibroblast growth factor, and transforming growth factor α), suggesting that the endothelium of CMs is not static but it proliferates.[17–19] These findings led some authors to hypothesize that CMs should be classified as slowly growing vascular neoplasms rather than true developmental vascular malformations.[17–19]

Table 20–1 Reported Overall Hemorrhage Rates of Cavernous Malformations

Author (Year)	Series Type	n	Hemorrhage Rates
Curling et al (1991)[12]	Retrospective	32	0.25%/patient-year
Robinson et al (1991)[15]	Prospective	66	0.7%/lesion-year
Kondziolka et al (1995)[11]	Retrospective arm of study below	122	1.3%/patient-year
Kondziolka et al (1995)[11]	Prospective arm of study above	122	2.6%/patient-year (4.5%/patient-year for rebleeding; 0.6%/patient-year for first bleed)
Kim et al (1997)[13]	Retrospective	62	2.3%/patient-year
Barker et al (2001)[14]	Retrospective	141	14% for first year after bleed, cumulative risk 56% after 5 years; 2%/month for first 2.5 years, then 1%/month

■ Familial Cavernous Malformations

Familial cases of cavernous malformations have been recognized to constitute 30 to 50% of all cases, although a referral bias may be responsible for exaggerating this frequency.[20] Familial cavernomas are believed to be transmitted as an autosomal dominant trait. The gene *Krit1*, located at the *CCM1* locus and responsible for familial cavernomas, has been localized to the long arm of chromosome 7.[21–24] It was initially characterized in patients of Hispanic descent.[20]

Compared with sporadic cases, familial patients more often harbor multiple lesions. In a series of familial cases only, 84% of patients had multiple lesions versus 10 to 15% of patients in sporadic cases.[5] A French study of 33 asymptomatic patients diagnosed with familial cerebral CMs followed prospectively showed appearance of a new lesion—de novo formation—in 30.3% of patients, confirming the dynamic nature of familial CMs as a hallmark of this variant.[25]

A report observed a 3.1% symptomatic hemorrhage rate per patient per year in a series of eight patients with 30% familial cases.[2] A study of only familial CMs reported a prospective hemorrhage rate of 1.1% per lesion-year (6.5% per patient-year).[5] The disparity in this familial series between lesion and patient hemorrhage rates underscores the high frequency of multiple lesions in familial cases. A study of 18 cases of multiple CMs and 200 lesions determined a hemorrhagic rate per lesion per year of <1%.[26] A Japanese case report described a patient not only with multiple congenital CMs but also with a thrombosed cerebral AVM.[27] Evaluation of congenital vascular anomalies needs to take into consideration the combination of other congenital vascular

anomalies and their familial occurrence. **Table 20–2** summarizes the hemorrhage rates for familial CMs and cases of multiple CMs already reported in the literature.

Sporadic and familial forms of these lesions behave similarly, or there is insufficient data to conclusively show a difference.[2]

■ Cavernous Malformations of the Brainstem

Cavernous malformations of the brainstem constitute a special entity and pose a challenge to neurosurgeons dealing with these lesions for different reasons. In view of their location, they rarely present incidentally. They produce more severe symptoms and neurological deficits than CMs in other locations. Clinically, these patients generally present with an ictus. The most common symptoms are headache, vertigo, nausea, and diplopia. The most common focal deficits are palsies of cranial nerves III to VII. One case report described cerebellar mutism after hemorrhage from a midbrain CM.[28] Another anecdotal report described a patient presenting with acute hydrocephalus from a hemorrhagic tectal CM.[29] Two cases of hemorrhagic brainstem CMs causing vestibular and auditory symptoms, such as sudden deafness, fluctuating hearing loss, and Meniere-like vertigo, have been reported.[30] In a series of 41 patients and a review of another 98 cases from the literature, none of the brainstem cavernomas presented as an incidental finding.[31]

Second, there is evidence in the literature that the hemorrhage rate of brainstem CMs is greater than in other locations. A series of 100 patients with CMs of the brainstem found a 5% per person annual risk of

Table 20–2 Reported Hemorrhage Rates in Familial and Multiple Cavernous Malformation (CM) Cases

Author (Year)	Series Type	n	Hemorrhage Rates
Zabramski et al (1994)[5]	Prospective	59	6.5%/patient-year and 1.1%/lesion-year (in familial cases)
Moriarity et al (1999)[2]	Retrospective	N/A	3.1%/patient-year (including 30% familial cases)
Perez Lopez et al (2002)[26]	Retrospective	18	<1%/lesion-year in cases of multiple CMs

Table 20–3 Reported Hemorrhage Rates of Brainstem Cavernous Malformations

Author (Year)	Series Type	n	Hemorrhage Rates
Fritschi et al (1994)[31]	Retrospective	134	2.7%/year without previous hemorrhage and 21%/year with previous hemorrhage
Portor et al (1999)[16]	Retrospective	100	5%/year
Kupersmith et al (2001)[32]	Retrospective	37	2.46%/year without previous hemorrhage & 5.1%/year with previous hemorrhage

hemorrhage.[16] Of 12 patients who were followed-up without surgical intervention for an average of 35 months, 7 were in the same condition or better (58%), 4 were worse (33%), and one died. Another study reported a 2.7% annual rate of hemorrhage in patients without previous hemorrhagic events, and 21% in those with previous hemorrhage.[31] A retrospective review of 37 patients[32] yielded a bleeding rate of 2.46% per year with brainstem CMs and a rebleeding rate of 5.1% per year; younger patients <35 years old and CMs >10 mm in diameter showed a greater propensity to bleed. The problem here is that this higher rate in the brainstem may be because hemorrhages in this location are usually symptomatic and therefore easier to identify than hemorrhage from lesions in less eloquent locations. **Table 20–3** summarizes the bleeding rates found in previously published reports for brainstem CMs.

Particularly in the brainstem, multiple bleeding episodes may increase the likelihood of a persistent neurological deficit. In the series of Porter et al, rebleeding caused debilitating and persistent deficits in 50% of patients with CMs of the brainstem and thalamus.[16]

■ Cavernous Malformations of the Thalamus

There are only rare reports of thalamic CMs. One Italian study examined the clinical course, treatment, and outcome of 12 patients with symptomatic thalamic CMs.[33] Sixty-six percent of patients presented with intracerebral hemorrhage; four patients underwent radical surgery, resulting in one death, one patient without change in neurological status, and two improved patients. One patient underwent radiosurgery that resulted in rehemorrhage 4 months after the procedure. Five patients underwent conservative treatment, with a 40% rate of rebleeding within 2 years.

■ Cavernous Malformations of the Third Ventricle

Patients with lesions in the region of the third ventricle presented with a more insidious onset of symptoms related to their mass effect rather than an acute hemorrhagic episode. None of these lesions were identified incidentally.[34,35]

Outcome is related to premorbid status, and preoperative cognitive difficulties are unlikely to resolve after surgery. Given the nature of the location of these lesions—suprachiasmatic region, the region of the foramen of Monro, the wall and floor of the third ventricle—surgery carries a significant risk of at least transient endocrinologic or neurological dysfunction.[2]

■ Cavernous Malformations of the Lateral Ventricles

Ventricular location is rare for CMs. Only 10 pediatric cases out of 46 previous cases of intraventricular CMs have been published.[36] Imaging features differ from intraparenchymal sites. Diagnosis is made only by histopathological examination due to the lack of classic magnetic resonance image (MRI) findings.[37]

■ Cavernous Malformations of the Spinal Cord

A descriptive study found four modes of clinical presentation in patients with CMs of the spinal cord.[38] These presentations relate directly to the degree of extralesional hemorrhage. Patients may present with an acute onset followed by a rapid decline, an acute onset followed by a gradual decline, a slow progressive decline, or discrete episodes of decline with intervening remission. The latter clinical picture of exacerbations and partial or complete remissions is also seen with CMs of the brainstem and accounts for the fact that CMs of the spinal cord and/or brainstem are frequently initially misdiagnosed as multiple sclerosis. The symptoms of spinal cord CMs generally consist of a painful myelopathy progressing to paraparesis or paraplegia.[39] As with cavernous malformations in the region of the third ventricle, there is little in the literature discussing hemorrhage rate in these lesions.

Outcomes in the most recent series are good, with almost all patients showing improvement in their symptoms following surgery.[38,39] Most authors advocate surgery for symptomatic patients and believe that postoperative outcome is related to preoperative status.[38,39] These authors also advocate following lesions found incidentally in asymptomatic patients.

■ Extra-axial Cavernous Malformations

The majority of these lesions grows within the cavernous sinus and expands it, stretching the third, fourth, and fifth cranial nerves over the pseudocapsule of the CM. The sixth cranial nerve is usually contained within the substance of the malformation.[40] Patients present with the acute or subacute onset of visual symptoms such as diplopia, ptosis, exophthalmos, and visual acuity disturbances.

In contrast to cerebral CMs, these lesions do not have a characteristic MRI appearance. However, a study reported MRI features of CMs of the cavernous sinus that may help in differentiation from meningiomas, such as a dumbbell shape with a small part in the suprasellar region and a large part in the cavernous sinus, as well as higher signal intensity on T2-weighted images.[41]

■ Conservative Management

Conservative management does not necessarily mean observation only. In some cases, microsurgical resection may actually be considered a more conservative route than expectant observation.

Supratentorial Cavernous Malformations

Surgical management does not appear to be indicated for the control of seizures unless intractable in nature. However, if a patient has a new-onset seizure and workup reveals a CM associated with a large hematoma, the most conservative approach may be to allow the hemorrhage to resorb, and once the patient is neurologically stable to excise the lesion.[42]

Brainstem Cavernous Malformations

There are two approaches to symptomatic brainstem CMs. For a first-time bleed, the most conservative approach is to follow the patient clinically. If the patient has a second neurological event from hemorrhage and the lesion is surgically accessible, then surgical excision may very well be the most conservative approach.

Multiple Cavernous Malformations

Multiple CMs should be treated as if the symptomatic lesion was the only lesion. Although there may be simultaneous bleeding in two or more lesions, surgical treatment should be undertaken for lesions jeopardizing critical structures or exerting mass effect.[43] All other lesions are to be followed expectantly like any other incidental CM.

Spinal Cord Cavernous Malformations

The potential for neurological devastation from a hemorrhage is very high. The question of whether this high potential warrants prophylactic surgery as the most conservative approach remains unanswered in clinical studies and anecdotal reports.

■ Microsurgery for Supratentorial Cavernous Malformations

Indications

The indications for microsurgical resection of supratentorial CMs are outlined by Shah and Heros[44]: (1) progressive neurological deficit, (2) documented episodes of recurrent hemorrhage, (3) medically intractable epilepsy, and (4) the need for tissue to establish a pathological diagnosis. In summary, accessibility, certainty of diagnosis, history of recurrent hemorrhage, and significance of focal neurological deficit are the main factors to weigh in the decision of whether to recommend surgical resection or not.

A mathematical analysis of surgical decision-making in cerebral CMs showed that for superficial lesions, permissible surgical risk ranged from 0.4 to 2.8% of combined morbidity and mortality.[45] The surgical gain of morbidity-free life expectancy was small (0 to 1.1 years). For deep lesions, permissible risk of surgery was larger, 64.1% for 20-year-olds and 31.4% for 60-year-olds. The gain in morbidity-free life expectancy was 17 to 35 years for 20-year-olds, but only 1.1 to 3.1 years for 60-year-olds. Hence, surgery is mathematically justified for younger patients with deep lesions.

Technical Pearls

The MRI is the principal imaging modality with its multiplanar capability. It is most helpful in planning operative approaches. There are limited indications for preoperative angiography: (1) extracerebral location, (2) hemorrhagic presentation, or (3) an atypical MRI or computerized tomography (CT) scan's appearance.[46] Stereoscopic angiography may help to identify sulci that can be used to approach deep lesions and minimize transcortical dissection. It is desirable to utilize intraoperative electrophysiologic functional mapping if the lesion is large and deep.

Surgical resection of supratentorial CMs in accessible areas is relatively straightforward, as there is no major arterial supply and subsequently no major blood loss. The most difficult part of the case, if any, is intraoperative localization. In addition to one's knowledge of topographic sulcal/gyral anatomy, the surgeon can usually be aided by CT- or MRI-based stereotactic guidance or intraoperative ultrasound.

A trans-sulcal approach is advocated by many because of its ability to minimize cortical resection.[47–50] However, whether disruption of the U-fibers in the trans-sulcal approach is less detrimental than disruption of the vertical fibers in the trans-gyral approach remains unknown.[49,51]

The CM is grossly identified as a well-circumscribed, blue or purple, lobulated mass resembling mulberries or grapes. As previously stated, bleeding is not a major problem. Occasionally, there are small feeding arteries that course with the sinusoidal spaces at the periphery of the lesion.[52] A well-defined gliotic plane allows for easy separation and complete removal of the lesion from the surrounding white matter; incomplete removal of the lesion incurs the risk of rebleeding that should be avoided. The hemosiderin-laden gliotic tissue comprising the capsule of the CM is epileptogenic and should be removed if not located in eloquent neural tissue.[53]

Overall Postoperative Outcomes

Bertalanffy et al reported excellent results and acceptable morbidity in a series of 72 patients with CMs surgically excised over 5 years.[3] There were 24 brainstems CMs, 18 in the deep white matter, 12 in the basal ganglia or thalamus, 11 supratentorial, and 7 in the cerebellar hemispheres. The perioperative morbidity was reported at 29.2%; however, the long-term morbidity fell to 5.5%. There were no mortalities is this series.

In another surgical series of 35 patients with 21 hemispheric CMs, 4 intraventricular, 4 brainstem, and 6 cerebellar, complete excision was achieved in 33 patients, with good outcome defined as improved seizure control or neurological deficit in 34 patients.[54] In a surgical series of 47 patients with CMs, only one mortality was reported with all other patients reaching satisfactory results—no recurrent hemorrhage, seizure-free survival, and low morbidity.[55] A pediatric surgical series of 24 children with cerebral CMs yielded good postop results, with one child that died and nine with persistence of preoperative neurological deficits.[56] An Italian surgical series of 74 cases and 76 CMs (57 hemispheric, 4 intraventricular, 1 middle cranial fossa, 2 brainstem, 5 cerebellar, and 7 orbital) reported good outcome in 66 patients, resulting in improved seizure control or lessened neurological deficit, and mortality in 2 cases.[57]

Postoperative Outcomes in Cavernous Malformations of the Cavernous Sinus

Surgery of CMs of the cavernous sinus carried a 36% mortality rate because of excessive bleeding. In fact, although histologically these cavernous sinus lesions look like typical CMs, at surgery they behave more like hemangioblastomas with a potential for catastrophic bleeding if the lesion itself is entered without previous maneuvers aimed at decreasing their vascularity, such as direct intralesional embolization. In 27 of the 53 cases reviewed, outcome for cranial neuropathies was analyzed. Twelve patients showed worsening after surgery, 11 patients showed improvement, and 4 patients showed no change.[40]

In another series of 13 patients who underwent an extradural approach for resection of CM of the cavernous sinus, there was no recurrence or growth of the residual lesion; however, the outcome of extraocular movements was poor.[58] Considering the benign nature of these lesions and the disability associated with an irreversible cranial neuropathy, less aggressive management may be advisable. **Table 20–4** summarizes the case series that provide either support for or against microsurgery for supratentorial CMs.

Postoperative Outcomes of Epilepsy and Cavernous Malformations

In a large series, 78.7% of patients showed good concordance between location of cortical CM and site of seizure focus. In cases of good concordance, complete lesionectomy resulted in disappearance of seizures.[59] Robinson et al reported a series of 32 patients with severe seizure disorder; 18 patients had medically intractable seizures.[15] Fourteen patients with seizures and an associated CM underwent surgical resection. Unfortunately, 50% continued to have seizures postop. A similar percentage and outcome was reported by McCormick et al.[60]

There still are anecdotal reports of good control of seizures following surgical excision of CMs in patients with previously uncontrolled seizures.[61] Three patients undergoing surgical treatment for intractable epilepsy

Table 20–4 Published Series for and against Microsurgery for Supratentorial Cavernous Malformations

For	Against
Bertalanffy et al (2002)[17]	Goel et al (2003)[58*]
Attar et al (2001)[54]	Linskey et al (1992)[40†]
Mahlah et al (1999)[55]	
Di Rocco et al (1997)[56*]	
Acciarri et al (1993)[57]	

*Pediatric series.
†Series of cavernous malformations of the cavernous sinus.

with CM in the dominant hemisphere had good results with a seizure-free postoperative course and no language or cognitive deterioration.[62] Another two patients with long-standing medically intractable epilepsy and CM were treated surgically, where the lesion and surrounding epileptogenic tissue were removed, resulting in seizure-free survival.[63] In a German series, 14 patients were operated on for CMs with seizures at presentation. Twelve of 14 patients improved; 10 of 14 had complete relief of epilepsy.[64] A series of 11 children undergoing surgical removal of CM causing epilepsy led to eight patients becoming seizure-free on the same preoperative drug therapy, one seizure-free on reduced drug dosage, and two seizure-free on no drug therapy.[65] A retrospective series of 36 patients suffering from epilepsy from cerebral CMs undergoing surgical treatment showed a complete cure in 25%, improved seizure control with decreased medication in 30.5%, and improved seizure control on the same preoperative drug regimen in 44.5%.[66]

A reduction of seizure frequency was seen in another series of surgically treated patients harboring CMs.[67] Four of seven patients were seizure-free after surgery. Six of six patients with focal deficits and intracerebral hemorrhage or mass effect due to CM improved postoperatively. **Table 20–5** summarizes the studies that demonstrate either good or poor postoperative seizure control.

■ Microsurgery for Infratentorial Cavernous Malformations

Indications

Infratentorial CMs cause symptoms, signs, and disability by bleeding and rebleeding. Seizures are not a feature of posterior fossa lesions. Kondziolka et al estimated the annual first-bleed rate in a series of 122 patients with CMs with a mean follow-up of 34 months to be 0.6% overall.[11] The rebleeding rate was estimated to be 4.5%. A brainstem location implied a first-bleed and rebleed rate of

2.4% and 5%, respectively. An infratentorial cavernous malformation represents a more aggressive lesion.[31,68–70]

A CM surrounded by highly eloquent brainstem tissue is clearly not resectable with low morbidity. A CM that has bled repeatedly and dissected a path to the ependymal or pial surface is an indication for surgical resection in the infratentorial compartment. It creates a slowly burrowed dissection path to the surface that obviates the need for a formal brainstem incision.[71]

Technical Pearls

Patients with acute brainstem hemorrhage may look devastated; however, they invariably improve to a large degree. Thus, the degree of preoperative morbidity does *not* predict the development of new postoperative deficits.[72] The general surgical techniques for CM resection in the infratentorial compartment are no different than for supratentorial CMs. The conventional imaging may be supplemented by stereotactic guidance for difficult-to-find lesions. Neurophysiologic monitoring should be used as a guide for where to place the parenchymal incision.

There is only one good way to remove a cavernoma: an all-or-none commitment.[72] Resection should be done by respecting the gliotic plane induced by hemorrhage. The brainstem has a low tolerance for spatial errors and technical mishaps. Small venous channels are often seen at the depth of the surgical cavity as anomalous veins or venous malformations. Nonetheless, they need to be preserved because they drain normal brainstem parenchyma.[73,74]

Postoperative Outcomes for Brainstem Cavernous Malformations

Because of their critical location, brainstem cavernous malformations represent a formidable challenge to neurosurgeons. The consensus among most neurosurgeons is that patients presenting with significant neurological deficits should be treated surgically if the lesion comes to an "accessible" pial/ependymal surface, such as

Table 20–5 Published Series Demonstrating Good (Improved or Complete) or Poor Postoperative Seizure Control

Good		*Poor*	
Series	*Control Rate*	*Series*	*Control Rate*
Muzumdar et al (2003)[61]	N/A	Robinson et al (1991)[15]	50%
Folkersma et al (2001)[67]	57.1%*	McCormick et al (1990)[60]	50%
Arita et al (2000)[62]	100%		
Siegel et al (2000)[63]	100%		
Braun et al (1996)[64]	85.7%		
Casazza et al (1996)[59]	78.7%		
Giulioni et al (1995)[65]	100%		
Acciarri et al (1995)[66]	100%		

*Represents seizure-free survival in a small series of seven patients.

the floor of the fourth ventricle or the lateral aspect of the brainstem. Patients with deeper lesions are generally monitored and surgically treated only if they exhibit severe progressive symptoms or if they develop permanent neurological deficits such as those that would be expected to result from surgery.

Several recent series have proven the feasibility of successful microsurgical resection of CMs from the brainstem in general.[75–86] Samii et al analyzed a series of 36 patients retrospectively who underwent surgical management of brainstem CMs.[86] Postoperative complications included new cranial nerve deficits in 17 patients, motor deficits in 3, and new sensory complaints in 12 postoperative Karnofsky Performance Scale scores ranged from 80 to 100, compared with an average preop KPS score of 70.3.[86]

The outcomes of patients who had been treated surgically and conservatively were compared retrospectively. Of the patients treated surgically, ~23% had no or only a slight deficit during the period of follow-up. This compared favorably with the 5% of patients with a similar outcome among those managed conservatively.[2] A Chinese study described a series of 14 patients with brainstem CMs—12 in the pons, 1 in the mesencephalon, and 1 in the medulla—who underwent surgical resection.[87] All of the brainstem CMs were totally excised, 66% of patients had improvement in neurological deficits following surgery, and one patient had a poor long-term neurological outcome.

On the other hand, a French study comparing a group of operated and non-operated patients with brainstem CMs showed that 38% of operated patients were permanently disabled postoperatively, whereas 38% improved; none in the non-operated group worsened at the end of the 47-month follow-up.[88] Only patients with multiple deficits and progressive neurological deterioration improved with surgery.

It is clear that successful surgical outcome depends on appropriate patient selection, optimal timing in relation to hemorrhage, careful surgical planning, meticulous surgical technique, and completeness of resection.[72] **Table 20–6** summarizes the surgical case series that voice support either for or against surgical excision of brainstem CMs.

■ Stereotactic Radiosurgery

Weil et al reported on a series of six patients that underwent gamma-knife radiosurgery for cavernous malformation.[89] At the end of 2 years, there was no change in size and in radiographic appearance. Two patients rebled during that period, and three patients suffered neurological deterioration from radiation-induced injury to surrounding brain parenchyma. These results

Table 20–6 Published Series for and against Microsurgery for Infratentorial/Brainstem Cavernous Malformations

For	Against
Mao et al (2001)[87]	Esposito et al (2003)[88]
Samii et al (2001)[86]	
Moriarity et al (1999)[2]	
Bricolo et al (1995)[76]	
Sakai et al (1992)[82]	
Sakai et al (1991)[81]	
LeDoux et al (1991)[80]	
Fahlbusch et al (1991)[78]	
Bertalanffy et al (1991)[75]	
Symon et al (1991)[83]	
Uede et al (1991)[84]	
Weil et al (1990)[89]	
Heffez et al (1990)[79]	

led the authors to conclude that stereotactic radiosurgery should not be recommended for treatment of CMs of the brainstem.

Similarly, another study was unable to conclude that radiosurgery protects patients with CMs against some future hemorrhage risk based on available data.[90] The risk of radiation-related complications after radiosurgery to treat cavernous malformations is greater than that found after radiosurgery in AVMs, even when adjusting for lesion size and location and for radiation dose.

A long-term study of 82 patients with CMs with previous hemorrhage showed a reduction of rehemorrhage rate from 33.9% prior to radiosurgery versus 12.3% for the first 2 years following radiosurgery and 0.76% per year thereafter; 13.4% developed radiation-induced neurological complications.[91] Yet another study showed that the retrospective bleeding rate in patients with evidence of previous hemorrhage receiving radiosurgery was reduced from 35.5% per year to 1.55% per year when compared with historical controls.[92] However, the rate of radiation-induced neurological complication was prohibitively high at 28%, with 50% of the lesions either remaining the same or increasing by MRI.

A European study of 26 patients with brainstem CMs undergoing gamma-knife radiosurgery after microsurgery was deemed too risky and showed a postoperative risk of rebleeding of 6.8% with rebleeding resulting in a 28% temporary morbidity, 8% permanent morbidity, and 2 deaths from rehemorrhage.[93] There were 33% of patients who showed a decrease in size in CM size on follow-up imaging. Gamma-knife radiosurgery has been used in a small series of patients with cavernous sinus and orbital CMs and resulted in a reduction of volume in three of four patients and no size progression in the fourth.[94] All four patients experienced symptomatic improvement, but one had persistent diplopia.

Annual hemorrhage rates fell from 13% before stereotactic radiosurgery to 3.7% after treatment; 17% of

Table 20–7 Complication Rates after Radiosurgery for Cavernous Malformations

Author (Year)	n	Complication Rates
Kim et al (2002)[92]	22	28% Radiation-induced neurological injury
Hasegawa et al (2002)[91]	82	13.4% Radiation-induced neurological injury
Liscak et al (2000)[93]	26	7.7% Mortality from rebleeding; 36% morbidity
Mitchell et al (2000)[95]	18	17% Radiation-induced neurological injury
Weil et al (1990)[89]	6	33% Rebleeding; 50% radiation-induced neurological injury

patients developed postradiosurgery complications.[95] In a French study, 49 patients with CMs and long-standing drug-resistant epilepsy were treated with gamma-knife radiosurgery; 53% were seizure-free at last follow-up, 20% with decrease in seizure frequency, while 26% remained with little or no improvement.[96] Complications of radiosurgery in or near eloquent brain regions remain prohibitive unless substantially reduced dosimetry is planned. However, any therapeutic benefit of such empirically reduced dosimetry is difficult to demonstrate.[97] **Table 20–7** summarizes the complication rates for various published series of patients receiving radiosurgery for CMs.

Most neurosurgeons do not currently recommend stereotactic radiosurgical treatment for CMs. The long-term efficacy and safety of radiosurgery in obliterating these lesions have not been demonstrated, and there are no series demonstrating even a 5-year follow-up in such patients. Evaluation of the significance of posttreatment MRI has been problematic, without clear evidence that lesions no longer represent a hemorrhagic potential. Cavernous malformations seem to react idiosyncratically to stereotactic radiosurgery. Edema and mass effect may occur after treatment, rather than obliteration of the malformation.[98] Although some centers claim that stereotactic radiosurgery for small CMs with deep location might be superior to microsurgical excision, recent studies of stereotactic radiosurgery have revealed that, generally, radiosurgery is not a useful treatment modality for prevention of hemorrhage from a CM.[90,95,99] In our view, consideration for radiosurgery for a presumed CM should be reserved for progressively symptomatic lesions in truly inoperable locations.[97]

■ Selecting the Right Surgical Approach

Once surgical resection is deemed appropriate, choosing the right angle of attack is the next decision point. We have discussed in a previous publication our 6-step conceptual approach to this problem.[72] It is an expansion of the "two-points method" advocated by Porter et al.[100] The infratentorial compartment is the location "par excellence" where approach selection is crucial.

Table 20–8 summarizes our biases in this selection process, based on exact lesion location. **Figures 20–1** and **20–2** demonstrate two case examples in the pons and midbrain, respectively. **Figures 20–3** to **20–5** illustrate a summary of common surgical approaches to the midbrain, pons, and medulla, respectively.

■ Conclusion

With increasing frequency, incidental (completely asymptomatic) CMs are being discovered during the work-up of several unrelated neurological symptoms. This is particularly true since the advent of MRI which, as discussed before, is very sensitive and specific for these lesions. However, it should be kept in mind that despite the great specificity of MRI for the diagnosis of these lesions, there are still occasions where a small tumor that has bled has an identical MRI appearance to that of a CM. For this reason (and to prevent future hemorrhage), we will generally recommend surgical excision of lesions that have the typical appearance of a CM, but that are located in such a site that excision is very unlikely to lead to morbidity. We are particularly aggressive in this respect with very young, healthy patients. On a few occasions, we have been unpleasantly surprised by finding a hemorrhagic tumor when, based on the preoperative MRI and a neuroradiologist's appraisal, we were expecting a CM.

It should be pointed out that in determining surgical morbidity for CMs, the important factor is the eloquence of the brain that has to be traversed to get to the lesion. As opposed to the case of cerebral AVMs, once the surgeon gets to the CM, excising the lesion itself is not problematic because these are very low flow lesions that can be removed essentially like a tumor without the risk of hemorrhage encountered with true cerebral AVMs. Most deep lesions, if they are not located in critical areas of the brain, can be reached through a safe trajectory with the help of intraoperative ultrasound or frame-based or frameless stereotactic guidance. The exceptions are lesions in the brainstem, basal ganglia, internal capsule, thalamus, and of course, lesions of the primary motor-sensory region and the visual cortex. Malformations in these locations should clearly be left alone if they are truly incidental. Clinical and MRI follow-up is indicated in these patients. Another

Table 20–8 Selection of Surgical Approaches Based on Location and Surface Representation

Location	Surface	Structures Represented	Surgical Approaches
Cerebellum	Occipital	Vermis (caudal); inferior semilunar, gracile, biventer lobules; tonsil (dorsal); deep cerebellar nuclei	Suboccipital transcerebellar approach
	Tentorial	Vermis (rostral); anterior and posterior quadrangular, superior semilunar lobules	1. Suboccipital supracerebellar infratentorial approach: Median (for medial half) Paramedian (for lateral half) 2. Occipital supratentorial trantentorial approach
	Petrous	Flocculus; middle cerebellar peduncle (posterior half); horizontal fissure; anterior and posterior cerebellar lobes (lateral half of ventral surface)	1. Lateral suboccipital (retrosigmoid) approach 2. Presigmoid combined subtemporal approach
Brain stem		Clival division: anterior and posterior medullary veli; tonsil (ventral); nodulus (ventral); lingula (ventral)	Suboccipital midline transcerebellar approach
		Petrous division: superior and inferior cerebellar peduncles; middle cerebellar peduncle (anterior half)	1. Suboccipital infratentorial supracerebellar, paramedian approach: For superior cerebellar peduncles 2. Lateral suboccipital (retrosigmoid), or far lateral partial transcondylar approach: For inferior cerebellar peduncles 3. Lateral suboccipital (retrosigmoid) approach, or presigmoid combined subtemporal, or supracerebellar infratentorial paramedian approach: For middle cerebellar peduncle (anterior half)
Medulla	Anterior	Pyramids; inferior olive	Far lateral partial transcondylar approach
	Lateral	Descending trigeminal tract and nucleus; tuberculum cinereum	Far lateral partial transcondylar approach
	Posterior	Gracile and cuneate fasciculi and nuclei; hypoglossal and vagal trigones; nucleus ambiguus; inferior salivatory nucleus; medial longitudinal fasciculus	Suboccipital midline transventricular approach
Pons	Anterior	Clival division: basis pontis (medial part)	1. Subtemporal transtentorial approach: For upper third of basis pontis 2. Subtemporal anterior transpetrous/Kawase approach: For middle third of basis pontis 3. Presigmoid (predominantly retrolabyrinthine) combined subtemporal approach: For any part of basis pontis 4. Transsigmoid approach: If presigmoid inadequate or not possible 5. "Combined–combined" approach: For lesions extending into medulla Same as above, but lateral suboccipital (retrosigmoid) approach may be adequate
		Petrous division: basis pontis (lateral part)	Suboccipital midline transventricular approach
	Posterior	Pontine tegmentum (facial colliculus; abducens nucleus; medial longitudinal fasciculus; superior salivatory nuclei; main trigeminal nucleus; spinothalamic tract; medial lemniscus; superior vestibular nucleus)	Suboccipital midline transventricular approach
Midbrain	Anterior	Interpeduncular fossa; crus cerebri (medial surface)	1. Transsylvian approach 2. Subfrontal interhemispheric lamina terminalis approach (only rarely)
	Anterolateral	Crus cerebri (most of)	1. Transsylvian combined pretemporal–temporopolar approach 2. Anterior subtemporal approach
	Posterolateral	Midbrain tegmentum (lateral lemniscus; medial and trigeminal lemnisci; medial longitudinal fasciculus; red nucleus; dorsal tegmental decussation)	1. Midsubtemporal approach 2. Supratentorial infraoccipital approach (as an alternative on dominant side)
	Posterior	Midbrain tectum (superior and inferior colliculi and their brachii; periaqueductal gray matter)	1. Suboccipital infratentorial supracerebellar approach: Median (for colliculi), paramedian (for brachii) 2. Occipital supratentorial transtentorial approach (if lesion above incisura and not bilateral)

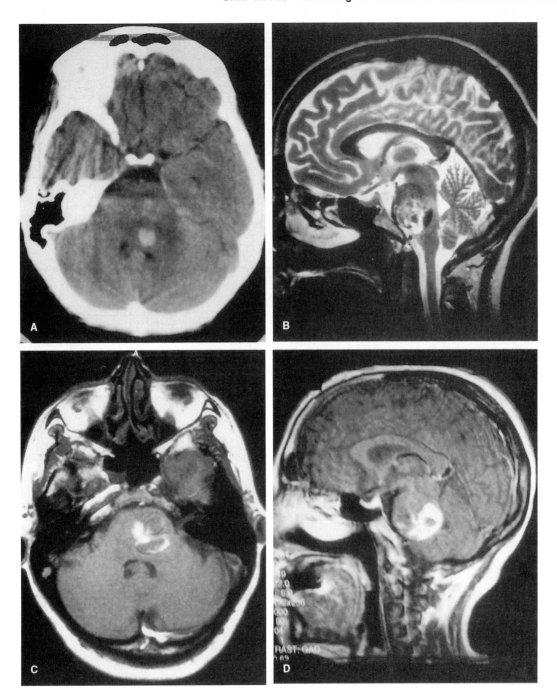

FIGURE 20–1 This is an extensive cavernous malformation of the basis pontis and pontine tegmentum predominantly on the left with rebleeding. A 34-year-old woman with intense headaches for several weeks followed by diplopia, then right arm and hand weakness and numbness of the entire right side of the body. Later, she started drooling and was unable to swallow her own saliva, her voice became hoarse, and she had difficulty maintaining her airway. Examination revealed severe right hemiparesis and marked impairment of pinprick sensation on the right side, along with a grade 5/6 peripheral left facial palsy, inability to conjugately gaze to the left, intention tremor of the left hand, and severe bulbar dysfunction. **(A)** A compuerized tomography (CT) scan showing subacute and acute hemorrhage in the pons. **(B, C)** Initial magnetic resonance images (MRIs) before transfer to our facility. She was placed on a gamma-knife treatment waiting list at another institution. **(D, E)** Subsequent MRIs taken 2 weeks later, confirming rebleeding with more acute blood posteriorly in the floor of the 4th ventricle (*Continued on page 216*).

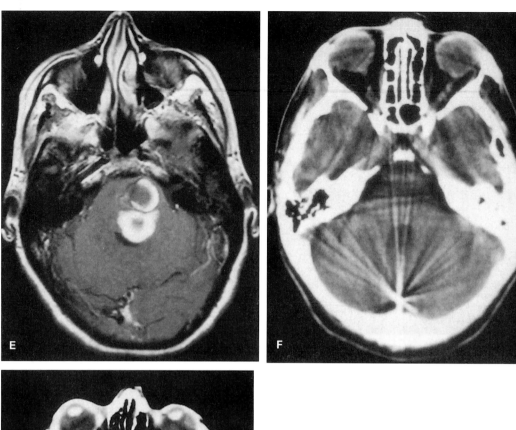

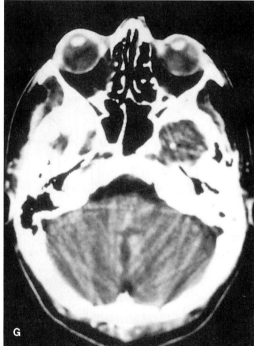

FIGURE 20–1 (*Continued*) **(F, G)** Postoperative CT scans showing complete resection. The surgery involved a midline suboccipital transvermian, transventricular approach, using intraoperative monitoring of somatosensory-evoked potentials and mapping of the 7th nerve. By 3 weeks after the operation, there was marked improvement in the strength of the right side, and the right eye was able to adduct. Speech and swallowing were much improved. The left 6th and 7th nerve palsies were complete.

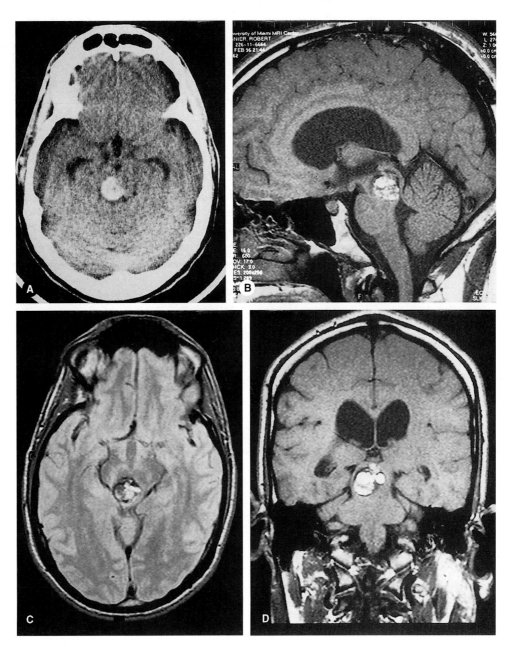

FIGURE 20–2 Shown is a cavernous malformation of midbrain tegmentum on both sides of a 30-year-old man with a 10-year history of multiple acute episodes of headaches, left face and arm numbness, and double vision. The most recent attack was 2 months prior, with uncontrollable movements of the left arm and unchanged numbness of the left face, arm, and trunk. On examination, he had a classic Benedikt syndrome. Pain and temperature were affected above T7 on the left including the face. Position sense was normal. There were gross choreiform movements and intention tremor of the left arm. **(A–D)** The lesion in the right midbrain tegmentum reaches the right posterolateral midbrain surface. (*Continued on pages 218 and 219*)

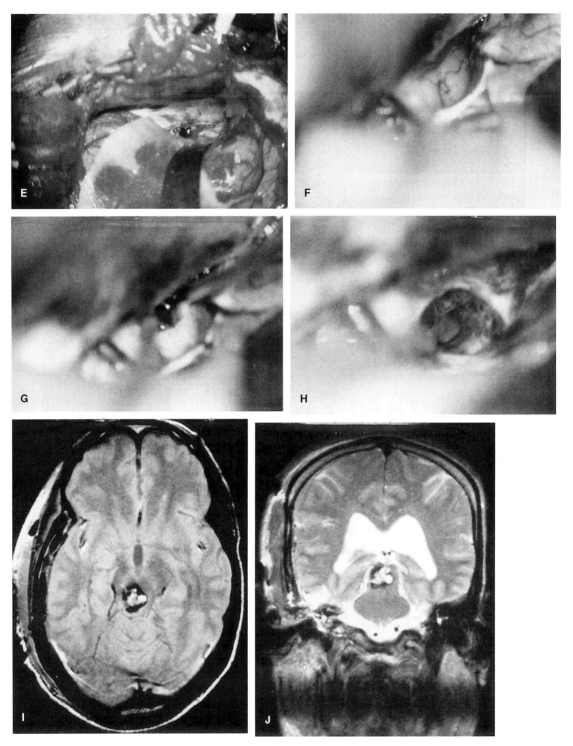

FIGURE 20–2 (*Continued*) **(E)** A right midsubtemporal approach is performed, exposing the midincisural space. **(F)** The hemosiderin discoloration is identified between the superior cerebellar and posterior cerebral arteries and dorsal to the lateral pontomesencephalic vein. **(G)** A small parenchymal incision is performed and dark red blood is encountered. **(H)** After a resection that was thought to be complete, an obvious venous angioma is encountered and preserved. **(I, J)** An MRI taken on postoperative day 3 shows predominantly postoperative blood but also a strong suspicion of a residual lesion most medially. Intraoperative somatosensory and brainstem-evoked potentials had shown no deterioration. The headaches and choreiform movements disappeared completely within days. He remained with a left-sided numbness but was fully independent. At 4 months, there was recurrence of severe headaches, gait difficulty, and worsening numbness of the left side. In addition, he had subjective difficulty breathing, with an uncontrollable urge to hyperventilate for at least 1 week.

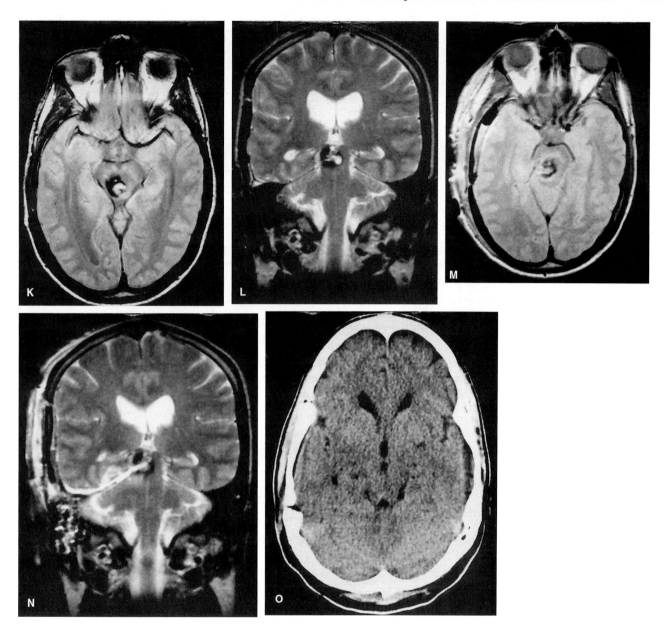

FIGURE 20–2 (*Continued*) **(K, L)** Although the early postoperative blood changed to hemosiderin, the residual lesion is more distinct. A repeat subtemporal approach was done with complete resection including full visualization of the aqueduct. The intraoperative somatosensory and brainstem evoked potentials were unaltered. **(M, N)** An MRI on postoperative day 1 showed total resection convincingly. **(O)** CT scan 6 weeks later confirms total resection. In the early postoperative period, his left hemisensory impairment worsened. He developed a mild left hemiparesis and a new partial right 3rd nerve palsy. At 6 weeks, the pupillary-sparing right 3rd nerve palsy was improving except for adduction movement. The left hemisensory numbness and left hand incoordination were unchanged.

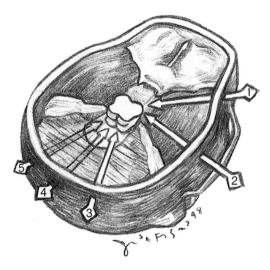

FIGURE 20–3 Surgical approaches to the midbrain. 1 = transsylvian and expanded transsylvian approaches; 2 = subtemporal; 3 = supratentorial infraoccipital; 4 = infratentorial supracerebellar, median; 5 = infratentorial supracerebellar, paramedian.

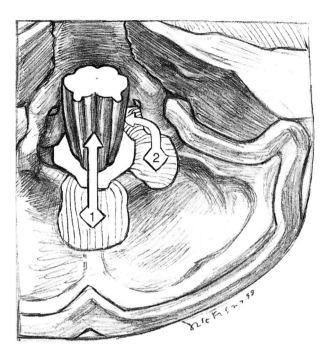

FIGURE 20–5 Surgical approaches to the medulla. 1 = midline suboccipital transventricular; 2 = far lateral partial transcondylar.

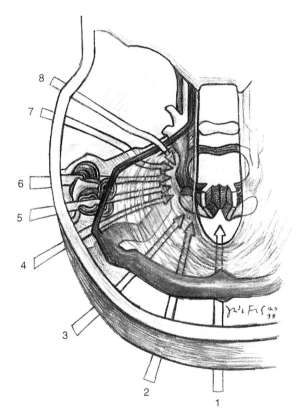

FIGURE 20–4 Surgical approaches to the pons. 1 = midline suboccipital transventricular; 2 = infratentorial supracerebellar, paramedian; 3 = retrosigmoid lateral suboccipital; 4 = retrolabyrinthine presigmoid combined subtemporal; 5 = translabyrinthine presigmoid combined subtemporal; 6 = transcochlear presigmoid combined subtemporal; 7 = subtemporal anterior petrosectomy/Kawase; 8 = subtemporal transtentorial.

group of patients that do not need surgery for incidental CMs are patients that have a clear-cut familial history (in these cases, the diagnosis is practically certain and there is no need to obtain pathologic confirmation) or patients with multiple CMs, whether familial or sporadic.

▪ References

1. Jafar JJ, Awad IA, Huang PP. Intracranial vascular malformations: clinical decisions and multimodality management strategies. In: Jafar JJ, Awad IA, Rosenwasser RH, eds. Vascular Malformations of the Central Nervous System. Philadelphia: Lippincott Williams and Wilkins; 1999:219–232
2. Moriarity JL, Clatterbuck RE, Rigamonti D. The natural history of cavernous malformations. Neurosurg Clin N Am 1999;10:411–417
3. Bertalanffy H, Benes L, Miyazawa T, Alberti O, Siegel AM, Sure U. Cerebral cavernomas in the adult. review of the literature and analysis of 11 surgically treated patients. Neurosurg Rev 2002;25:1–53
4. Elmaci I, Ates G, Kurtkaya O, Necmettin Pamir M. Chiasmal cavernous malformation: a rare cause of acute visual loss. J Neurosurg Sci 2000;44(4):226–229
5. Zabramski JM, Wascher TM, Spetzler RF, et al. The natural history of familial cavernous malformations: Results of an ongoing study. J Neurosurg 1994;80:422–432
6. Maraire JN, Awad IA. Intracranial cavernous malformations: lesion behavior and management strategies topic review. Neurosurgery 1995;37:591–605
7. Porter PJ, Willinsky RA, Harper W, Wallace MC. Cerebral cavernous malformations: natural history and prognosis after clinical deterioration with or without hemorrhage. J Neurosurg 1997;87:190–197
8. Robinson JR, Awad IA. Clinical spectrum and natural course. In: Awad IA, Barrow DL, eds. Cavernous malformations. Park Ridge, IL: American Association of Neurological Surgeons; 1993:25–36

9. Xie J, Ma Z, Luo S. The clinical features and treatment of cerebral cavernous angiomas in children. Zhonghua Yi Xue Za Zhi 2002; 82(6):407–409

10. Mottolese C, Hermier M, Stan H, et al. Central nervous system cavernomas in the pediatric age group. Neurosurg Rev 2001;24(2–3): 55–71

11. Kondziolka D, Lunsford LD, Kestle JR. The natural history of cerebral cavernous malformations. J Neurosurg 1995;83:820–824

12. Del Curling Jr O, Kelly Jr DL, Elster AD, et al. An analysis of the natural history of cavernous angiomas. J Neurosurg 1991;75:702–778

13. Kim DS, Park YG, Choi JU, et al. An analysis of the natural history of cavernous malformations. Surg Neurol 1997;48:9–17

14. Barker FG II, Amin-Hanjani S, Butler WE, et al. Temporal clustering of hemorrhages from untreated cavernous malformations of the central nervous system. Neurosurgery 2001;49(1):15–24

15. Robinson JR, Awad IA, Little JR. Natural history of cavernous angioma. J Neurosurg 1991;75(5):709–714

16. Porter RW, Detwiler PW, Spetzler RF, et al. Cavernous malformations of the brainstem:experiences with 100 patients. J Neurosurg 1999;90:50–58

17. Bertalanffy H, Benes L, Miyazawa T, Alberti O, Siegel AM, Sure U. Cerebral cavernomas in the adult. Review of the literature and analysis of 11 surgically treated patients. Neurosurg Rev 2002; 25:1–53

18. Sonstein WJ, Kader A, Michelsen WJ, et al. Expression of vascular endothelial growth factor in pediatric and adult cerebral arteriovenous malformations: an immunocytochemical study. J Neurosurg 1996;85:838–845

19. Sure U, Butz N, Schlegel J, et al. Endothelial proliferation, neoangiogenesis and potential de novo generation of cerebral vascular malformations. J Neurosurg 2001;94:972–977

20. Rigamonti DR, Hadley MN, Drayer BP, et al. Cerebral cavernous malformations: incidence and familial occurrence. N Engl J Med 1988;319:343–347

21. Hayman AL, Evans RA, Ferrell RE, et al. Familial cavernous angiomas: natural history and genetic study over a 5-year period. Am J Med Genet 1982;11:147–160

22. Dubovsky J, Zabramski JM, Kurth J, et al. A gene responsible for cavernous malformations of the brain maps to chromosome 7q. Hum Mol Genet 1995;4:453–458

23. Gunel M, Awad IA, Finberg K, et al. A founder mutation as a cause of cerebral cavernous malformation in Hispanic Americans. N Engl J Med 1996;334:946–951

24. Reich P, Winkler J, Straube A, et al. Molecular genetic investigations in the CCM1 gene in sporadic cerebral cavernomas. Neurology 2003;60(7):1135–1138

25. Labauge P, Brunereau L, Laberge S, Houtteville JP. Prospective follow-up of 33 asymptomatic patients with familial cerebral cavernous malformations. Neurology 2001;57(10):1825–1828

26. Perez Lopez C, Isla Guerrero A, Gomez Sierra A, et al. Management of the multiple cerebral cavernomatosis. Rev Neurol 2002;35(5): 407–414

27. Hayashi Y, Tohma Y, Mouri M, et al. Congenital multiple cavernous angiomas associated with thrombosed arteriovenous malformation of the brain—case report. Neurol Med Chir (Tokyo) 2002;42(2): 67–72

28. Wang MC, Winston KR, Breeze RE. Cerebellar mutism associated with a midbrain cavernous malformation: case report and review of the literature. J Neurosurg 2002;96(3):607–610

29. Fujiwara S, Ohta M, Takeda T, et al. A surgical case of tectal cavernous malformation presented by hydrocephalus. No Shinkei Geka 2002;30(1):81–85

30. Dumas G, Schmerber S, Boulat E, Lavieille JP. Cavernous angiomas of the brainstem: auditory and vestibular manifestations. Rev Laryngol Otol Rhinol (Bord) 2001;122(2):103–110

31. Fritschi JA, Reulen HJ, Spetzler RF, et al. Cavernous malformations of the brainstem: a review of 139 cases. Acta Neurochir (Wien) 1994;130:35–46

32. Kupersmith MJ, Kalish H, Epstein F, et al. Natural history of brainstem cavernous malformations. Neurosurgery 2001;48(1):47–53

33. Pozzati E. Thalamic cavernous malformations. Surg Neurol 2000;53(1):30–39

34. Katayama Y, Tsubokawa T, Maeda R, et al. Surgical management of cavernous malformations of the third ventricle. J Neurosurg 1994;80:64–72

35. Sinson G, Zager EL, Grossman RI, et al. Cavernous malformations of the third ventricle. Neurosurgery 1995;37:37–42

36. Nieto J, Hinojosa J, Munoz MJ, et al. Intraventricular cavernoma in pediatric age. Childs Nerv Syst 2003;19(1):60–62

37. Tatsui CE, Koerbel A, Prevedello DM, et al. Magnetic resonance imaging of the intraventricular cavernomas: diagnostic aspects. Arq Neuropsiquiatri 2003;61(1):79–82. Epub 2003 Apr 16. Portuguese

38. Ogilvy CS, Louis DN, Ojemann RG. Intramedullay cavernous angiomas of the spinal cord: Clinical presentation, pathological features, and surgical management. Neurosurgery 1992;31:219–229

39. Anson JA, Spetzler RF. Surgical resection of intramedullary spinal cord cavernous malformations. J Neurosurg 1993;78:446–451

40. Linskey ME, Sekhar LN. Cavernous sinus hemangiomas: a series, a review, and a hypothesis. Neurosurgery 1992;30:101–108

41. Suzuki Y, Shibuya M, Başkaya MK, et al. Extracerebral cavernous angiomas of the cavernous sinus in the middle fossa. Surg Neurol 1996;45:123–132

42. Michelson WJ. Conservative management. In: Awad IA, Barrow DL, eds. Cavernous Malformations. Park Ridge, IL: American Association of Neurological Surgeons; 1993:81–85

43. Chanda A, Nanda A. Multiple cavernomas of brain presenting with simultaneous hemorrhage in two lesions: a case report. Surg Neurol 2002;57(5):340–344

44. Shah M, Heros RC. Microsurgical treatment of supratentorial lesions. In: Awad IA, Barrow DL, eds. Cavernous Malformations. Park Ridge, IL: American Association of Neurological Surgeons; 1993:101–116

45. Chang HS, Hongo K, Nakagawa H, Tsuge T. Surgical decision-making on cerebral cavernous malformations. J Clin Neurosci 2001;8(5):416–420

46. Maruoka N, Yamakawa Y, Shimauchi M. Cavernous hemangioma of the optic nerve: case report. J Neurosurg 1988;69:292–294

47. Davis DH, Kelly PJ. Stereotactic resection of occult vascular malformations. J Neurosurg 1990;72:698–702

48. Kelly PJ, Goerss SJ, Kall BA. The stereotactic retractor in computer-assisted stereotaxic microsurgery. Technical note. J Neurosurg 1988; 69:301–306

49. Harkey HL, Al-Mefty O, Haines DE, et al. The surgical anatomy of the cerebral sulci. Neurosurgery 1989;24:651–654

50. Yasargil MG. Microsurgical anatomy of the brain. In: Microsurgery, Vol I. New York, NY: Thieme Medical Publishers; 1984:284–320

51. Heros RC. Brain resection for exposure of deep extracerebral and paraventricular lesions. Surg Neurol 1990;34:188–195

52. Yasargil MG. Arteriovenous malformations of brain, history, embryology, pathological considerations, hemodynamics, diagnostic studies, microsurgical anatomy. In: Microneurosurgery Vol IIIA. Stuttgart, West Germany: George Thiems Verlag; 1987:45–49

53. Wilson CB. Cryptic vascular malformations. In: Selman W, ed. Clinical Neurosurgery. Baltimore, MD: Williams and Wilkins; 1992:49–84

54. Attar A, Ugur HC, Savas A, et al. Surgical treatment of intracranial cavernous angiomas. J Clin Neurosci 2001;8(3):235–239

55. Mahla K, Rizk T, Fischer C, et al. Intracranial cavernoma: surgical results of 47 cases. Neurochirurgie 1999;45(4):286–292

56. Di Rocco C, Iannelli A, Tamburrini G. Surgical management of paediatric cerebral cavernomas. J Neurosurg Sci 1997;41(4): 343–347

57. Acciarri N, Padovani R, Giulioni M, et al. Intracranial and orbital cavernous angiomas: a review of 74 surgical cases. Br J Neurosurg 1993;7(5):529–539

58. Goel A, Muzumdar D, Sharma P. Extradural approach for cavernous hemangioma of the cavernous sinus: experience with 13 cases. Neurol Med Chir (Tokyo) 2003;43(3):112–118

59. Casazza M, Broggi G, Franzini A, et al. Supratentorial cavernous angiomas and epileptic seizures: preoperative course and postoperative outcome. Neurosurgery 1996;39(1):26–32

60. McCormick PC, Michelson WJ. Management of intracranial cavernous and venous malformations. In: Barrow DL, ed. Intracranial Vascular Malformations. Park Ridge, IL: American Association of Neurological Surgeons 1990:197–217

61. Muzumdar DP, Bhatjiwale MG, Goel A. Giant cerebral cavernous haemangioma: a case report and review of literature. J Clin Neurosci 2003;10(3):348–351

62. Arita K, Kurisu K, Iida K, et al. Surgical treatment for intractable epilepsy caused by cavernous angioma in the temporal lobe of the dominant hemisphere—three case reports. Neurol Med Chir (Tokyo) 2000;40(8):439–445

63. Siegel AM, Roberts DW, Harbaugh RE, Williamson PD. Pure lesionectomy versus tailored epilepsy surgery in treatment of cavernous malformations presenting with epilepsy. Neurosurg Rev 2000;23(2):80–83

64. Braun V, Antoniadis G, Rath S, Richter HP. Cavernoma: indications for surgical removal and outcome. Nervenarzt 1996;67(4):301–305

65. Giulioni M, Acciarri N, Padovani R, Galassi E. Results of surgery in children with cerebral cavernous angiomas causing epilepsy. Br J Neurosurg 1995;9(2):135–141

66. Acciarri N, Giulioni M, Padovani R, et al. Surgical management of cerebral cavernous angiomas causing epilepsy. J Neurosurg Sci 1995;39(1):13–20

67. Folkersma H, Mooij JJ. Follow-up of 13 patients with surgical treatment of cerebral cavernous malformations: effect on epilepsy and patient disability. Clin Neurol Neurosurg 2001;103(2):67–71

68. Aiba T, Tanaka R, Koike T, et al. Natural history of intracranial cavernous malformations. J Neurosurg 1995;83:56–59

69. Isamat F, Conesa G. Cavernous angiomas of the brainstem. Neurosurg Clin N Am 1993;4:507–518

70. Pozzati E, Acciarri N, Tognetti F, et al. Growth, subsequent bleeding and de novo appearance of cerebral cavernous angiomas. Neurosurgery 1996;38:662–670

71. Wowra B, Layer G, Schad LR, et al. Three-dimensional time-of-flight MR-angiography and the surgical indication of brainstem cavernomas. Acta Neurochir (Wien) 1991;112:77–82

72. Morcos JJ, Heros RC, Frank DE. Microsurgical treatment of infratentorial malformations. Neurosurg Clin N Am 1999;10(3):441–474

73. Bogucki J, Gielecki J, Czernicki Z. The anatomical aspects of a surgical approach through the floor of the fourth ventricle. Acta Neurochir (Wien) 1997;139:1014–1019

74. Fahlbusch R, Strauss C, Huk W, et al. Surgical removal of pontomesencephalic cavernous hemangiomas. Neurosurgery 1990;26:449–457

75. Bertalanffy H, Gilsbach JM, Eggert HR, et al. Microsurgery of deep-seated cavernous angiomas: report of 26 cases. Acta Neurochir (Wien) 1991;108:91–99

76. Bricolo A, Turazzi S. Surgery for gliomas and other mass lesions of the brainstem. In: Advances and Technical Standards in Neurosurgery, Vol. 22. New York: Springer-Verlag; 1995:262–341

77. Fahlbusch R, Strauss C. Surgical significance of cavernous hemangioma of the brainstem. Zentralbl Neurochir 1991;52:25–32

78. Fahlbusch R, Strauss C, Huk W. Pontine-mesencephalic cavernomas: indications for surgery and operative results. Acta Neurochir Suppl (Wien) 1991;53:37–41

79. Heffez DS, Zinreich SJ, Long DM. Surgical resection of intrinsic brainstem lesions: an overview. Neurosurgery 1990;27:789–798

80. LeDoux MS, Aronin PA, Odrezin GT. Surgically treated cavernous angiomas of the brainstem: report of two cases and review of the literature. Surg Neurol 1991;35:395–399

81. Sakai N, Yamada H, Tanigawara T, et al. Surgical treatment of cavernous angioma involving the brainstem and review of the literature. Acta Neurochir (Wien) 1991;113:138–143

82. Sakai N, Sakai H, Gotoh Y, et al. Surgical treatment of brainstem lesions with reference to cavernous angioma. No To Shinkei 1992;44:983–988

83. Symon L, Jackowski A, Bills D. Surgical treatment of pontomedullary cavernomas. Br J Neurosurg 1991;5:339–347

84. Uede T, Nonaka T, Takigami M, et al. Cavernous malformation of the brainstem: clinical symptoms and its surgical indication. No Shinkei Geka 1991;19:27–34

85. Weil SM, Tew JM Jr. Surgical management of brainstem vascular malformations. Acta Neurochir (Wien) 1990;105:14–23

86. Samii M, Eghbal R, Carvalho GA, Matthies C. Surgical management of brainstem cavernomas. J Neurosurg 2001;95(5):825–832

87. Mao Y, Zhou L, Du G. Brain-stem cavernous hemangioma: surgical indications and approaches. Zhonghua Wai Ke Za Zhi 2001;39(9): 672–674

88. Esposito P, Coulbois S, Kehrli P, et al. Place of the surgery in the management of brainstem cavernomas: results of a multicentric study. Neurochirurgie 2003;49(1):5–12

89. Weil S, Tew Jr JM. Surgical management of brain stem vascular malformations. Acta Neurochir (Wien) 1990;105:14–23

90. Pollock BE, Garces YI, Stafford SL, Foote RL, Schomberg PJ, Link MJ. Stereotactic radiosurgery for cavernous malformations. J Neurosurg 2000;93:987–991

91. Hasegawa T, McInerney J, Kondziolka D, et al. Long-term results after stereotactic radiosurgery for patients with cavernous malformations. Neurosurgery 2002;50(6):1190–1197

92. Kim DG, Choe WJ, Paek SH, et al. Radiosurgery of intracranial cavernous malformations. Acta Neurochir (Wien) 2002;144(9): 869–878

93. Liscak R, Vladyka V, Simonova G, et al. Gamma knife radiosurgery of the brain stem cavernomas. Minim Invasive Neurosurg 2000; 43(4):201–207

94. Thompson TP, Lunsford LD, Flickinger JC. Radiosurgery for hemangiomas of the cavernous sinus and orbit: technical case report. Neurosurgery 2000;47(3):778–783

95. Mitchell P, Hodgson TJ, Seaman S, Kemeny AA, Forster DMC. Stereotactic radiosurgery and the risk of hemorrhage from cavernous malfotrmations. Br J Neurosurg 2000;14:96–100

96. Regis J, Bartolomei F, Kida Y, et al. Radiosurgery for epilepsy associated with cavernous malformation: retrospective study in 49 patients. Neurosurgery 2000;47(5):1091–1097

97. Awad IA, Barrow DL. Editorial comment: radiosurgery. In: Awad IA, Barrow DL, eds. Cavernous Malformations. Park Ridge, L: American Association of Neurological Surgeons; 1993:202–203

98. Frim DM, Scott RM. Management of cavernous malformations in the pediatric population. Neurosurg Clin N Am 1999;10:513–518

99. Karlsson B, Kihlstrom L, Lindquist C, Ericson K, Steiner L. Radiosurgery for cavernous malformations. J Neurosurg 1998;88: 293–297

100. Porter RW, Detwiler PW, Spetzler RF. Surgical approaches to the brain stem. Operative Techniques in Neurosurgery, 2000;3: 114–123

21

Observation of Cavernous Malformations

DARYL R. GRESS AND VINEETA SINGH

Objectives: After reading this chapter, the reader should be able to select patients appropriately for conservative management, and describe all facets of medical management and clinical surveillance.

Accreditation: The AANS* is accredited by the Accreditation Council for Continuing Medical Education (ACCME) to sponsor continuing medical education for physicians.

Credit: The AANS designates this educational activity for a maximum of 15 credits in Category 1 credit toward the AMA Physician's Recognition Award. Each physician should claim only those hours of credit that he/she spent in the educational activity.

The Home Study Examination is online on the AANS Web site at: http://www.aans.org/education/books/controversy.asp

* The acronym AANS refers to both the American Association of Neurological Surgeons and the American Association of Neurosurgeons.

Cerebral cavernous malformations (CCMs) are known to be associated with intracerebral hemorrhage.[1-4] They are commonly recognized on computerized tomography (CT) and magnetic resonance imaging (MRI) scans in both asymptomatic and symptomatic patients.[5] The diagnosis of CCMs can often be made on an MRI scan based on the characteristic morphology of the subacute and chronic blood products. An atypical appearance of a CCM in the setting of a recent hemorrhage requires follow-up imaging to confirm the diagnosis.[3,5]

At pathological examination CCMs are rounded or lobulated collections of dilated single-cell-layer endothelium-lined vascular channels.[6-10] Calcification and thickened collagen can be observed in association with some thrombosis.[11,12] By definition, there is no smooth muscle and no elastin in these vascular channels. There is no intervening neural tissue, and gliosis and hemosiderin staining are common at the periphery of these lesions. Small arteries and veins enter and exit the lesion at the periphery. In biological terms, it is likely that the mechanisms of origin and growth are different for CCMs than other vascular anomalies. Efforts at characterizing the particular vascular growth factors that may underlie these differences will help provide an understanding of the biological differences.

■ Epidemiology

The prevalence of CCMs in the general population is not known[2,13-22]; however, the frequency of occurrence has been reported to be 0.02 to 0.5% based on autopsy studies.[2,19,23] Detection rates of 0.39 to 0.9% are based on a retrospective review of MRI scans.[3,5,24,25] Cerebral cavernous malformations do not appear to be more prevalent in females. Some have suggested that males under the age of 30 have a higher rate of detection, while the rate of detection is higher in women aged between 30 to 60 years. At 60+ years, the frequency is similar for both men and women.[3,26] In children, a bimodal age presentation has been described, with increased detection at age 3 and 11 years.[21,27] Late presentation in elderly individuals is rare. It is likely that lesions invariably become symptomatic in life or not at all, or that aging may be associated with regression of CCM.

■ Anatomical and Biological Characteristics

These lesions present in a broad spectrum of size from several millimeters to 4 to 5 cm in diameter. The frequency of occurrence appears to correspond with the volume of various central nervous system (CNS) compartments, with 80% found supratentorially and 20% infratentorially (**Table 21–1**). Cerebral cavernous malformations can occur with other vascular anomalies. Cavernous malformations are commonly juxtaposed to deep venous malformations. This association has likely confounded the interpretation of the natural history of venous malformations. In a retrospective review, patients with CCMs associated with vascular malformations were more likely to be female patients who suffered symptomatic hemorrhage with lesions in the posterior fossa. They were also less likely to present with seizures or to have familial histories when compared with patients with CCMs alone.[28] As documented in imaging studies, CCMs enlarge over time with de novo appearance of new lesions by MRI criteria.[8,29–31] Precursor lesions such as capillary telangiectasias have been postulated, but origins remain obscure. It has been speculated that growth factors such as basic fibroblast growth factor (bFGF) and vascular endothelial growth factor (VEGF) are involved in the growth of these lesions[32]; their presence has been demonstrated by the immunostaining of surgical specimens. Ultrastructural studies suggest that abnormalities of the blood–brain barrier are important in the pathophysiology of cavernous malformations.[33,34]

Cerebral cavernous malformations occur in two forms: sporadic, generally producing a single, isolated lesion, and the autosomal dominant, frequently producing multiple lesions.[12,31,35,36] The inherited form accounts for up to 50% of all cases of cavernous malformation. Familial cavernous malformation is genetically heterogenous, with at least three disease-causing loci. So far, CCM loci have been assigned to chromosomes *7q* (*CCM1*), *7p* (*CCM2*), and *3q* (*CCM3*) and have been identified in 40%, 20%, and 40%, respectively, of families with CCM. Loss-of-function mutations have been identified in *CCM1/KRIT1*, the sole CCM gene identified to date.[37–41]

The loss of *CCM1* leads to primary vascular defects and disrupts the molecular pathway regulating arterial identity.[42–44] The gene responsible for *CCM2* was recently discovered and named malcavernin or *MGC4607*.[37,45] The gene(s) responsible for *CCM3* still await identification.

■ Clinical Presentations

A cerebral cavernous malformation presents clinically as a seizure (60%), focal deficit (40%), or headache (30%), or without symptoms (15%) (**Table 21–2**). Seizures in CCM are related to brain irritation, neural compression, and local hemorrhages with exposure of the local brain parenchyma to blood products, particularly iron and later local gliotic reaction.[8,26] The possible pathophysiological mechanisms of epileptogenesis include neuronal cell loss, glial proliferation and abnormal glial physiology, altered neurotransmitter levels, free radical formation, and aberrant second messenger physiology.[46] In CCMs, temporal lobe location, heavy calcification, and extensive hemosiderin deposition are more likely to have epileptic presentation rather than gross hemorrhage.[47,48]

With the more liberal use of magnetic resonance imaging, the incidental or asymptomatic category will come to represent a larger percentage of the lesions identified. Given that one of the defining MRI characteristics is evidence of hemosiderin, it is important to emphasize that clinical hemorrhage associated with these lesions should be accompanied by frank hematoma and clear clinical symptoms.

■ Diagnostic Evaluation

Definition by imaging studies has become most common in the era of magnetic resonance imaging. Cerebral cavernous malformations are rounded or lobulated lesions with a mixed signal core surrounded by low signal rim. Susceptibility sequences and high-resolution blood oxygenation level–dependent venography detect more lesions than conventional MRI sequences (**Fig. 21–1**).[49–51] No definitive feeding artery or a draining vein can be identified by MR angiography or conventional contrast

TABLE 21–1 Anatomical Locations of Cavernous Malformations

Compartments	Most Common Locations	Number of Cases (%)
Supratentorial	Temporal lobes Frontal and parietal lobes Occipital lobes	80%
Infratentorial	Pons cerebellum	20%

TABLE 21–2 Clinical Presentations of Cerebral Cavernous Malformations

Clinical Symptoms	No. of Cases (%)
Seizures	60
Focal Deficits	40
Headache	30
Asymptomatic	15

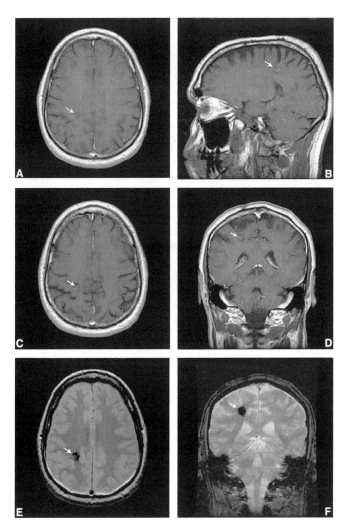

FIGURE 21–1 This 54-year-old man presented with a history of chronic daily headaches and two brief episodes of tingling involving his left hand. An abnormality seen on a head CT "offered" to him during a cardiac imaging session showed an abnormality, prompting a visit to the neurologist. His neurological examination was nonfocal. **(A, B)** Pregadolinium T1-weighted images demonstrate intrinsic T1 shortening with a surrounding rim of hypointensity. **(C, D)** Postgadolinium images demonstrate minimal enhancement. **(E)** This T2-weighted image has a prominent low signal caused by hemosiderin. **(F)** The multi-planar gradient (MPGR) sequences clearly show focal ovoid area of susceptibility in the right frontoparietal region right adjacent to the central sulcus.

angiography. The clinician rarely has all of this information available for the classification of a particular lesion. This leads to difficulty in the evaluation of a suspected CCM (**Fig. 21–2**). It is not possible based on imaging studies alone to exclude a small thrombosed arteriovenous malformation; some clinicians therefore prefer to use a less-specific term of cryptic vascular malformation. The administration of gadolinium contrast is unnecessary for the diagnosis but may help identify venous malformations that frequently coexist with these lesions.[49–51]

▪ Hemorrhage Risk

Combining various magnetic resonance series, 27,000 patients have been studied with respect to the clinical presentation and natural history of CCM.[3,12,18,52] In the series reported by Robinson et al there were 66 patients with 77 CCM. Six of those patients had presented with clinically significant hemorrhage at the time of their initial study. This group provided 143 lesion years of follow-up, during which time one clinical hemorrhage occurred, leading to an estimated annualized risk of 0.7%.

Many clinicians believe that while the risk of incidental CCM is quite low, a clinically significant hemorrhage presents a significantly increased risk of recurrent bleeding. A study reported by Kondziolka et al provides some of the most useful natural history data to date. A registry of CCM enrolled 162 patients with follow-up available on 122 patients. Half of these patients had no history of symptomatic hemorrhage. In the group with no prior hemorrhage, the annualized risk was 0.6%. However, in patients with prior hemorrhage, there was an annual risk of 4.5%, thus supporting prior clinical impressions.

▪ Long-Term Outcomes

The long-term outcome in patients with CCM has been studied in 84 patients.[4] In this study, female gender was associated with neurological disability, but this was not significant after controlling for location and previous hemorrhage. There was more neurological disability associated with infratentorial lesions and those with previous frank hemorrhage. The lesion size or the multiplicity did not have an impact on disability. In another review,[53] 30 patients were followed for an average of 35.7 months; 66.6% had no or minimal deficit, 6.7% had moderate disability, 6.7% were completely dependent, and 20% died. There were no deaths related to neurological events among 110 patients followed; 22 recovered partially, and 16 had no significant improvement.[52]

▪ Medical Management

Expectant Follow-Up

Patients with CCMs comprise separate clinical scenarios that correlate with their risk of hemorrhage and neurological disability. To predict the natural risk of a CCM for an individual patient, one must consider the morphological and functional specifications of the CCM as known statistical data and the life expectancy of the patient. Theoretically, earlier detection of a CCM can influence the natural risk in as much as a longer life expectancy increases the probability of bleeding.

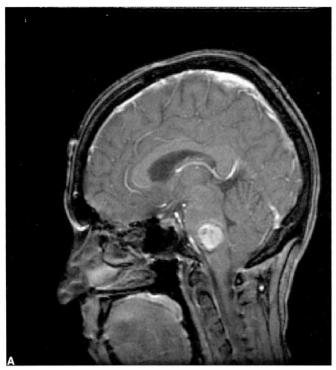

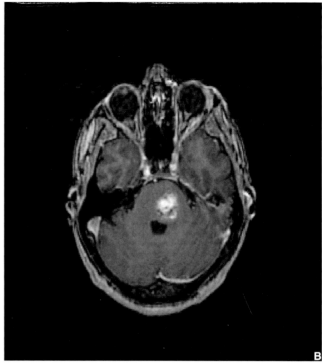

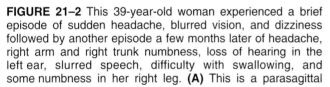

FIGURE 21–2 This 39-year-old woman experienced a brief episode of sudden headache, blurred vision, and dizziness followed by another episode a few months later of headache, right arm and right trunk numbness, loss of hearing in the left ear, slurred speech, difficulty with swallowing, and some numbness in her right leg. **(A)** This is a parasagittal

T1-weighted postgadolinium MRI scan of the brain showing a 2.2 × 2.1 cm mass extending from the medulla to the mid-and left pons and has heterogeneously increased signal on the postcontrast images. **(B)** This MRI scan is of the same patient with an axial view of the brain showing pontine cavernous malformation.

Patients who present without any symptoms or non-specific symptoms like headache and dizziness in the absence of neurological deficits are at a very low risk of disabling hemorrhage. Despite the fact that surgery for solitary lesions is low risk and eliminates the risk of any future bleeding,[54] the current data does not support the surgical approach. These patients should be followed clinically and have sequential MRI scans. In young patients, solitary lesions should be watched closely, with lesion resection at the first manifestation of increase in the size or exacerbation of symptoms. The threshold for lesion resection should be higher in patients with inaccessible lesions.

Management of Seizures

Cerebral cavernous malformations frequently present with seizures of various subtypes including generalized, complex partial and simple partial seizures. The lesion is usually located in the supratentorial compartment, frequently in the temporal lobe. It is important to localize the seizure focus satisfactorily, before ascribing the seizures to a CCM. Unfortunately, in a significant number of patients, it is not possible to localize the

seizure focus by surface electroencephalogram (EEG).[26] In these cases, prolonged video EEG monitoring and interictal as well as ictal positron emission tomography (PET) scans may enhance the accuracy of the localization. In some cases, invasive electrode monitoring may be necessary for adequate mapping of the seizure focus.[26] Some have suggested that the occurrence of a seizure in the presence of a CCM is higher than that associated with other vascular malformations. In a series of vascular malformations excised for refractory seizures, 74.7% were CCMs, while only 14.8% were arteriovenous malformations (AVMs).[55] In the majority of patients, a good seizure control can be achieved with anticonvulsants.[55,56]

Hormonal Factors

Prospective studies show the incidence of cavernous malformation to be ~0.50%.[3] Cavernous malformations occur with equal prevalence in both sexes, although the risk of hemorrhage is higher in females.[54] Familial occurrence is observed in 25 to 54% of cases.[8] Pregnancy may increase the risk of hemorrhage in some women.[21,54,57–59] During pregnancy, an occult lesion such as a cavernous angioma should be considered with a new-onset seizure.[57] A case of recurrent bleeding from a CCM in a woman on hormonal treatment has been reported; this case lends support for the role hormonal factors may play in the biological behavior of CCM.[60] In a case of the de novo development of a CCM, the immunohistochemistry of the resected lesion demonstrated strong expression of β FGF but a lack of expression of hormone receptors.[61] Cerebral cavernous malformations have shown aggressive behavior in young patients and in women of child-bearing age. It is likely that such changes are mediated by sex hormone receptors. The potential link between hormonal factors and cavernous malformations is an important issue that needs to be resolved with additional studies.

■ Future Directions

Prognostication

The behavior of CCMs remains highly unpredictable, and it is clear that host, environmental, and gene susceptibility factors affect the disease progression. Better definition of these factors should allow screening for patients harboring a particular lesion who are more likely to have a hemorrhagic presentation or refractory seizures. There may be risk factors predicting individual lesion progression, and clinicians should learn to characterize the clinical features in individual patients. With advances in the molecular characterization of CCMs, better correlations are expected between a genotype and phenotype.

Genetic Counseling

Advances in the identification of genes and the gene products involved in the pathogenesis of CCM have influenced the clinical management of these patients. Multifocal CCM now calls for a thorough family history; this helps to detect previously unrecognized cases. Familial clustering has helped to diagnose unrecognized CCMs in cases presenting with myelopathy of unknown cause and others mislabeled as multiple sclerosis. The management of epilepsy in the setting of CCM is vastly different if lesions are solitary or multiple on gradient echo MRI.[62] The presence of an associated venous anomaly calls for special surgical considerations aimed at preserving the venous angioma.[28] The counseling of women of childbearing age with a CCM about pregnancy, management options before and during pregnancy, and screening regarding possibly affected children has alleviated many patients' anxiety.

With the great advances in our understanding of these lesions in relation to genetic susceptibility and the biochemical pathways involved in the disease process, novel therapeutic strategies will soon emerge for the treatment of CCM.

■ References

1. Margolis G, Odom GL, Woodhall B, et al. The role of small angiomatous malformations in the production of intracerebral hematomas. J Neurosurg 1951;8:564–575

2. Otten P, Pizzolato GP, Rilliet B, et al. 131 Cases of cavernous angioma (cavernomas) of the CNS, discovered by retrospective analysis of 24,535 autopsies. Neurochirurgie 1989;35:82–83, 128–131. French

3. Robinson JR, Awad IA, Little JR. Natural history of the cavernous angioma. J Neurosurg 1991;75:709–714

4. Robinson JR Jr, Awad IA, Magdinec M, et al. Factors predisposing to clinical disability in patients with cavernous malformations of the brain. Neurosurgery 1993;32:730–736

5. Del Curling O Jr, Kelly DL Jr, Elster AD, et al. An analysis of the natural history of cavernous angiomas. J Neurosurg 1991;75:702–708

6. Davis R, Robertson DM. Textbook of Neuropathology, 3rd ed. Baltimore, MD: Williams and Wilkins; 1997

7. Hoang TA, Hasso A. Intracranial vascular malformations. Neuroimaging Clin N Am 1994;4:823–842

8. Rigamonti D, Hadley MN, Drayer BP, et al. Cerebral cavernous malformations. Incidence and familial occurrence. N Engl J Med 1988;319:343–347

9. Robinson JR Jr, Awad IA, Masaryk TJ, et al. Pathological heterogeneity of angiographically occult vascular malformations of the brain. Neurosurgery 1993;33:547–554

10. Zabramski JM, Henn JS, Coons S. Pathology of cerebral vascular malformations. Neurosurg Clin N Am 1999;10:395–410

11. Maraire JN, Awad IA. Intracranial cavernous malformations: lesion behavior and management strategies. Neurosurgery 1995;37:591–605

12. Zabramski JM, Wascher TM, Spetzler RF, et al. The natural history of familial cavernous malformations: results of an ongoing study. J Neurosurg 1994;80:422–432

13. Abe T, Singer RJ, Marks MP, et al. Coexistence of occult vascular malformations and developmental venous anomalies in the central nervous system: MR evaluation. AJNR Am J Neuroradiol 1998;19:51–57

14. Dubovsky J, Zabramski JM, Kurth J, et al. A gene responsible for cavernous malformations of the brain maps to chromosome 7q. Hum Mol Genet 1995;4:453–458

15. Gunel M, Awad IA, Anson J, et al. Mapping a gene causing cerebral cavernous malformation to 7q11.2-q21. Proc Natl Acad Sci USA 1995;92:6620–6624

16. Gunel M, Awad IA, Finberg K, et al. A founder mutation as a cause of cerebral cavernous malformation in Hispanic Americans. N Engl J Med 1996;334:946–951

17. Horowitz M, Kondziolka D. Multiple familial cavernous malformations evaluated over three generations with MR. AJNR Am J Neuroradiol 1995;16:1353–1355

18. Kondziolka D, Lunsford LD, Kestle JR. The natural history of cerebral cavernous malformations. J Neurosurg 1995;83:820–824

19. McCormick WF, Boulter TR. Vascular malformations ("angiomas") of the dura mater. J Neurosurg 1966;25:309–311

20. Moriarity JL, Clatterbuck RE, Rigamonti D. The natural history of cavernous malformations. Neurosurg Clin N Am 1999;10:411–417

21. Pozzati E, Acciarri N, Tognetti F, et al. Growth, subsequent bleeding, and de novo appearance of cerebral cavernous angiomas. Neurosurgery 1996;38:662–670

22. Pozzati E, Musiani M. Cavernous hemangioma. J Neurosurg 1998;89:498–499

23. Berry RAB, White J. The Site, Structure and Frequency of Intracranial Aneurysms, Angiomas, and Arteriovenous Abnormalities. Baltimore, MD: Williams and Wilkins; 1996

24. Kim DS, Park YG, Choi JU, et al. An analysis of the natural history of cavernous malformations. Surg Neurol 1997;48:9–18

25. Sage MR, Brophy BP, Sweeney C, et al. Cavernous haemangiomas (angiomas) of the brain: clinically significant lesions. Australas Radiol 1993;37:147–155

26. Awad IA, Robinson JR. Comparison of the clinical presentation of symptomatic arteriovenous malformations (angiographically visualized) and occult vascular malformations. Neurosurgery 1993;32:876–878

27. Sakai N, Yamada H, Nishimura Y, et al. Intracranial cavernous angioma in the 1st year of life and a review of the literature. Childs Nerv Syst 1992;8:49–52

28. Abdulrauf SI, Kaynar MY, Awad IA. A comparison of the clinical profile of cavernous malformations with and without associated venous malformations. Neurosurgery 1999;44:41–47

29. Kim DS, Park YG, Choi JU, Chung SS, Lee KC. An analysis of the natural history of cavernous malformations. Surg Neurol 1997 Jul;48(1):9-18

30. Labauge P, Brunereau L, Coubes P, et al. Appearance of new lesions in two nonfamilial cerebral cavernoma patients. Eur Neurol 2001;45:83–88

31. Labauge P, Brunereau L, Laberge S, et al. Prospective follow-up of 33 asymptomatic patients with familial cerebral cavernous malformations. Neurology 2001;57:1825–1828

32. Rothbart D, Awad IA, Lee J, et al. Expression of angiogenic factors and structural proteins in central nervous system vascular malformations. Neurosurgery 1996;38:915–924

33. Clatterbuck RE, Eberhart CG, Crain BJ, et al. Ultrastructural and immunocytochemical evidence that an incompetent blood-brain barrier is related to the pathophysiology of cavernous malformations. J Neurol Neurosurg Psychiatry 2001;71:188–192

34. Wong JH, Awad IA, Kim JH. Ultrastructural pathological features of cerebrovascular malformations: a preliminary report. Neurosurgery 2000;46:1454–1459

35. Gil-Nagel A, Wilcox KJ, Stewart JM, et al. Familial cerebral cavernous angioma: clinical analysis of a family and phenotypic classification. Epilepsy Res 1995;21:27–36

36. Siegel AM. Familial cavernous angioma: an unknown, known disease. Acta Neurol Scand 1998;98:369–371

37. Denier C, Goutagny S, Labauge P, et al. Mutations within the MGC4607 gene cause cerebral cavernous malformations. Am J Hum Genet 2004;74:326–337

38. Denier C, Labauge P, Brunereau L, et al. Clinical features of cerebral cavernous malformations patients with KRIT1 mutations. Ann Neurol 2004;55:213–220

39. Gault J, Sarin H, Awadallah NA, et al. Pathobiology of human cerebrovascular malformations: basic mechanisms and clinical relevance. Neurosurgery 2004;55:1–17

40. Laurans MS, DiLuna ML, Shin D, et al. Mutational analysis of 206 families with cavernous malformations. J Neurosurg 2003;99:38–43

41. Reich P, Winkler J, Straube A, et al. Molecular genetic investigations in the CCM1 gene in sporadic cerebral cavernomas. Neurology 2003;60:1135–1138

42. Marchuk DA, Srinivasan S, Squire TL, et al. Vascular morphogenesis: tales of two syndromes. Hum Mol Genet 2003;12 Spec No 1:R97–112

43. Tille JC, Pepper MS. Hereditary vascular anomalies: new insights into their pathogenesis. Arterioscler Thromb Vasc Biol 2004;24:1578–1590

44. Whitehead KJ, Plummer NW, Adams JA, et al. Ccm1 is required for arterial morphogenesis: implications for the etiology of human cavernous malformations. Development 2004;131:1437–1448

45. Liquori CL, Berg MJ, Siegel AM, et al. Mutations in a gene encoding a novel protein containing a phosphotyrosine-binding domain cause type 2 cerebral cavernous malformations. Am J Hum Genet 2003;73:1459–1464

46. Kraemer DL, Awad IA. Vascular malformations and epilepsy: clinical considerations and basic mechanisms. Epilepsia 1994;35(Suppl 6): S30–S43

47. Simard JM, Garcia-Bengochea F, Ballinger WE Jr, et al. Cavernous angioma: a review of 126 collected and 12 new clinical cases. Neurosurgery 1986;18:162–172

48. Steiger HJ, Markwalder RV, Reulen HJ. Is there a relationship between the clinical manifestations and the pathologic image of cerebral cavernomas? Neurochirurgie 1989;35:84–88. French

49. Atlas SW, Mark AS, Fram EK, et al. Vascular intracranial lesions: applications of gradient-echo MR imaging. Radiology 1988;169:455–461

50. Lee BC, Vo KD, Kido DK, et al. MR high-resolution blood oxygenation level-dependent venography of occult (low-flow) vascular lesions. AJNR Am J Neuroradiol 1999;20:1239–1242

51. Rigamonti D, Drayer BP, Johnson PC, et al. The MRI appearance of cavernous malformations (angiomas). J Neurosurg 1987;67:518–524

52. Porter PJ, Willinsky RA, Harper W, et al. Cerebral cavernous malformations: natural history and prognosis after clinical deterioration with or without hemorrhage. J Neurosurg 1997;87:190–197

53. Fritschi JA, Reulen HJ, Spetzler RF, et al. Cavernous malformations of the brain stem. A review of 139 cases. Acta Neurochir (Wien) 1994;130:35–46

54. Awad I, Barrow DL. Cavernous Malformations. Park Ridge, IL: American Association of Neurological Surgeons; 1993

55. Awad I, Robinson J. Cavernous Malformations and Epilepsy. Park Ridge, IL: American Association of Neurological Surgeons; 1993

56. Weber M, Vespignani H, Bracard S, et al. Intracerebral cavernous angioma. Rev Neurol (Paris) 1989;145:429–436. French

57. Awada A, Watson T, Obeid T. Cavernous angioma presenting as pregnancy-related seizures. Epilepsia 1997;38:844–846

58. Hayashi S, Kondoh T, Morishita A, et al. Congenital cavernous angioma exhibits a progressive decrease in size after birth. Childs Nerv Syst 2004;20:199–203

59. Hoeldtke NJ, Floyd D, Werschkul JD, et al. Intracranial cavernous angioma initially presenting in pregnancy with new-onset seizures. Am J Obstet Gynecol 1998;178:612–613

60. Gazzaz M, Sichez J, Capelle L, et al. Recurrent bleeding of thalamic cavernous angioma under hormonal treatment: a case report Neurochirurgie 1999;45:413–416

61. Ludemann W, Ellerkamp V, Stan AC, et al. De novo development of a cavernous malformation of the brain: significance of factors with paracrine and endocrine activity: case report. Neurosurgery 2002;50:646–650

62. Vives KPAI. Vascular Malformations and Epilepsy. New York: Raven Press; 1998

The Practice of Neurovascular Medicine

22

The Departmental Model for Practice

CHRISTOPHER S. OGILVY, BOB S. CARTER,
CHRISTOPHER M. PUTMAN, AND COLIN T. MCDONALD

Objectives: After completing this chapter, the reader should be able to describe how neurosurgeons, interventional neuroradiologists, and neurologists can collaborate from within their separate departments.

Accreditation: The AANS* is accredited by the Accreditation Council for Continuing Medical Education (ACCME) to sponsor continuing medical education for physicians.

Credit: The AANS designates this educational activity for a maximum of 15 credits in Category 1 credit toward the AMA Physician's Recognition Award. Each physician should claim only those hours of credit that he/she spent in the educational activity.

The Home Study Examination is online on the AANS Web site at: http://www.aans.org/education/books/controversy.asp

* The acronym AANS refers to both the American Association of Neurological Surgeons and the American Association of Neurosurgeons.

In this text, separate chapters are devoted to the various "practice models" that have been developed over time by various institutions for the efficient evaluation and management of neurovascular patients. We will describe the "departmental model." In this model, physicians from several neurovascular specialties work together to evaluate, treat, and manage patients. However, each remains an employee of his or her department. We will review the structured framework for patient care and will note the financial implications of the departmental model. We will highlight some of the potential advantages and disadvantages of this structure.

■ The Evolution and Structure of the Departmental Model: The Massachusetts General Hospital Brain Aneurysm/AVM Neurovascular Center

Many of the currently existing tertiary care programs that offer care of complicated neurovascular problems have evolved over time and within institutions, depending on the preexisting arrangements of the various departments involved. This is certainly true for the situation at the Massachusetts General Hospital (Boston, MA). The Massachusetts General Hospital Brain AVM/Aneurysm Neurovascular Center was formally developed in conjunction with the hospital administration in 1991. The Center was proposed based on collaborations that were emerging between neuroradiology (specifically, the evolving section of interventional neuroradiology), vascular neurology, and vascular neurosurgery. This "Center of Excellence" was conceptualized as a distributed network of caregivers without the need for a specific physical location within the hospital. The Center was developed with partial support from each department involved, as well as a financial commitment from the hospital.

In the development of the Center, we agreed that physician members of the Center would remain employed by their respective department. The member is directly responsible to their respective chief of service. There is no "fee for service" remuneration for any members of the physician staff involved with the Center, and each member receives a salary. **Figure 22–1** shows how the Center concept relates to the various members involved. As can be seen, the specialists from vascular neurology, neurointensive care, interventional neuroradiology, radiation oncology, and vascular neurosurgery all combine expertise to care for a patient with a neurovascular problem.

■ The Logistics of How the Center Operates in a Non-Emergency Situation

The offices of the Center physicians are dispersed throughout the hospital; therefore, an initial challenge was to find a time point every week for Center physicians to gather and efficiently discuss issues regarding the management of new patients. Thus, we scheduled a weekly morning neurovascular conference. The various Center physicians are free to place cases on the agenda. In some cases, one or another of the Center physicians has already met the patient. Physicians throughout the country send in other cases for review and recommendations.

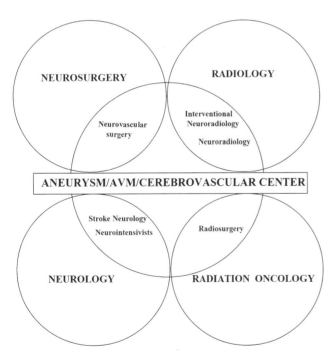

FIGURE 22–1 The AVM/Aneurysm/Cerebrovascular Center unites physicians from the departments of neurosurgery, radiology, neurology, and radiation oncology. These physicians remain salaried employees of their respective departments but collaborate in the management of patients with cerebrovascular diseases.

The conference takes place within the neuroradiology suite. The neurovascular problem is presented in a bulleted point format, and the relevant radiological images are reviewed. We then discuss the merits and methods of treatment in an open environment and reach a consensus on a treatment plan. The Center physicians leave the meeting with an understanding of their roles in follow-up. Nurse coordinators consolidate the patient information prior to the conference. Following the conference, they inform the support staff of the various Center physicians what appointments need to be scheduled. Each week, as many as 20 cases can be discussed over a 2-hour period.

The weekly conference also provides a forum to discuss current cases in the hospital. The Center physicians benefit from the cross-disciplinary research updates provided by colleagues. Such a conference also provides a focused learning opportunity for physicians in training. This conference also consistently attracts attending physicians who, while not specifically members of the Center, may have similar interests (e.g., neuroradiologists).

■ The Logistics of How the Center Operates in an Emergency

Usually one member of the neurovascular team is notified about a patient with a neurovascular problem. For instance, an outside physician requesting transfer of a patient with a subarachnoid hemorrhage may call the vascular neurosurgeon. The other members of the team are given a "heads up" warning that a patient is in transfer. The patient is examined and stabilized upon arrival in the emergency department or the neurointensive care unit. Diagnostic studies are rapidly obtained. The involved Center physicians review and discuss the studies. They then decide on the need to treat and the modality of treatment. The treating physician provides the treatment and primary care of the patient; other Center physicians may be called in for input. Several Center members are expert in the delivery of neurointensive care and aid the primary treating physician in the medical management of these complicated patients.

■ The Financial Aspects of the Departmental Model

What are the financial implications of this departmental model, and how do they bear on the care of the patient? One important aspect of this model is that budget allocations and salary designations are made at the departmental level. All Center physicians are salaried by their individual departments; there are no direct fee-for-service arrangements. This allows objective decision-making without financial influence on the process. We feel that if one or more of the treating physicians are compensated personally for treating the patient, then the decision-making may be influenced by this factor. The respective department performing the procedure bills for the procedures performed to treat a patient. Part of the financial support used to maintain the neurological intensive care unit comes from the neurosurgical and radiology departments because of the care given by the neurointensivists on behalf of these departments.

■ The Admitting Policies of the Center

In this model, any Center physician can individually admit patients with neurovascular disease. While Center members from interventional neuroradiology have admitting privileges, most acutely ill patients are admitted to the neurology service (primarily patients with ischemic cerebrovascular disease) or the neurosurgical service (primarily patients with hemorrhagic cerebrovascular disease). The attending staff physicians see the patients each day from each service involved. While attending physicians have overall responsibility, residents and fellows provide invaluable assistance in the day-to-day management of these patients.

To illustrate this multidisciplinary approach, imagine a patient with subarachnoid hemorrhage initially accepted by and admitted to the neurosurgical service. After review and discussion of the diagnostic studies by Center physicians, all agree that treatment is indicated and that an intravascular treatment is most appropriate for this patient. The interventional neuroradiology team coils a ruptured intracranial aneurysm. The neurosurgical team maintains overall responsibility for the patient and may place a ventriculostomy for hydrocephalus. The neurointensivists provide specific consultation on medical issues including ventilator management. The vascular neurologists provide diagnostic support by performing daily transcranial Dopplers to assess for vasospasm. The group as a whole will come to consensus regarding the institution and weaning of hyperaugmentation therapy or endovascular treatment of vasospasm.

■ The Political Aspects of the Departmental Model

In the arrangement described above, there are several "political" implications. For the system to work effectively, each department and each department chairperson must supply complete financial support of the Center physicians. Each department must work toward the mutual goal of maintaining an active interdisciplinary system for caring for neurovascular patients. Sometimes, this means that department chairs may relieve certain Center physicians of duties normally undertaken by other department physicians. For example, neurointensivists may be excused from coverage of patients without neurovascular issues or critical illness, as well as from outpatient duties. Further, these individuals may focus their outpatient encounters solely on neurovascular patients. This has the danger of creating "departments within departments." Our institution has addressed this issue by having the neurointensivists infrequently attend on the general neurology service.

For this model to work, all involved disciplines must be equally valued. The interventional neuroradiologists are not simply "procedurists" but are integral members of the neurovascular team; their input is needed at the time of diagnostic workup and treatment decision as well as when post-procedure management questions arise.

We have found that a practical way to foster collegiality is to view the Center as a research as well as a clinical tool. We encourage collaborative projects between the Center members that will foster the academic advancement of all. Ongoing collaborative research projects include neurosurgeons and neurointensivists investigating factors such as fever that might influence outcome in subarachnoid hemorrhage patients. Vascular neurologists with interventional neuroradiologists continue to look prospectively at the effects of different interventions and treatments for acute large vessel stroke.

■ Conclusion

In the end, a Center physician is identified by his or her ongoing interest in the management of patients with neurovascular disease and concomitant willingness to work as part of a distributed team. Departments recruit physicians individually, while the Center provides a means for neurovascular specialists to treat greater numbers of patients more efficiently in an environment that remains collegial and academic in orientation.

We have shown the main benefit of the departmental model is in the area of clinical decision-making. Because no one physician benefits in a direct financial way from a decision to treat or not treat a patient, that decision may more likely be made on strictly clinical grounds. This model requires a willingness of individual specialists to defer on occasion to the consensus of the team.

■ Future Directions

With new recognition of formalized training programs that will allow physicians from neurology, neurosurgery, and radiology to gain expertise in endovascular therapy, we may rightfully ask what is the future of the departmental model for the care of cerebrovascular patients. As training becomes more integrated across specialties, will the academic and financial models follow a similar integration? Will separate departments of neurovascular therapy develop? While training is often integrated and general, the *practice* of medicine tends to be specialized. Specialization occurs on two axes: disease-based and technical skill-based. In the near future we will have neurologists qualified in endovascular therapy but unable to perform open surgery; neurosurgeons trained in catheter techniques and open surgery; surgeons who specialize in one type of open surgery but without skills in catheter techniques; and a large cadre of interventionalists who perform catheter techniques but are not able to perform open surgery. We propose that each of these types of practitioners can be accommodated in a Center model as we have described, bringing the best of disease- and procedure-based specialization to the care of the patient.

23

The Institutional Model for Practice: An Interventional Neurovascular Program within an Academic Neurological Surgery Department

T. C. ORIGITANO, HARISH N. SHOWNKEEN,
MARY T. FITZGERALD, AND PATRICIA CASSIDY

Objectives: After completing this chapter, the reader should be able to explain how to integrate an endovascular surgeon into an academic neurosurgical department.

Accreditation: The AANS* is accredited by the Accreditation Council for Continuing Medical Education (ACCME) to sponsor continuing medical education for physicians.

Credit: The AANS designates this educational activity for a maximum of 15 credits in Category 1 credit toward the AMA Physician's Recognition Award. Each physician should claim only those hours of credit that he/she spent in the educational activity.

The Home Study Examination is online on the AANS Web site at: http://www.aans.org/education/books/controversy.asp

* The acronym AANS refers to both the American Association of Neurological Surgeons and the American Association of Neurosurgeons.

"The secret of success in an institution . . . is to blend the old with the new, the past with the present in due proportion, and it is not difficult if we follow Emerson's counsel: 'We cannot overstate', he says, 'our debt to the past, but the moment has the supreme claim; the sole terms on which the past can become ours are its subordination to the present.'"

—Sir William Osler[1]

■ Background

With this reminder from a brilliant innovator of modern medicine, we detail a single institution's effort to establish and maintain a state-of-the-art interventional neurovascular program. Like politics in Chicago, everything is local. The local politics may facilitate or hamper the success of one program's model.

Loyola University Medical Center and the Loyola Health System in Maywood, Illinois is a Catholic, tertiary/ quaternary healthcare provider. The Center/System consists of a 523-bed acute care hospital (ranked in the top 20 nationally among academic institutions for patient acuity), 22 ambulatory sites, and a 600-person faculty; it is affiliated with a major rehabilitation facility and long-term ventilation care hospital. The Health System and the Loyola University Physician Foundation (which includes the 600-person faculty) are highly aligned and share many common resources and liabilities including a joint malpractice subsidiary. The common

235

relationship of the entire faculty within one foundation circumvents issues related to the Stark Law[*], while providing a single billing and collection agent. Financially, each department within the Physician Foundation is an independent cost center responsible for its expenses as well as faculty management, compensation, and bonuses. The departments of neurological surgery, neurology, otolaryngology, and psychiatry participate in the neuroscience service line within the health system and function as a unit for marketing services' purchases, hospital budget and management, and resource allocation. It is within the framework of this environment that the interventional neurovascular program was launched.

■ History

It was apparent by the mid-1990s that interventional management of cerebrovascular disease was here to stay.[2] Technological advances in delivery systems and embolic devices such as the Guglielmi detachable coil (GDC) system had improved efficacy. A social milieu reflected more toward minimally invasive procedures. Issues of informed consent relating to treatment alternatives were on the malpractice horizon. Cerebrovascular programs providing the full spectrum of treatment (surgical and interventional) were changing patient–physician referral patterns.[3]

It Takes a Vision: Groundwork

In the fall of 1997, the Department of Neurological Surgery with the consent of the Department of Radiology approached the Health System administration through the Vice President of Service Lines with a proposal for a joint interventional neurovascular program. A key element for programmatic success was to identify an administrative champion who would partner with the physician leaders to shepherd the program through the complex financial and organizational review process. This process was data driven; it required access to sensitive Health System, as well as local–regional health care data, which was accessible through the office of the Senior Vice President of System Development. In the health care economic environment, where margins can be 1 to 2%, there is substantial economic risk when establishing a new program. Interventional neurovascular programs have substantial facility, technology,

marketing, and personnel start-up costs. The administrator champion understands the language of financial productivity and method of formatting the data for senior administrator evaluation.

An initial SWOT (strengths/weaknesses/opportunities/threats) analysis provided a framework for the establishment of a Health System task force to assess the feasibility and viability of the proposal. The administrator champion headed the task force, which consisted of representatives from relevant clinical departments (Neurological Surgery, Radiology, Neurology, Cardiology, Cardiovascular Surgery, Peripheral Vascular Surgery, Anesthesia, Pharmacy, and Emergency Room), Health System and hospital administration (including Marketing and Finance), Nursing, and Support Services.

The task force initiated a quality planning process that encompassed a comprehensive analysis of financial, operational, and clinical outcomes and indicators. A detailed financial analysis was performed based on patient volumes, payer mix, and procedural codes. The analysis included an examination of ICD-9 (*International Classification of Diseases, 9th Edition/Revision*),[4] DRG (diagnosis-related group), and CPT (the American Medical Association's current procedural terminology) codes, and the institution's historic payer mix. It is important to understand the economic realities: (1) the difference between fee schedule and payer reimbursement, (2) the difference between physician reimbursement and hospital reimbursement, (3) the difference of payer mix and profit, and (4) the difference between charge and cost as it relates to the revenue statement for your program.

The clinical and operational analysis included facilities, technology, personnel, and system coordination needs. The establishment of the program coordinated both existing and anticipated resource needs. Existing resources included a dedicated 13-bed neuroscience intensive care unit, a 40-bed neuroscience medical–surgical floor, monitoring equipment, transcranial Doppler and cerebral blood flow technology, and a biplane angiographic suite. The required resources included a second 3D biplane angiographic suite; an interventional team of dedicated technologists and nurses; a database for tracking volumes, outcomes, and resource utilization; vendor meetings to establish price and stock; patient education/discharge and social work interface; and a marketing plan. The quality planning process took ~6 to 9 months and resulted in a comprehensive business and operational plan. The program opened in July 1998.

---

[*]Briefly, the Stark Law prohibits physicians from making referrals for a designated health service (DHS), payable to Medicare of Medicaid, to any entity with which the physician or a member of the physicians immediate family has a direct or indirect financial relationship.

■ Key Philosophical Considerations: It Is Not What You Get but What You Are Willing to Give Up That Counts

The most comprehensive and viable business plan is all for naught if core philosophical issues are not resolved. One of the key rules to success is to face reality as it is, not as it was or you wish it were. This program's success is based in part on the melding of two unique and quite different specialties—Neurological Surgery and Radiology.

Neurological Surgery and Radiology: Perspectives

To begin with, a strong neurosurgical chair can direct policy regarding "the rites of first attempt." Much can be learned from microcatheter analysis and even attempted coiling regarding operative surgical anatomy.

Neurosurgical residency and practice is rich in critical care, inpatient floor management, and outpatient clinics. Traditionally, radiologists have limited exposure and experience in these areas. The interventional patients are often sick or can become so quickly. The vast majority of patient management and complications fall to neurosurgery to manage.

The cerebrovascular surgeon must view the neurointerventionalist as a partner, not a competitor. The cultures must meet at the patient. The interventionalist and the neurosurgeon must make their rounds of their patients together, talk to the families, and make the treatment decisions together. Neurosurgeons should attend their patients' neurointerventional procedures to participate in decisions, intervene if necessary, or proceed to surgery. Interdiction cannot happen after the fact. Calling for neurosurgical support in a crisis is a "no-win" situation; making the decision together permits sharing in the joys of success and the burden of complications. Likewise, the interventionalist should attend all operative interventions and participate in the intraoperative angiography. These shared experiences enrich mutual respect and mutual understanding of programmatic capabilities and limitations. The result of this is that the interventionalist is a first-class citizen in both departments and provides each patient with optimal care.

The neurointerventionalist in our case is a radiologist. He has a joint appointment in neurological surgery and a physical office in both departments. He is fully integrated into the neurosurgery faculty and educational program. Our residents participate in a 3- to 6-month interventional rotation where they perform and participate in catheter angiography, interventional vertebroplasty, and diagnostic interpretation. Residents acquire an understanding of the capacity and capabilities of interventional procedures, which aids in clinical judgment. This experience can also count toward their interventional fellowship. A monthly joint cerebrovascular conference for neurosurgery, radiology, neurology, and medicine is held. The neurointerventionalist attends all faculty meetings and morbidity and mortality conferences and interviews resident applicants.

■ Core Financial Philosophy

It is not about the money—it is about the money. Many interdepartmental relationships and, for that matter, marriages fail due to finances. The environment at Loyola, being a unified practice plan with a single billing agent, simplifies the matter greatly. Collected dollars are paid to the Physician Foundation, which can distribute them by negotiated formulae.

In collaboration with the chairman of the radiology department, the following financial formula was arranged. Base salary is split 60/40 radiology/neurological surgery to reflect the additional non-angiographic neurodiagnostic work. Each department pays their bonuses according to their individual policy: radiology has a set, shared department plan; neurosurgery has an incentive plan based on individual productivity above expense. The practical application of this formula is accomplished by providing three separate physician billing codes: (1) non-angiodiagnostic (100% to radiology), (2) transcranial Doppler/cerebral blood flow (TCD/CBF) readings (100% to neurosurgery), and (3) interventional and catheter diagnostic work (50/50 split radiology/neurosurgery). Historical tracking of collections demonstrates a 60/40 (radiology/neurological surgery) return. This formula removes financial competition. Its justification, in part, comes from the concept of the CPT code, which embodies a technical component, an administration component, and a patient care component. The distribution of collections honors each program member's contribution.

■ Philosophical Summary

The removal of financial concerns changes the "mine–mine" to an "ours" concept of turf. "Win–win" does not mean one department wins twice but, rather that both departments win. Most importantly, the patient benefits from programmatic expansion of treatment options. Viewing each other as partners, not competitors, consolidates the turf and gives the program a competitive advantage. The lessons are:

- It's not about the money—if you are willing to share.
- "Win–win" does not mean you win twice but, rather that the patient wins all the time.

- The rites of first attempt go to the interventionalist; valuable information and experience are gained even from a failed attempt.
- Extract the best of each culture. Neurosurgeons have a robust clinical acumen. Use it. Neurosurgery residents must have exposure to hands-on training in neurointerventional techniques. It is part of the future of cerebrovascular neurosurgery.
- The neurosurgeon should attend at least the decision-making part of an interventional procedure. It enhances understanding, builds teamwork, and can avoid complications.

■ Selling the Vision

"Even if you're on the right track, you'll get run over if you just sit there."

—Will Rogers

All the planning and programmatic analysis is for naught if you cannot sell the program to referring physicians, patients, payers, and key senior administrators. Communication is the key: Communicate early and often. An effective marketing plan is essential. The components of the plan must read the internal market (600-person practice plan, 5,000 medical center/health system employees, senior administrators, board of directors), and external market (outside referring physicians/group practices; patients in immediate, primary, secondary and tertiary service area; and third-party payers).

It is important to create an identity that differentiates your program. This can, as in our case, draw on and augment the overall institutional branding. There are several tools that can be utilized, including annual departmental reports, health system reports, medical center brochures, CD-ROMS, direct mail, TV and radio commercials, CME events, capabilities brochures, and hospital grand rounds (both your own and outside hospitals).

Early-on internal marketing, especially to key supporting administrators, is important to reinforce the benefit of their investment in the program. Take to their office copies of key X-rays that demonstrate a successful procedure, especially if it is a system first. Invite them to watch a procedure. Take them to see a patient who received treatment and introduce them as the administrator who helped make the new procedure possible by facilitating the program. Remember they are your partners; share the success with them.

■ Turn the Vision into Reality: Results

Prior to the establishment of the program in July 1998, the institution averaged 105 cerebral angiograms per year over the previous 4 years (**Fig. 23–1**). With the institution of the interventional program, that number grew

to 355 the first year. Even with the financial formula in place, the department of radiology nearly doubled its collectibles. Additionally, patients participating in this program averaged an additional four imaging examinations in the form of computed tomography and magnetic resonance imaging scans. The program has continued to

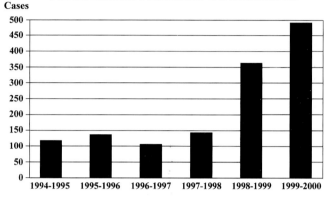

Figure 23–1 The growth in neuroendovascular procedures at Loyola University Medical Center from 1994 through 2000 is depicted. Overall procedures increased ~500%.

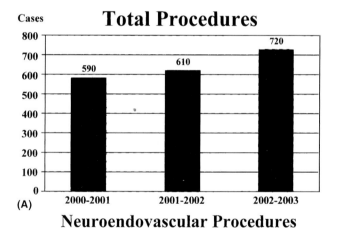

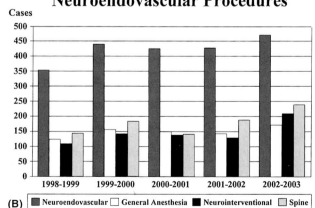

Figure 23–2 (A) The growth in neuroendovascular procedures at Loyola University Medical Center from 2000 through 2003 is shown. **(B)** This profile of neuroendovascular procedures shows growth from the inception of program in 1998 to 2003.

Patient Discharges with Principal Diagnosis of:
Subarachnoid Hemorrhage 430 or
Nonruptured Brain Aneurysm 437.3

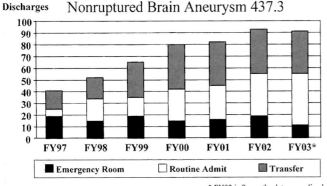

* FY03 is 9 months data annualized

Figure 23–3 This chart shows the growth in the number of treated patients with subarachnoid hemorrhage. Primary growth was seen in transfers and nonruptured aneurysm referrals.

Neuroendovascular Procedures

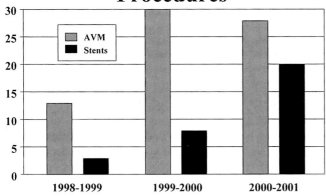

Figure 23–4 This figure charts the growth and exposure to arteriovenous malformations and extracranial cerebrovascular disease from 1998 to 2001.

grow each year, reaching 720 cases in 2002–2003 year (**Figs. 23–2A and 23–2B**).

Two particular classes of cases can be utilized to benchmark the growth: aneurysms and arteriovenous malformations (AVMs). From 1996/1997 to 2002/2003 the number of aneurysms treated increased 2.15-fold (**Fig. 23–3**). This increase was seen in both ruptured and unruptured aneurysms. It also reflected a stable emergency room admission rate with growth in routine and transfer admissions. The number of open operations that actually fell rebounded to above pre-interventional levels. There was also a significant increase in AVM cases with a conservative rise in open operations and radiosurgical treatments (**Fig. 23–4**).

From the educational standpoint, neurosurgical residents had access to extracranial-occlusive vascular

Table 23–1 Resident Neuroendovascular Exposure during a 3-Month Rotation

Assisted in the Following Cases:	
Cerebral Angiograms	61
Embolization of Arteriovenous Malformation	16
Embolization of Aneurysm	8
Vertebroplasty	4
Embolization of Head and Neck Tumor	4
Embolization of Intracranial Tumor	3
Embolization of Epistaxis	3
Embolization of Spinal Tumor	2
Carotid Stent Placement	2
Balloon Occlusion Test	2
WADA Test	2
Angioplasty	1
Tissue Plasminogen Activator Therapy	1
Inferior Petrosal Sinus Sampling	1
	111
Performed most of the Following:	
Cerebral Angiograms	39
Aortic Arch and Carotid Angiograms	3
Intraoperative Angiogram	2
Vertebroplasty	1
	45

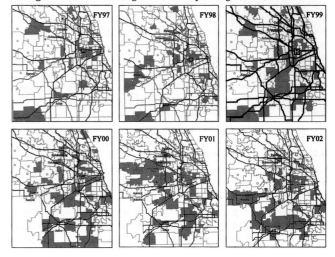

Figure 23–5 This figure maps the growth in demographic referral for aneurysm and subarachnoid hemorrhage from 1997 to 2002.

disease through the angioplasty/stenting cases. Each resident participating in a 3- to 6-month rotation performed or assisted in over 100 neuroendovascular cases (**Table 23–1**). This intimate interaction has given trainees entering practice a perspective on capabilities and capacities of neuroendovascular procedures that will influence their patients' treatment paradigms.

The influence of the program is reflected in the referral demographics for cerebroaneurysms, as demonstrated in **Fig. 23–5**. This region has five major academic medical centers and 130 neurological surgeons.

■ Conclusion

The establishment of an interventional neurovascular program enhances the academic neurological surgery cerebrovascular program. It expands treatment options for patients with aneurysms, AVMs, extra- and intracranial occlusive vascular disease, vasospasm, and stroke. Secondary areas of expansion include functional testing for epilepsy and tumor resection, supra-selective drug delivery programs, and vertebroplasty/kyphoplasty treatments. Enhancements in open surgical management are associated with the increased number of diagnostic angiograms with interventional/surgical views, microcatheter analysis, and intraoperative angiography.

Success Factors

1. There must be cooperative planning between health care and clinical departments. This is a partnership between departments and health care. Find an administrative champion and partner with that individual. Your success is their success, and their success is the institution's success.
2. The single most important aspect concerns philosophy: Peace is not the absence of conflict but a sense of tranquility in the midst of it.

"Progress is a nice word. But change is the motivator. And change has its enemies."

—Robert F. Kennedy

Neurological surgery must be willing to compromise, to grow, and to diversify. Resolve the financial issue. Keep medicine at heart but business on your mind. This program is a marriage of cultures. To be successful, realize that and embrace the best of each. Neurosurgical leadership must set the example. Lead, do not manage; change before you have to. If you do not have a competitive advantage, do not compete. Control your destiny, or someone else will.

3. This program cuts across the entire health system. Immediate and ongoing access to, and analysis of, financial demographic and clinical data are vital for ongoing success.

■ References

1. Cushing H. The Life of Sir William Osler. Oxford: Clarendon Press; 1925;177
2. Ausman JI. The future of neurovascular surgery. Part I: Intracranial aneurysms (comment) Surg Neurol 1997;48(1):98–100
3. Ausman JI. The death of cerebral aneurysm surgery. Surg Neurol 2001;56(5):348
4. Practice Management Information Corporation. International Classification of Diseases, 9th Edition/Revision. Los Angeles, CA: Practice Management Corporation; 2003

24

The Neurovascular Center Model for Practice

EDWIN J. CUNNINGHAM AND MARC R. MAYBERG

Objectives: After completing this chapter, the reader should be able to describe how to organize neurosurgeons, interventional neuroradiologists, and neurologists into a specialized group outside of their different departments.

Accreditation: The AANS* is accredited by the Accreditation Council for Continuing Medical Education (ACCME) to sponsor continuing medical education for physicians.

Credit: The AANS designates this educational activity for a maximum of 15 credits in Category 1 credit toward the AMA Physician's Recognition Award. Each physician should claim only those hours of credit that he/she spent in the educational activity.

The Home Study Examination is online on the AANS Web site at: http://www.aans.org/education/books/controversy.asp

* The acronym AANS refers to both the American Association of Neurological Surgeons and the American Association of Neurosurgeons.

The Neurovascular Center Model is an integrated multidisciplinary program of excellence designed to advance state-of-the-art care for patients with cerebrovascular disorders. The Center consists of physicians, nurses, and researchers from multiple specialties (Neurosurgery, Interventional Neuroradiology, Neurocritical Care, Neurology, and Basic Research) who comprise an autonomous clinical and research unit. In this chapter, we address the structure, benefits, and prerequisites for the establishment of successful neurovascular centers.

■ Benefits of the Center Model

Foremost among the benefits of an integrated neurovascular center is improved patient outcome. Randomized clinical trials and prospective observational studies suggest that organized stroke centers deliver better care and achieve better outcomes for patients suffering acute ischemic stroke.[1–4] The results of these studies led to the recent publication of *Recommendations for the Establishment*

of Primary Stroke Centers by the Brain Attack Coalition.[5] The authors cite several reasons for the development of the recommendations:

1. There are a large number of strokes per year (~750,000).
2. Many patients with stroke do not receive optimal therapy as defined by established guidelines.[6-11]
3. It is important to make new therapies available efficiently and safely to patients with strokes.

The need for such centers is underscored by a study demonstrating that only 1.8% of patients suffering acute ischemic stroke in the Cleveland area received FDA-approved intravenous tissue-type plasminogen activator (tPA).[12] Nationally, only 2 to 3% of patients with acute ischemic stroke receive tPA.[13,14] Reasons for the low rate of thrombolytic therapy include the inability of some medical systems to triage and evaluate such patients rapidly, patient presentation beyond the 3-hour treatment window, and clinician concerns about cerebral hemorrhage. Hemorrhage complicating intravenous tPA administration for acute ischemic stroke appears to be related to clinician expertise and experience in managing stroke. The Cleveland study also found that the rate of symptomatic intracranial hemorrhage following tPA administration was 15.7%, but for 50% of patients treated, national treatment protocols were violated. In a separate multicenter study, the rate of intracranial hemorrhage following tPA administration was 3.3%, with only 15% of treated patients having violations of treatment protocols.[15] These studies and others suggest that regional centers with expertise and experience in stroke management treat a higher proportion of acute stroke patients more aggressively, follow detailed protocols more closely, and achieve better results. Other expected clinical benefits of stroke centers are summarized by the Brain Attack Coalition in **Table 24–1**. It is likely that stroke centers will be certified in the near future, using credentialing methods analogous to that used to designate trauma centers.[16]

Aside from improving the level of care for stroke patients, there are other advantages of a neurovascular center. Education of medical students, residents, and fellows benefits from the center model. The integrated neurovascular team is especially advantageous for senior-level residents and neurovascular fellows in neurology, neurosurgery, and radiology. In the center model of multispecialty management, trainees acquire a working knowledge of diagnostic and therapeutic options that may be outside their primary discipline. This occurs during daily rounds, in weekly neurovascular meetings, and during interdisciplinary rotations.

Basic and clinical research of neurovascular diseases should improve in the multidisciplinary approach of the neurovascular center model. Under the leadership of a single director of cerebrovascular research, clinicians and postdoctoral researchers from multiple specialties collaborate on projects and provide critical feedback to one another on proposed and ongoing research. This collaborative process will focus efforts on the most clinically relevant areas in need of research, will assist in refining the objectives and methodology of planned research, and will eliminate overlapping projects.

A final advantage of the center model is consolidation of administrative, financial, and operational functions. Physician, nursing, and secretarial duties and inpatient

and outpatient services are combined. There are reduced operational costs, and patient management is streamlined. For example, since the establishment of a center model at the Cleveland Clinic Foundation in 2001, there has been a significant increase in inpatient (11%) and outpatient (19%) procedures and a 16% increase in gross revenues (unpublished data).

■ Prerequisites for Center Model

The elements of a center model as summarized by the Brain Attack Coalition are shown in **Table 24–2**. Other prerequisites are detailed below:

1. State-of-the-art facilities in surgery, radiology, intensive care, outpatient care, and education
2. Financial incentives for multidisciplinary care
3. A commitment to advancing patient care through education and research (including residency training, postgraduate fellowships, and continuing medical education)
4. Focused clinical and basic research in cerebrovascular and vascular biology
5. An integrated regional health care system to serve as referral base
6. An advanced information system enabling precise tracking of patient demographics, costs, utilization, and outcomes

■ Organizational Structure of the Center Model

The organization of the center model is based on the following premises:

Physical proximity—Care providers share common offices, outpatient facilities, administrative/secretarial support, inpatient wards, and intensive care units.

Table 24–1 Expected Benefits of Primary Stroke Centers

Improved Efficiency of Patient Care
Fewer Peristroke Complications
Increased Use of Acute Stroke Therapies
Reduced Morbidity and Mortality
Improved Long-Term Outcome
Reduced Costs to Health Care System
Increased Patient Satisfaction

Source: From Brain Attack Coalition. JAMA 2000;283(23):3102–3109. Reprinted by permission.

Table 24–2 Major Elements of a Primary Stroke Center

Patient Care Areas
    Acute Stroke Teams
    Written Care Protocols
    Emergency Medical Services
    Emergency Department
    Stroke Unit
    Neurosurgical Services

Support Services
    Commitment and Support of Medical Organization;
        a Stroke Center Director
    Neuroimaging Services
    Laboratory Services
    Outcome and Quality Improvement Activities
    Continuing Medical Education

Source: From Brain Attack Coalition. JAMA 2000;283(23):3102–3109. Reprinted by permission.

Neurovascular Center

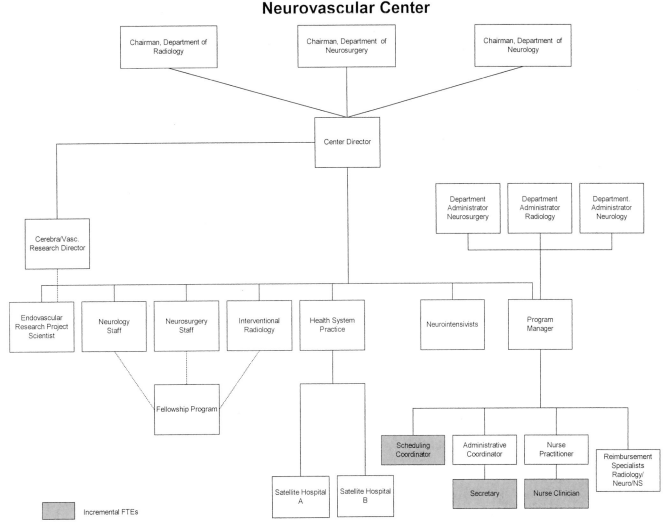

FIGURE 24-1 This diagram shows the organizational structure of the Neurovascular Center as set up at the Cleveland Clinic Foundation.

Cost accounting—Professional and technical (hospital) revenues and total expenses (personnel, equipment, supplies, outpatient, and hospital costs) can be accurately accounted for each diagnosis or procedure category.

Marketing—The concepts of multidisciplinary care, quality of care, cost effectiveness, and technology application can be effectively marketed to patients, physicians, and payers.

Care pathways—Clinical pathways are implemented to standardize treatment, improve outcome, and increase cost efficiency through improved utilization.

Outcome analysis—A centralized database provides continuous outcome data for academic research and marketing to payers.

Clinical research—Research protocols are efficiently implemented to facilitate technology development, early and rapid enrollment, and regulatory compliance

Basic and translational research—Focus group of clinician–scientists in the fields of cerebrovascular physiology and vascular biology facilitate creative and innovative translational experiments directed toward current clinical problems.

The structure of a planned center will have to conform to specific requirements of the institution. We provide a working example of the Neurovascular Center at the Cleveland Clinic as a guide (**Fig. 24–1**).

■ References

1. Collaborative systematic review of the randomized trials of organized inpatient (stroke unit) care after stroke. Stroke Unit Trialists' Collaboration. BMJ 1997;314(7088):1151–1159
2. Alberts MJ, Chaturvedi S, Graham G, et al. Acute stroke teams: results of a national survey. National Acute Stroke Team Group. Stroke 1998;29(11):2318–2320

3. Gomez CR, Malkoff MD, Sauer CM, Tulyapronchote R, Burch CM, Banet GA. Code stroke. An attempt to shorten inhospital therapeutic delays. Stroke 1994;25(10):1920–1923

4. Webb DJ, Fayad PB, Wilbur C, Thomas A, Brass LM. Effects of a specialized team on stroke care. The first two years of the Yale Stroke Program. Stroke 1995;26(8):1353–1357

5. Alberts MJ, Hademenos G, Latchaw RE, et al. Recommendations for the establishment of primary stroke centers. Brain Attack Coalition. JAMA 2000;283(23):3102–3109

6. Ad Hoc Committee of the American Heart Association. Guidelines for the management of transient ischemic attacks. Stroke 1994;25(6):1320–1335

7. Ad Hoc Committee of the American Heart Association. Guidelines for the management of patients with acute ischemic stroke. Stroke 1994;25:1901–1914

8. Ad Hoc Committee of the American Heart Association. Management of patients with acute ischemic stroke. Circulation 1994; 90:1588–1601

9. Ad Hoc Committee of the American Heart Association. guidelines for carotid endarterectomy—a multidisciplinary consensus statement. Stroke 1995;26:188–201

10. Adams HP Jr, Brott TG, Furlan AJ, et al. Guidelines for thrombolytic therapy for acute stroke: a supplement to the guidelines for the management of patients with acute ischemic stroke. A statement for health professionals from a special writing group of the Stroke Council American Heart Association. Stroke 1996;27(9):1711–1718

11. Adams HP Jr, Brott TG, Furlan AJ, et al. Guidelines for thrombolytic therapy for acute stroke: a supplement to the guidelines for the management of patients with acute ischemic stroke. A statement for health professionals from a special writing group of the Stroke Council American Heart Association. Circulation 1996;94(5):1167–1174

12. Katzan IL, Furlan AJ, Lloyd LE, et al. Use of tissue-type plasminogen activator for acute ischemic stroke: the Cleveland area experience. JAMA 2000;283(9):1151–1158

13. Alberts MJ. tPA in acute ischemic stroke: United States experience and issues for the future. Neurology 1998; 51(3, Suppl 3)S53–S55

14. Alberts MJ. Hyperacute stroke therapy with tissue plasminogen activator. Am J Cardiol 1997;80(4C):29D–34D discussion 35D–39D

15. Albers GW, Bates VE, Clark WM, Bell R, Verro P, Hamilton SA. Intravenous tissue-type plasminogen activator for treatment of acute stroke: the Standard Treatment with Alteplase to Reverse Stroke (STARS) study. JAMA 2000;283(9):1145–1150

16. Adams R, Acker J, Alberts M, et al. Recommendations for improving the quality of care through stroke centers and systems: an examination of stroke identification options: multidisciplinary consensus recommendations from the Advisory Working Group on Stroke Center Identification Options of the American Stroke Association. Stroke 2002;33(1):e1–e7

25

Regionalization of Neurovascular Medicine

E. SANDER CONNOLLY JR, MITCHELL F. BERMAN, AND ROBERT A. SOLOMON

Objectives: After completing this chapter, the reader should be able to identify the options for managing a cavernous malformation patient, and the appropriate indications and approaches for surgical resection.

Accreditation: The AANS* is accredited by the Accreditation Council for Continuing Medical Education (ACCME) to sponsor continuing medical education for physicians.

Credit: The AANS designates this educational activity for a maximum of 15 credits in Category 1 credit toward the AMA Physician's Recognition Award. Each physician should claim only those hours of credit that he/she spent in the educational activity.

The Home Study Examination is online on the AANS Web site at: http://www.aans.org/education/books/controversy.asp

* The acronym AANS refers to both the American Association of Neurological Surgeons and the American Association of Neurosurgeons.

A quiet revolution has been taking place over the past 25 years in the treatment of cerebral vascular diseases. The era of delayed aneurysm surgery is history. Prophylaxis and therapy for cerebral vasospasm have changed the face of the management of aneurysmal subarachnoid hemorrhage (SAH). Guglielmi detachable coil (GDC) embolization of aneurysms, introduced less than 10 years ago, has become an integral component of the arsenal for the treatment of cerebral aneurysms. N-butyl-cyano-acrylate (NBCA) glue embolization and stereotactic radiosurgery have so completely altered the landscape in the area of cerebral arteriovenous malformations that treatment approaches and outcomes bear little resemblance to the paradigms expounded by the current generation of retiring leaders in the field. The "Decade of the Brain" that has just passed has impressed on the national consciousness the need for emergency treatment of "brain attack." This concept has dramatically altered the approach to patients with ischemic stroke and intracranial hemorrhagic diseases. Intravascular thrombolysis, neurological intensive care units, and critical care neurology are terms not found in textbooks of a quarter century ago.

It is intuitively evident that with the explosion of supportive technology and modern treatment paradigms for vascular disease that every medical center in the country cannot be ideally equipped for treating cerebrovascular diseases. Within the field of neurosurgery, similar advances are occurring in spine treatments, oncology, epilepsy, etc. The task of remaining current and technologically up to date in all areas is a daunting task.

■ The Case for Regionalization

Regionalization of neurovascular medicine is an eventuality that cannot be denied. The underlying premise behind regionalization is that optimal outcomes are achieved at greatest efficiency if patient care is restricted to relatively few dedicated cerebrovascular centers. The first issue is that the majority of practicing physicians in this country were trained in an era when the approach to neurovascular medicine bore little resemblance to the state of the art at the dawn of the 21st century. Change continues at a rapid and accelerating pace. Obviously, many physicians have kept up with progress and have constantly modernized treatment approaches. Many have not. Substandard treatment is not only tolerated, it has been well-documented.

The central problem lies not only with physicians who are inadequately trained or have not kept up with their medical education but with facilities that do not possess the core resources necessary to deliver a modern standard of care to patients with cerebrovascular diseases. The technological revolution of the last quarter century has changed the face of treatment of cerebrovascular diseases. These changes, however, have added tremendous cost by way of modern imaging facilities required, advanced treatment modalities that are indicated, and the required personnel. Hospital administrators, struggling to keep their hospitals profitable in an era of declining reimbursements, have not been able to make the investment required when only small groups of patients are involved.

Meanwhile, economics and local politics have led the medical staff of small hospitals to be reluctant to transfer patients to regional centers, even when the modern infrastructure for the treatment of cerebrovascular diseases does not exist. Unfortunately, numerous studies show significant differences in morbidity and mortality for the management of cerebrovascular diseases in high-volume centers with high-volume surgeons compared with low-volume surgeons and hospitals.[1–9] Mortality has also been demonstrated to be significantly lower at high-volume hospitals for elective abdominal aortic aneurysm repair, carotid endarterectomy, lower extremity arterial bypass surgery, coronary artery bypass surgery, coronary angioplasty, heart transplantation, pediatric cardiac surgery, pancreatic cancer surgery, esophageal cancer surgery, trauma care, and treatment of human immunodeficiency virus (HIV)/acquired immunodeficiency syndrome (AIDS).[3–5,10–12] The inference is inescapable: The management of cerebrovascular diseases is safer and less expensive at regional medical centers with specialized facilities and medical personnel.

Solomon et al demonstrated that in New York State hospitals from 1987 to 1993 there was a 43% reduction in mortality for aneurysm surgery in hospitals performing more than 30 craniotomies per year for cerebral aneurysm compared with the lower-volume hospitals ($p < 0.01$).[8] Taylor et al analyzed Medicare patients over an 8-year period from 1984 through 1991.[9,13] The mortality rate for patients treated surgically for aneurysmal SAH was inversely correlated with the annual number of craniotomies performed at a given institution. Johnson et al studied individual California hospital experiences and overall treatment volume of cerebral aneurysms as a predictor of outcome.[7] The data on both endovascular treatment and surgical treatment was retrieved from a California statewide database of hospital discharges from

January 1990 through December 1998. Hospital treatment volume was divided into quartiles to distribute patients into four groups of equal size (quartile 1: 0 to 15.7 cases per year; quartile 4: 68 to 107 cases per year). Adverse outcomes for unruptured aneurysms decreased with increasing hospital volume (from 33% in quartile 1 to 14% in quartile 4; $p < 0.005$).

Despite some of the inherent weaknesses associated with retrospective database-based studies, we recently took a second look at the New York State discharges database, this time focusing on patients treated between 1995 and 2000.[14–17] For each 10 additional procedures performed per year, hospital volume was associated with fewer adverse outcomes and lower in-hospital mortality for both unruptured cerebral aneurysms (adverse outcome odds ratio [OR] 0.89, $p < 0.0001$; mortality OR 0.94, $p = 0.002$) and aneurysmal subarachnoid hemorrhage (adverse outcome OR 0.94, $p = 0.03$; mortality OR 0.95, $p = 0.005$). Indeed, even among the top 10 hospitals in New York State, there was a surprising residual effect of volume on outcome. In the top hospitals, which treated nearly 50% of the state's cases, the beneficial effect of institutional volume on adverse outcomes following treatment for both unruptured and ruptured aneurysms was about as large as it was for the overall state dataset. We also found that outcome following embolization of cerebral aneurysms is less affected by overall hospital volume than is clipping of cerebral aneurysms. This is not surprising given the fact that many have posited that aneurysm clipping may be more dependent on operator experience than aneurysm coiling. Although direct support for this contention has been difficult to demonstrate, data from the Cleveland Clinic does at least show that the number of aneurysm operations performed by each individual surgeon is a robust predictor of functional outcome ($r = 0.99$, $p = 0.05$).[18]

Armed with the data from New York State, we then looked to see what the effect would be of regionalizing aneurysm care in New York State by referring patients to the top 10 busiest centers (≥35 cases/year [35 to 133]). For unruptured aneurysms, there we predicted a 27% annual improvement in the adverse outcome rate and a 14% improvement in mortality. For aneurysmal subarachnoid hemorrhage, the reductions would be 12% and 11%, respectively. In absolute numbers, the reduction in poor outcome or death per year would 18 patients with unruptured aneurysms and 50 patients with ruptured aneurysms. If fewer centers were used with even higher volume, the predicted reductions in suffering would be even greater. If one extrapolates these data to the United States as a whole, regionalization of cerebral aneurysm treatment alone would eliminate 5700 poor outcomes or deaths each year in the United States.[2,19] One could only guess at the potential cost savings. Add stroke, carotid artery disease, and arteriovenous malformations to the mix, and the case for a serious national health care initiative is on the table.

In addition to the historical data supporting regionalization of cerebrovascular services, there are additional factors on the horizon that make regionalization even more important. One of these factors is the shrinking number of aneurysms, carotid stenoses, and arteriovenous malformations available for training and maintenance of open surgical skill sets because of the rapid proliferation of technologies such as coiling, stenting, and gamma knife radiosurgery. For instance, in New York State alone, the percentage of aneurysms treated with open surgery has fallen from 91% in 1995 to 77% in 2000. In the next 10 years alone, we expect to see this fall to somewhere around 35%. The combination of a shrinking number of "open" cases and a diminished workforce of experienced cerebrovascular surgeons will make it increasingly important to develop referral centers to provide the younger generation of open surgeons with the volume necessary to develop and maintain competency.

Given the rapidity of the projected growth in endovascular procedures, without regionalization, there will be a real shortage of qualified neuroendovascular surgeons. Even as the number of these specialists grows, the main driving force will be the treatment of acute stroke rather than orphan diseases such as aneurysms and arteriovenous malformations (AVMs). Therefore, as the field of endovascular surgery matures, individual practitioners will treat fewer and fewer aneurysms and AVMs in much the same way as the neurosurgical workforce as a whole has come to treat less and less intracranial disease. Eventually, it is possible that only those endovascular surgeons in busy centers will be able to demonstrate the lowest complication rates for rarer diseases. Currently there is no direct evidence that this will be the case for endovascular coiling, but only 19 (7%) of New York State's 257 hospitals actually coil aneurysms, compared with 113 (44%) in which clipping is performed. In California from 1990 to 1998, only 11 centers performed GDC coiling, whereas 167 centers provided open surgical services for these lesions.[7] As endovascular techniques filter to the community, it will obviously be necessary to examine whether results with common diseases such as cerebral ischemia vary to the same degree as results with less-common diseases like aneurysms. What is certain is that there will likely be a need for several types of cerebrovascular referral centers as time goes on. There will be quaternary centers treating low-frequency diseases that can stand minor delays in therapy related to transportation, and there will be tertiary centers where services are provided for common diseases that cannot bear any delay at all in referral. Even a large state like New York might have 10 centers treating aneurysms, but 100 centers providing acute pharmacologic and mechanical thrombolysis.

■ Cerebrovascular Disease Center

The heart of a modern center for the treatment of cerebrovascular diseases is a neuroscience intensive care unit (NICU). Ideally, the ICU will focus only on patients with neurological diseases. This type of focus guarantees that the medical staff is trained and devoted to treating neurological illness. Such a unit could also be part of a more general ICU but there would have to be staff commitment to the clinical neurosciences. Physicians trained in critical care neurology staffing the unit 24 hours/day are an essential component. These physicians could be neurology residents, neurosurgery residents, trained intensive care specialists, or other physicians attuned to the cardiopulmonary management of patients with central nervous system diseases. The most successful models of NICUs are in major medical centers with full-time neurology and neurosurgery residents, and thus the capacity to staff the unit on a 24-hour basis with involved, well-trained physician support staff. This staffing usually consists of a resident on call at night with backup from a fellow and senior staff member. Resident work hours' restrictions, the movement among neurology training programs to limit clinical inpatient experiences in favor of outpatient and laboratory training, and the growing evidence that ICU patients should be continuously, visually observed by attending-level physicians make the NICU an increasingly complex and expensive program to administer.

Nursing is also an essential aspect of the NICU. Nurses at the bedside are the ones that have to be able to recognize the earliest signs of neurological deterioration that often initiate a chain reaction of treatment that can make the difference between a good and poor outcome. General ICU nurses without a special interest in neurological diseases usually are not well trained in recognizing important subtle changes in the neurological examination. These nurses may also not be able to institute critical therapy even before the physician staff becomes available. With national nursing shortages and the increasing opportunities open to nurses in management, public health and as inpatient and outpatient physician extenders, nursing turnover in ICUs has increased in the last decade, making the experienced neuroscience ICU nurse an endangered species. Assembling and maintaining teams of these nurses is increasingly complicated and expensive.

Neuroradiological facilities have obvious implications for the management of cerebrovascular diseases. 24-hour access to sophisticated computerized tomography (CT) scanning (CT angiography [CTA], CT perfusion [CTP], Xenon-CT etc.), magnetic resonance imaging (MRI), and cerebral angiography are essential components of any fully equipped modern cerebrovascular center.

Availability also includes radiology technicians and fully trained neuroradiologists capable of performing invasive diagnostic procedures, reconstructing critical data sets, and reading the films as they become available at all hours of the day and night.

Finally, the equipment needs for running a state-of-the-art NICU are evolving at an increasingly rapid pace. Cerebral microdialysis catheters, intracerebral pressure (ICP) monitors, LICOX monitors, near-infrared spectroscopy pads, continuous electroencephalogram (EEG) monitoring, and round-the-clock access to transcranial Doppler ultrasonography have all become commonplace. In addition to minute-to-minute maintenance of ventriculostomies, the ICU of the future may be involved in neuroperfusion and cerebrospinal fluid (CSF) filtration, in addition to providing a whole host of temperature-managing devices including intravenous, intraarterial, transcutaneous, and transcalvarial. When ordered in quantity, the price of these devices becomes manageable. In addition, all of these devices have a finite complication rate; this is reduced with repetitive use.

Once a properly staffed and equipped NICU has been assembled, the final critical pieces of a modern neurovascular service can be developed. Neurosurgeons, skilled and experienced in the surgical treatment of intracranial vascular disease, have to staff the center and have access to high-quality operating room facilities. The operating microscope, intraoperative angiography, and an image-based frameless stereotactic guidance system are minimal requirements for modern cerebrovascular surgery. Similarly, endovascular neurosurgeons or interventional neuroradiologists must be available to provide endovascular therapies for aneurysm patients, AVM patients, and stroke victims. These services have to be on-site and consistently available for maximum benefit. Angioplasty for vasospasm after SAH, thrombolysis for acute arterial occlusion, and coil embolization of ruptured aneurysms are often emergency procedures. It is rare that emergency embolization of AVMs is also required. The provision of surgical services at one institution with transfer to another institution if endovascular services are required will result in an unnecessary delay in treatment, with unnecessary morbidity and mortality. Similarly, surgeons skilled in and available to perform decompressive craniotomies, clot evacuations, and a variety of CSF diversion procedures need to be available at a moment's notice.

All of these services have to be provided not only 24 hours a day and 7 days a week, but 365 days a year; therefore, a significant staff of experts (often three deep in each area) has to be assembled. To maintain competence in such a staff, a critical volume of clinical material has to be available. Regionalization makes sense by identifying institutions capable of providing high-level service and directing appropriate patients and resources to that center. The high patient volume will attract the best clinicians and ensure that those clinicians are highly experienced. The net result is high-quality care for patients, significant reduction in morbidity and mortality, and huge cost savings to society.

■ The Case against Regionalization

Perhaps one of the arguments most often voiced against regionalization is that in relegating the treatment of patients to a few centers, the care of patients in these centers may become inbred and innovation might be undermined. While this is of theoretical concern, history does not support this contention, with the vast majority of medical advances being initiated and developed in large quaternary referral centers. Another criticism is that regionalization requires many patients to travel far from their homes and social support systems often when they are the sickest. While this is of concern, the overwhelming majority of those who have made such a sacrifice say they would do so again in similar circumstances. Moreover, many of these patients can transfer back to local facilities within a short time period. Finally, others have argued that centralization of care might undermine the financial health of community hospitals that provide important local services that could never be provided by quaternary or even tertiary centers. While this argument may hold some water with other disease states, this does not appear to be the case with cerebrovascular disease, especially if the local hospital were required to possess the same infrastructure as the regional center. Even as it stands now, with aneurysms treated in the community with no specialized expertise or equipment whatsoever, the high morbidity with attendant length of stay associated even with unruptured aneurysm surgery probably results in little economic benefit to these facilities. Most of the centralization effort would effect a movement of cases from those hospitals providing care for less than one patient a month to centers treating 10 times that number.

■ The Future

The preponderance of evidence suggests that centralization of care for complex cerebrovascular diseases, especially aneurysms and arteriovenous malformations, is likely to result in a great savings in lost lives. The reasons for this are multifactorial but include physician- as well as hospital-related factors. Despite the likely benefit to society in terms of cost and suffering, centralization is unlikely without the direct insistence of both private and public third-party payers.

■ References

1. Bardach NS, Zhao S, Gress DR, Lawton MT, Johnston SC. Association between subarachnoid hemorrhage outcomes and number of cases treated at California hospitals. Stroke 2002;33:1851–1856

2. Becker KJ. Epidemiology and clinical presentation of aneurysmal subarachnoid hemorrhage. Neurosurg Clin N Am 1998;9:435–444

3. Dudley RA, Johansen KL, Brand R, Rennie DJ, Milstein A. Selective referral to high-volume hospitals: estimating potentially avoidable deaths. JAMA 2000;283:1159–1166

4. Epstein AM. Volume and outcome—it is time to move ahead. N Engl J Med 2002;346:1161–1164

5. Hamilton SM, Johnston WC, Voaklander DC. Outcomes after the regionalization of major surgical procedures in the Alberta Capital Health Region (Edmonton). Can J Surg 2001;44:51–58

6. Johnston SC, Dudley RA, Gress DR, Ono L. Surgical and endovascular treatment of unruptured cerebral aneurysms at university hospitals. Neurology 1999;52:1799–1805

7. Johnston SC, Zhao S, Dudley RA, Berman MF, Gress DR. Treatment of unruptured cerebral aneurysms in California. Stroke 2001;32:597–605

8. Solomon RA, Mayer SA, Tarmey JJ. Relationship between the volume of craniotomies for cerebral aneurysm performed at New York state hospitals and in-hospital mortality. Stroke 1996; 27:13–17

9. Taylor CL, Yuan Z, Selman WR, Ratcheson RA, Rimm AA. Mortality rates, hospital length of stay, and the cost of treating subarachnoid hemorrhage in older patients: institutional and geographical differences. J Neurosurg 1997;86:583–588

10. Birkmeyer JD, Siewers AE, Finlayson EV, et al. Hospital volume and surgical mortality in the United States. N Engl J Med 2002;346: 1128–1137

11. Hannan EL, Siu AL, Kumar D, Kilburn H Jr, Chassin MR. The decline in coronary artery bypass graft surgery mortality in New York State. The role of surgeon volume. JAMA 1995;273:209–213

12. Silber JH, Rosenbaum PR, Williams SV, Ross RN, Schwartz JS. The relationship between choice of outcome measure and hospital rank in general surgical procedures: implications for quality assessment. Int J Qual Health Care 1997;9:193–200

13. Taylor CL, Yuan Z, Selman WR, Ratcheson RA, Rimm AA. Cerebral arterial aneurysm formation and rupture in 20,767 elderly patients: hypertension and other risk factors. J Neurosurg 1995; 83:812–819

14. Johnston SC. Combining ecological and individual variables to reduce confounding by indication: case study–subarachnoid hemorrhage treatment. J Clin Epidemiol 2000;53:1236–1241

15. New York Statewide Planning and Research Cooperative System (SPARCS). Inpatient and Outpatient Data. Albany, NY: New York State Department of Health; 1999

16. New York Statewide Planning and Research Cooperative System (SPARCS). Inpatient Output Data Dictionary. Albany, NY: New York State Department of Health; 2001

17. Berman MF, Solomon RA, Mayer SA, Yung P. The impact of hospital related factors on outcome following treatment for cerebral aneurysms. Stroke 2003;34:2200–2207

18. Chyatte D, Porterfield R. Functional outcome after repair of unruptured intracranial aneurysms. J Neurosurg 2001;94:417–421

19. Census 2000. Washington, DC: US Census Bureau, US Dept. of Commerce; 2001

26

Resolving Controversy and Uncertainty with Evidence in Neurovascular Medicine

S. CLAIBORNE JOHNSTON

Objectives: After reading this chapter, the reader should be able to describe the types of clinical studies (case series, case-control studies, cohort studies, and randomized trials) and judge the quality of data derived from those studies.

Accreditation: The AANS* is accredited by the Accreditation Council for Continuing Medical Education (ACCME) to sponsor continuing medical education for physicians.

Credit: The AANS designates this educational activity for a maximum of 15 credits in Category 1 credit toward the AMA Physician's Recognition Award. Each physician should claim only those hours of credit that he/she spent in the educational activity.

The Home Study Examination is online on the AANS Web site at: http://www.aans.org/education/books/controversy.asp

* The acronym AANS refers to both the American Association of Neurological Surgeons and the American Association of Neurosurgeons.

If every clinical decision was supported by solid, irrefutable evidence, there would be little controversy in clinical practice. Appropriate treatment decisions would be obvious. In reality, treatment decisions are based on imperfect evidence. Physicians receive bits of data from a variety of sources, including study results, expert opinion, and experience. These data must be combined and applied to a specific clinical situation.[1]

Ideally, every decision should be based on the highest standard of evidence available—the results of a randomized trial. However, very few informative randomized trials are undertaken. They are expensive and may be impractical, with delayed results.[2] Further, the results of a randomized trial apply to the average patient enrolled in the study; they may not apply readily to the particular patient for whom a treatment decision is being made.[3] In the foreseeable future, it still will not be possible to base clinical decisions entirely on the results of randomized trials. Therefore, it is important to understand the strengths and limitations of other sources of evidence.

Entirely rational clinical decision-making is not achievable. Subjectivity is unavoidable. Among other influences, our instinct for self-preservation is too powerful and important. For example, the decision to delay endovascular repair of a ruptured aneurysm may be influenced by a child's Saturday morning birthday party. Personal financial gain also influences physician behavior.[4] Some degree of physician self-interest is natural and essential. Few would join or survive the practice of medicine if every decision made were entirely altruistic. Our current monkish lifestyle would become intolerable. Nonetheless, it is essential to examine personal motivations in clinical decision-making and to view our interpretation of evidence with suspicion, always on the lookout for our own biases.[5]

In this chapter, I provide a framework for interpreting and generating evidence, with the goal of focusing attention on key sources of bias. Such a framework may be useful in identifying the boundaries between objective evidence and subjective bias to improve the quality of clinical decision-making.

■ Levels of Evidence

Clinical decisions generally involve synthesizing data from a variety of sources. Quality of the data source should influence the weight of the data in the final decision.[1,6] Quality is dependent on the study type—case series, case-control study, cohort study, or randomized trial—and on the details of its execution. Standard methods for ranking quality of data have been proposed and are often used in developing clinical guidelines (**Table 26-1**).[7,8] These rankings provide a rough template for assessing evidence.

■ Physician Experience and Opinion

The experience of the treating physician may be the most influential evidence used in making clinical decisions. Others may rely on the experience and opinions of experts to guide decisions. Textbooks frequently contain phrases such as "our experience has shown…" and "It is quite clear from our experience…."

Generally, this is the least reliable level of evidence. Any individual's observations are subject to biases, regardless of years of experience and prominence in the field. These biases may be completely unrecognized by the individual.

Experience and opinion may be the only source of data. In this instance, developing consensus based on opinions of practitioners from various backgrounds may reduce the influence of bias. The loudest voice may have the greatest influence, so it is important to ensure that the opinions of a dominating personality are not weighted disproportionately. The RAND Corporation (Santa Monica, CA) has developed standardized methods for combining the experience and opinions of multiple practitioners.[9] The method incorporates expert opinions with respect to specific, well-defined cohorts of patients.

■ Case Series

The next level of evidence is the description of a series of cases. A case series may produce more reliable evidence than opinion because the details of the experience are explicitly described. The opinion drawn from the cases can be questioned because its source can be examined by the reader.

Case series are particularly susceptible to bias, and details of study design must be considered carefully. Case selection is one major source of bias; designs that establish systematic methods of inclusion reduce this risk. For example, a study may describe five patients with unruptured aneurysms who died after coil embolization, and this may influence physicians by suggesting that endovascular treatment is unsafe. However, these five patients may have part of a series of 500 patients. Then the selection of only those cases that died has produced a misleading impression of the safety of coil embolization.

Choosing a consecutive series of cases may reduce the risk of bias in case selection. However, a bias can still be introduced if the beginning or ending of the collection period is influenced by outcome. For example, the occurrence of a death with coil embolization could trigger the initiation of a prospective study period, and the occurrence of five deaths among 15 treated patients could trigger preparation of a manuscript and publication. However, these 15 patients may not be representative of the entire experience at the center. Similarly, describing the initial experience with a technique and comparing it to prior results with a different technique may also be misleading because expertise will not be developed with the new procedure.

Practitioners with greater experience and prominence often publish case series. Further, those with poor results of treatment are less likely "to air the dirty laundry." Therefore, case series tend to be biased toward underreporting of adverse events from treatment. This form of publication bias is not unique to case series and may influence reporting of all study designs.

Table 26–1 Levels of Evidence and Grading of Recommendations[9A,9B]

Level of Evidence	
Level I	Data from randomized trials with low false-positive (α) and low false-negative (β) errors
Level II	Data from randomized trials with high false-positive (α) or high false-negative (β) errors
Level III	Data from nonrandomized concurrent cohort studies
Level IV	Data from nonrandomized cohort studies using historical controls; data from case-control studies
Level V	Data from anecdotal case series
Strength of Recommendation	
Grade A	Supported by Level I evidence
Grade B	Supported by Level II evidence
Grade C	Supported by Level III, IV, or V evidence

Case series often do not include a comparison group. Centers with expertise in surgical clipping report a series of surgically treated unruptured aneurysms. Centers with experience in endovascular surgery report results for coil embolization. Comparing therapies described in different case series is problematic. First, outcome measures are variable and their assessment is influenced by the method of ascertainment, as discussed below. A poor outcome may be defined as death or vegetative state in one study, and as inability to return to work in another, and these results are not readily comparable. Second, the patients selected for treatment in different case series may not be comparable. For example, a surgical series may be derived from a referral population with a disproportionate number of giant aneurysms, and an endovascular series may be more representative of the community. Comparing these series could produce the misleading impression that differences in outcome are because of the greater safety of coil embolization.

Case series are a mainstay of the surgical and interventional literature. They are required to recognize priorities for further study but are seldom useful for establishing standards of care.

■ Case-Control Studies

Case-control studies are rarely used to evaluate treatment. By definition, a case-control study first classifies subjects by the outcome—such as dead/not dead—and compares all other characteristics in the two outcome groups. The design is useful when the outcome is rare and when it is difficult to define the study group prior to treatment. For example, if an investigator were interested in the risk factors for rerupture after coil embolization and had not been keeping track of details of all treated patients, a case-control study could be useful. A collection of 20 cases with rerupture could be compared with a random sample of 20 patients who had been treated but did not rerupture. A difference in aneurysm neck size in the two groups could implicate this characteristic as a risk factor for rerupture. The case-control design is more efficient than collecting neck size for all treated patients (which would be a cohort study): there would be fewer films to review with only marginal loss of statistical power. However, the case-control design is susceptible to biases if controls are not representative of the population from which the cases arose. For example, smoking may appear to be a risk factor for rerupture, but this could be due to a greater likelihood of refusal to participate in a control group with smokers, a phenomenon that is well-recognized. Difficulty in identifying an appropriate control group severely limits the utility of the case-control design.

■ Cohort Studies

Cohort studies are simply systematic case series. All patients are studied who meet specified entry criteria. Contrary to case series, cohort studies are always fully inclusive of all qualifying patients treated over a given time period. Contrary to case-control studies, subjects are identified by characteristics at the time of or prior to treatment rather than by the outcome, and outcomes are compared between groups treated in different ways. Though it is possible to study only a single therapy in a cohort study, the method is frequently used to compare therapies. The cohort study is a great improvement over case series when comparing therapies because it guarantees that outcomes are measured on the same scale and, preferably, by the same investigators.

The inclusion criteria of a cohort study must be explicit and should be established before outcomes are tallied. If the outcome influences the decision to include a case, bias will result. For example, if we are comparing surgery and endovascular therapy of unruptured aneurysms, and in preliminary analyses, we discover that new disability occurred in 5 of 10 middle cerebral artery (MCA) aneurysms treated by coil embolization, we would introduce a bias if we redefined entry criteria to restrict the cohort to aneurysms in other locations. It would be reasonable to report that outcomes were different with MCA aneurysms, but it would be misleading to omit them from the analysis after noting the outcomes. Establishing inclusion criteria prior to tallying outcomes prevents this form of bias. If we are convinced that MCA aneurysms should be treated with surgery, we can make the decision to omit this subgroup a priori, but we cannot alter our initial hypothesis and entry criteria once the outcomes have been evaluated.

The validity of cohort studies is strengthened by their standardized and explicit entry criteria established a priori. Further, the entry criteria can be used to define a group that could have received either therapy. This is essential because the appropriate treatment decision is known for those who could only receive one of the two therapies being compared, and these patients would not be included in a randomized trial. Including results of patients who could only receive one of the therapies could result in bias because their outcomes may be entirely different from those who could receive either therapy—the group in whom treatment decisions are made. Systematic inclusion criteria can be crafted to reduce the likelihood of including those who are not candidates for both procedures.[10] For example, it might be reasonable to exclude cavernous carotid aneurysms from a study of unruptured aneurysm treatment because many would not be appropriate candidates for surgical clipping. When indications for treatment are unclear, physicians can be asked to determine whether a case could receive both treatments; blinding the reviewing physicians to actual treatment assignment and outcome further reduces the potential for bias when selecting cases that are candidates for both procedures.[11]

Applying identical entry criteria to both treatments does not ensure that there are no systematic differences in the risk profiles of the treatment groups. For example, a hospital may triage older patients to endovascular therapy because of the perception that the elderly do poorly with surgery. Unless the cohort is limited to patients in a certain age group, there will be an imbalance in age in the treatment groups, and this may result in poorer outcomes in the endovascular group. Evaluating and reporting other risk factors for the outcome of interest is essential in any cohort study. In this way, systematic differences in known risk factors can be identified.

Identifying systematic differences in risk profile between treatment groups does not invalidate a study. Multivariable analysis is one tool for reducing the potential for imbalances in risk that influence the relative outcomes of the compared treatments. Logistic regression is the standard form of multivariable analysis used to evaluate binary outcomes (such as dead/alive), and linear regression is used for continuous outcomes (such as infarct volume). By adjusting for other risk factors, multivariable analysis isolates the independent effect of treatment on outcome. However, multivariable analysis only adjusts for other risk factors that are measured. If there are unmeasured factors that may be different in the treatment groups, a difference in outcome could still be due to risk profile rather than actual treatment. For example, the configuration of certain aneurysms may result in more-difficult procedures, and we may not be able to capture this in a standard multivariable analysis because configuration is too poorly defined to measure. One solution is to have physicians review the films and judge the difficulty in treatment, reducing the potential for bias by blinding to actual treatment selection and outcome.[11] Then, normally immeasurable factors can be incorporated into multivariable models. Such an analysis prevents one group from later blaming poorer outcomes on a patient-risk profile. However, it is always possible that a risk factor of either procedure, unknown to practitioner, is unbalanced between the treatment groups. This is the greatest inherent limitation of cohort studies and of all other studies in which treatment assignment is not random.

■ Randomized Trials

Randomized trials generally produce the most reliable evidence. Because only the randomization determines which treatment is received, all other risk factors are generally balanced between the treatment groups as long as the study sample size is adequate.[12] Even unmeasured factors should be distributed evenly between treatments.

Double blinding is the ideal in randomized trials. By blinding the patient to treatment assignment, one reduces the likelihood that the patients' preconceived notions of treatment will bias their responses when outcomes are assessed. This is important because patients tend to favor newer and more technical therapies and receive psychological benefit from these.[13] Blinding the physician or the assessor of outcome reduces the likelihood that subject biases will influence assessment of outcomes. Though blinding is straightforward for most medical therapies, which can be compared with placebo, it is much more difficult with invasive therapies. Sham surgeries are used, but some argue that they are unethical because an unnecessary risk and discomfort are undertaken. An alternative approach is to blind the assessor of outcome to treatment assignment and to choose an outcome measure that is as objective as possible. Such an approach is common in modern trials of neurosurgical interventions.[14]

Randomized trials are difficult to perform.[2] They require extensive planning and substantial resources, and results are often delayed. Some clinical questions cannot be ethically studied with randomized trials. For these reasons, most clinical decisions are made without the benefit of randomized trials. The results of randomized trials should always be considered in making clinical decisions, but other sources of evidence are essential.

■ Elements of Study Design

Prospective versus Retrospective

Studies are defined as prospective if patients are identified before the outcome has occurred and are retrospective otherwise.[15] Case-control studies are always retrospective because outcome defines the groups being compared. Randomized trials are always prospective because inclusion and randomization occur before the outcome. Case series and cohort studies can be either prospective or retrospective.

Prospective studies have several advantages. First, it is not possible for outcome to influence inclusion of a case because outcomes are unknown when the study begins. Second, baseline factors can be assessed more completely to evaluate changes with therapy and to ensure a more complete balance. For example, a prospective study may allow measurement of cognitive function prior to treatment so that change with therapy can be assessed. Third, some pretreatment variables may be inaccurately or incompletely recalled, and these factors can be measured before treatment in a prospective study. For these reasons, prospective studies are often more likely to produce valid results.

However, prospective studies are inefficient. Often results are delayed for years while an adequate number of cases are generated. The results of a retrospective study are generated as rapidly as an analysis is performed. This is a tremendous advantage, but only if the potential pitfalls of retrospective studies are overcome by mimicking the design of prospective studies. First, to reduce the likelihood of outcome influencing case inclusion, strict entry criteria should be established before beginning the analysis, as discussed above. Second, the outcome chosen should be robust without a measure of pretreatment condition. For example, a retrospective study of unruptured aneurysm treatment with a cognitive test score as an outcome may be acceptable because patients are often unimpaired prior to treatment, but a similar outcome measure in a study of subarachnoid hemorrhage would be much more problematic in a retrospective study. Third, retrospective studies should only be undertaken if the measurable pretreatment risk factors are expected to allow for adequate adjustment of prognostic differences between treatment groups. Although we may have a Hunt and Hess score in a retrospective study of subarachnoid hemorrhage, this measure could not be expected to capture important differences in pretreatment prognosis in a study of subarachnoid hemorrhage treatment. In this instance, even a prospective study may not allow complete adjustment for important differences in prognosis. Compared with prospective studies, retrospective studies are clearly more efficient and, if performed carefully, are not necessarily more susceptible to bias.

Size and Power

Study size is often determined by convenience—the number of available cases. This strategy does not produce bias in a retrospective study because the size is fixed. In prospective studies, bias is produced if the results are evaluated at intervals and the study is stopped when a significant effect is seen. This strategy is more likely to produce significant results when the treatments are the same.

Study size determines the power to find a significant effect if one is truly present. Studies that are too small may fail to find clinically important differences in outcomes but should not be interpreted as showing no difference. A recent small, randomized trial of clipping versus coiling of ruptured aneurysms included 109 patients.[16] Severe disability or worse occurred in 25% of surgical cases and 21% of endovascular cases, and the difference was not significant. However, the 95% confidence intervals were consistent with a threefold lower risk with coil embolization or a twofold lower risk with surgery, which demonstrates the limitations of study power. The International Subarachnoid Aneurysm Trial

(ISAT) will include 2500 patients to answer the same question and was designed to detect a 25% difference in outcome between the two therapies.[17]

Necessary sample size and power can be calculated from tables, equations, or software programs (such as Epi-Info, which is available without charge from the Centers for Disease Control and Prevention Web site: www.cdc.gov). All prospective studies should include some calculation and consideration of power if the goal is to generate significant results when a true, clinically important difference is present. Further, all studies should acknowledge the limitations in the precision of treatment effect estimates. This can be done most readily by reporting the 95% confidence intervals.

Measuring Outcomes

Choosing the outcomes of a study requires careful consideration. The measure used by colleagues in recent publications may not be the ideal measure. Before beginning a study, it is preferable to define a single primary outcome measure for the main study hypothesis. Any number of secondary outcome measures can be evaluated, but committing to a single primary measure prevents bias produced by "cherry-picking" the outcome that happens to be significant. For example, if the Glasgow Outcome Scale,[18] Barthel Index,[19] and Rankin Scale[20] are measured as outcomes but only the Rankin Scale shows a significant effect, an investigator is likely to focus on the Rankin Scale results to stress the importance of the findings. However, it is more likely that a single outcome will be positive if more outcomes are measured. Therefore, a study that measures multiple outcomes and does not commit to a primary outcome measure is more likely to find an effect even when none exists. If the Glasgow Outcome Scale results were defined a priori as the primary outcome measure, the study would be negative, though other results from secondary outcome measures could suggest that a smaller or more specific effect was present. If a primary outcome measure is not chosen a priori, all the study results should be examined carefully to confirm that findings are consistent in all the outcomes measured.

Outcome measures should be reproducible, valid, measure clinically meaningful results, and allow comparison of results between studies. The simplest way to define such an outcome measure is to utilize an existing scale. Many investigators bow to the temptation to create a new scale—such as excellent, fair, poor outcome—but this creates several problems. First, such a scale is not generalizable. What one physician calls an excellent outcome, another may define as unacceptable. This makes it impossible to compare results of one study with another. Second, vague definition of the outcome states encourages bias. It increases the likelihood that classification will be subjective with the potential to underrepresent the true impact of therapeutic complications. Third, home-made scales do not necessarily measure outcomes that are important to patients or to the health care system in general. For example, an excellent outcome may be defined as anything better than a vegetative state. However, patients may have significant and important disabilities that would not be captured in this scale. Fourth, a nonstandard scale may be difficult to repro-duce over time or between investigators, introducing random misclassification that reduces the likelihood of finding an effect when one is present. If two patients with identical outcomes are classified differently because the scale definitions are vague, this introduces random varia-tion that makes it harder to find a true effect.

Mortality is perhaps the cleanest outcome measure. There is little argument about whether an event has occurred or whether the outcome is important. How-ever, mortality may be rare, which results in reduced power. Important differences in outcomes may be ignored if mortality is chosen as the primary outcome measure. For example, two therapies may have identical mortality rates but disability may be quite different. The difference in the therapies would be missed if only mor-tality were measured.

Scales with additional gradations increase the likeli-hood of finding a significant effect if one is present and may more accurately reflect the health impact of the therapies being studied. There are many standard, validated, and reproducible outcome measures available. These scales can measure functional states (such as the Barthel Index, Rankin Scale, Glasgow Outcome Scale, cognitive scales[21]), quality of life (such as the Sickness Impact Profile[22]), or health perceptions (such as the SF-36[23]).

Choosing between these and other scales can be diffi-cult. From the perspective of statistical power, the best outcome measure is one that spreads out results evenly. For a binary outcome, this means that 50% of patients are in each category. The Glasgow Outcome Scale and Barthel Index do not measure minor deficits well. They are weighted toward differentiating very poor functional states. Therefore, in a study in which poor functional states are uncommon, such as a study of treatments for unruptured aneurysms, only a few patients would be expected to show impairment in these scales, and power would be low relative to a scale that included cognitive impairment. This was illustrated in the International Study of Unruptured Intracranial Aneurysms in which the inclusion of cognitive impairment nearly doubled the number of patients classified as disabled.[24] If surgery and endovascular therapy were compared in this study, including cognitive impairment would increase the like-lihood that a significant difference would be detected if one were truly present.

It is important to standardize a chosen outcome scale's or scales' measure to reduce the potential for bias. First, it is best to define a specific time point for assessment of the outcomes. In this way, differences in the timing of the evaluation between groups will not influence the results. For example, if an outcome is measured at hospi-tal discharge and length of stay is longer for one therapy than another, one group will have longer to recover from treatment, potentially introducing a bias. Determining the timing of measurement requires careful consideration. The outcome should be measured after recovery is largely complete if differences in lifelong outcomes are expected but could be measured sooner if the rate of recovery is important in distinguishing thera-pies. Further, if patients have other medical problems, a delayed measure of outcome could introduce additional random variation or bias due to complications from other diseases unrelated to the therapies studied.

Second, who will be measuring the outcome must be carefully considered. The assessor can affect the sensitiv-ity and reproducibility of the outcome measure. For example, studies have shown that neurologists detect complications much more frequently after carotid endarterectomy than neurosurgeons.[25] In case series, this may affect the perceived risks of treatment. The assessor can also introduce his or her own biases into the assessment. For example, it is not realistic to expect a neurointerventional radiologist to evaluate outcomes of surgery in a study comparing clipping to coil emboliza-tion unless he is blinded to the actual treatment received. Even the best intentions and the highest integrity are challenged by subtle biases to favor one's own practice. Therefore, it is best to obtain outcomes blinded to the actual treatment received. If this is not possible, other alternatives include choosing an assessor with no clear bias, such as a study nurse, or choosing a team of assessors with equal representation from both the procedures being compared.

■ Conclusion

Medical knowledge is constantly evolving. Physicians are responsible for integrating information of varying quality from multiple sources with varying applicability to a given clinical situation. The task is impossible to perform without error. Understanding and addressing biases in our own integration of evidence is important in making the most rational clinical decisions and in improving the quality of the evidence. There is a natural tendency to defend one's own current practice, and this may influ-ence the acceptance of new evidence and performance of studies. Recognizing potential sources of bias in clini-cal studies is important in weighing the evidence and improving it.

■ References

1. Guyatt GH, Haynes RB, Jaeschke RZ, et al. Users' Guides to the Medical Literature: XXV. Evidence-based medicine: principles for applying the Users' Guides to patient care. Evidence-Based Medicine Working Group. JAMA 2000;284(10):1990–1996

2. Feinstein AR. Current problems and future challenges in randomized clinical trials. Circulation 1984;70(5):767–774

3. Dans AL, Dans LF, Guyatt GH, Richardson S. Users' guides to the medical literature: XIV. How to decide on the applicability of clinical trial results to your patient. Evidence-Based Medicine Working Group. JAMA 1998;279(7):545–549

4. Swedlow A, Johnson G, Smithline N, Milstein A. Increased costs and rates of use in the California workers' compensation system as a result of self-referral by physicians. N Engl J Med 1992;327(21):1502–1506

5. Cabana MD, Rand CS, Powe NR, et al. Why don't physicians follow clinical practice guidelines? A framework for improvement. JAMA 1999;282(15):1458–1465

6. Guyatt GH, Sinclair J, Cook DJ, Glasziou P. Users' guides to the medical literature: XVI. How to use a treatment recommendation. Evidence-Based Medicine Working Group and the Cochrane Applicability Methods Working Group. JAMA 1999;281(19):1836–1843

7. Wilson MC, Hayward RS, Tunis SR, Bass EB, Guyatt G. Users' guides to the Medical Literature. VIII. How to use clinical practice guidelines. B. what are the recommendations and will they help you in caring for your patients? The Evidence-Based Medicine Working Group. JAMA 1995;274(20):1630–1632

8. Adams HP Jr, Brott TG, Crowell RM, et al. Guidelines for the management of patients with acute ischemic stroke. A statement for healthcare professionals from a special writing group of the Stroke Council, American Heart Association. Stroke 1994;25(9):1901–1914

9. Normand SL, McNeil BJ, Peterson LE, Palmer RH. Eliciting expert opinion using the Delphi technique: identifying performance indicators for cardiovascular disease. Int J Qual Health Care 1998;10(3):247–260

9A. Cook DJ, Guyatt GH, Laupacis A, et al. Rules of evidence and Clinical recommendations on the use of antithrombotic agents. Chest 1992;102(suppl 4):S305–S311.

9B. Mayberg MR, Batjer HH, Dacey R, et al. Guidelines for the management of aneurysmal subarachnoid hemorrhage: a statement for healthcare professionals from a special writing group of the stroke council, American Heart Association Stroke 1994;25:2315–2328.

10. Horwitz RI, Viscoli CM, Clemens JD, Sadock RT. Developing improved observational methods for evaluating therapeutic effectiveness. Am J Med 1990;89(5):630–638

11. Johnston SC, Wilson CB, Halbach VV, et al. Endovascular and surgical treatment of unruptured cerebral aneurysms: comparison of risks. Ann Neurol 2000;48:11–19

12. Piantadosi S. Clinical Trials A Methodologic Perspective. New York, NY: John Wiley & Sons; 1997

13. Kaptchuk TJ, Goldman P, Stone DA, Stason WB. Do medical devices have enhanced placebo effects? J Clin Epidemiol 2000;53(8):786–792

14. Executive Committee for the Asymptomatic Carotid Atherosclerosis Study. Endarterectomy for asymptomatic carotid artery stenosis. JAMA 1995;273(18):1421–1428

15. Kleinbaum DG, Kupper LL, Morgenstern H. Epidemiologic Research: Principles and Quantitative Methods. New York, NY: Van Nostrand Reinhold; 1982

16. Koivisto T, Vanninen R, Hurskainen H, Saari T, Hernesniemi J, Vapalahti M. Outcomes of early endovascular versus surgical treatment of ruptured cerebral aneurysms: a prospective randomized study. Stroke 2000;31:2369–2377

17. Molyneux A, Kerr R, Bacon F, Shrimpton J. The need for health technology assessment in the management of unruptured intracranial aneurysms [abstract]. Annu Meet Int Soc Technol Assess Health Care 1999;15(1):129

18. Jennett B, Bond M. Assessment of outcome after severe brain damage. A practical scale. Lancet 1975;1:480–484

19. Mahoney FI, Barthel DW. Functional evaluation: the Barthel Index. Md State Med J 1965;14:61–65

20. Rankin J. Cerebral vascular accidents in patients over the age of 60: II Prognosis. Scott Med J 1957;2:200–215

21. Folstein MF, Folstein SE, McHugh PR. "Mini-mental state." A practical method for grading the cognitive state of patients for the clinician. J Psychiatr Res 1975;12(3):189–198

22. Buck D, Jacoby A, Massey A, Ford G. Evaluation of measures used to assess quality of life after stroke. Stroke 2000;31(8):2004–2010

23. Ware JE Jr, Sherbourne CD. The MOS 36-item short-form health survey (SF-36). I. Conceptual framework and item selection. Med Care 1992;30(6):473–483

24. The International Study of Unruptured Intracranial Aneurysms Investigators. Unruptured intracranial aneurysms—risk of rupture and risks of surgical intervention. N Engl J Med 1998;339(24):1725–1733

25. Rothwell PM, Slattery J, Warlow CP. A systematic review of the risks of stroke and death due to endarterectomy for symptomatic carotid stenosis. Stroke 1996;27(2):260–265

27

Developing the Neurovascular Surgical Specialists of the Future

CHARLES Y. LIU, MICHAEL Y. WANG, ARUN P. AMAR, AND STEVEN L. GIANNOTTA

Objectives: After completing this chapter, the reader should be able to identify the personal characteristics, residency training environment, and fellowship standards needed to gain competency in microsurgical techniques required to treat neurovascular diseases.

Accreditation: The AANS* is accredited by the Accreditation Council for Continuing Medical Education (ACCME) to sponsor continuing medical education for physicians.

Credit: The AANS designates this educational activity for a maximum of 15 credits in Category 1 credit toward the AMA Physician's Recognition Award. Each physician should claim only those hours of credit that he/she spent in the educational activity.

The Home Study Examination is online on the AANS Web site at: http://www.aans.org/education/books/controversy.asp

* The acronym AANS refers to both the American Association of Neurological Surgeons and the American Association of Neurosurgeons.

The field of neurovascular surgery was born with Walter Dandy's description of the treatment of an intracranial aneurysm with surgical clip ligation.[1] Since its genesis, numerous advances have propelled the evolution the field of neurovascular surgery. For example, the assimilation of the operating microscope has allowed improved visualization and understanding of the anatomic substrate. A further result of magnifying and illuminating the microvascular surgical field are the advances in the ergonomics and design effectiveness of instruments. The recent focus on outcomes has led to the codification of a set of psychomotor skills that are essential for the successful operative treatment of neurovascular disorders. In the current sports parlance, the microscope has caused us to focus on our "short game." Indeed, common terms associated with this skill set include among others "touch" and "soft hands." The long tee shot may be analogous to the postoperative angiogram showing obliteration of the aneurysm, whereas low scores (good neurologic outcome) result from that delicate touch around perforators and short temporary clip times.

Although some of the basic underlying mechanisms of neurovascular physiology are yet to be completely elucidated at the cellular or molecular levels, concurrent advances in science and medicine have led to modern concepts of the field, including brain ischemia, stroke, cerebral vasospasm, and cellular and molecular mechanisms of neuronal injury and death. However, neurovascular surgery, and indeed neurosurgery itself, continues to change at an escalating pace driven by technological, social, and economic progress.[2-5] Indeed, these changes have called into question the very definition of the neurovascular surgeon. It follows that the training paradigm for the modern and future neurovascular surgeon must be similarly reexamined and restructured to reflect these changes to remain effective. In this chapter, we review the elements that characterize the effective training and development of the traditional microvascular neurosurgeon. From this starting point, the major forces that are driving the evolution of neurovascular surgery are examined, including the changing paradigms and scope of practice of the field, the forces affecting neurosurgical training within the context of residency education generally, and the evolving issues that relate to credentialing and fellowship accreditation. Consideration of these issues raises many important questions, the answers of which will no doubt impact the training of the modern neurovascular surgical specialist into the future.

■ Developing the Microvascular Neurosurgeon: The Traditional Paradigm

The development of the microvascular neurosurgeon ideally begins with the identification of suitable individuals to undergo the training process.[6] We have yet to specifically define the aptitudes necessary for cerebrovascular surgery; thus, we must rely on the process that generates the entire pool of neurosurgical residents. For the most part, cerebrovascular practitioners are self-selected, as are other neurosurgical subspecialists. The criterion for that selection is solely based on interest, which frequently is dependent on association with a role model. Assuming the self-selection process works, the burden is then on the training program to develop the competencies that produce a satisfactory level of performance. The success of any training program can be considered to be measured by achieving competency in the following areas: (1) patient care, (2) medical knowledge, (3) practice-based learning and improvement, (4) interpersonal and communication skills, (5) professionalism, and (6) systems-based practice.

The Ideal Characteristics of a Microvascular Neurosurgeon

The ideal characteristics of a microvascular neurosurgeon are similar to those demanded of other highly technical disciplines that involve a high level of risk.[6] A consensus conference on surgical education has developed a set of personality traits that correlate with an agreed-upon ideal. Emotional control is a key characteristic of a microvascular surgeon. The ability to remain even-tempered and maintain flexibility during stressful situations exemplifies that control. A strong sense of self-efficacy is integral; this promotes the decisiveness needed to enable the kind of prioritization necessary for complex tasks. Aggression tempered by compassion allows for the ideal balance between "pushing the envelope" of skill maximization while remaining cognizant of some safety limits. Of course, individual personality traits will ultimately serve as the basis for the development of important interpersonal and communication skills for effective practice.

Given the level of risk often associated with neurovascular operations, a high degree of integrity is absolutely required; honest self-assessment is required throughout the development of the neurovascular surgeon to ultimately ensure the delivery of compassionate patient care. Improvement in patient care occurs through practice-based learning that involves investigation and an honest evaluation of an individual's own patient care and appraisal and assimilation of scientific evidence. Integrity is also critical for the trainee to develop an understanding of the practice and implications of cerebrovascular surgery in the larger context of the health care system in general.

Along with ideal personality traits, aptitude for cerebrovascular surgery includes superior manual dexterity with multilimb coordination.[6] There are few areas of surgery where maneuvers spanning less than a millimeter can result in such devastating disability. However, vascular procedures by nature can be long and complex, so efficiency and coordination of subtasks is equally important to good outcomes. The technology to select for these skills is lacking; hence, they must be inferred from other information. To the extent that at the medical student level, some operating room (OR) experience has been witnessed or a research experience has been gained that included some psychomotor surgical skills, evidence of aptitude may be forthcoming. In its absence, inference of bimanual skills can conceivably be gained by the candidates' performance in athletics or musical instrumentation, endeavors where individual performers with special potential are similarly identified for training.[7] Indeed, during a recent lecture by the senior author to a group that can be considered "experts" in microvascular neurosurgery, the majority had engaged in either or both music performance or athletics at a high level. Elite athletes and musicians, by virtue of the preparation needed for their performances develop or inherently manifest both a resistance to boredom and physical and mental stamina. Given the nature of surgical training, which still amounts to apprenticeship, it is easy to see how these two characteristics would be highly valued in a cerebrovascular trainee. Finally, the intellectual endowment of the trainee that is critical to the conceptualization, ordering, and execution of complex cerebrovascular treatment plans must be established through academic performance in credible institutions, awards, board scores, leadership roles, letters of recommendation, research, and personal motivation as reflected in personal statements.

Training Environment

Mentor

The crucial elements that characterize good neurovascular training programs include mentorship from a skillful, respected role model with integrity, good outcomes, and honest appraisal of skills. Psychomotor skills are learned through mimicry. Thus, the teacher must have first mastered the movements for them to serve as a model. If those movements are performed in an efficient manner, learning is compressed in time and is therefore more effective. Empathy, patience, and a strong ego allow the mentor to hand over the tasks to the trainee facilitating the rapid attainment of relevant skills. Prolonged observation of a mentor will also guide the trainee to develop a sense of professionalism, manifested by a commitment to carrying out professional responsibilities, adherence to ethical principles, and sensitivity to a diverse patient population. A good mentor with awareness of and responsiveness to the larger context and system of health care will all help the trainee learn to develop the ability to call on resources effectively to provide care that is of optimum value. Finally, the mentor plays a central role in the development of critical interpersonal and communication skills that result in effective information exchange and teaming with patients, families, and other health professionals.

Volume

In addition, large numbers of complex clinical material of wide scope must be available. Mastery of skills requires repetition. Most graduating senior neurosurgery residents average ~45 aneurysm surgeries during their training. It can be inferred that this is adequate to establish competence for this procedure. Proficiency with advanced skill development would require further "experience."

Technologies

There should be the opportunity for trainees to assume primary responsibility within a center environment with wide availability of support from synergistic services such as neurology and neurocritical care. Those services should be supported by an array of the latest techniques to monitor and assay physiological data for advanced decision-making. Endovascular support technologies are necessary for satisfactory outcomes and are rapidly becoming a standard of care. Such an environment allows the trainee to witness the incorporation of adjunctive and competing technologies to build judgment.

Research

Ideally, an active research effort related to cerebrovascular disorders on a clinical or basic order should be a component. This certainly would be true of a program that offers a fellowship. Such an effort stimulates original thinking and promotes a critical viewpoint toward the published literature.

Curriculum

Within the context of the training program, the neurovascular trainee should gain skills and acquire the necessary medical knowledge by progression of graded responsibilities and attainment of learning goals. The Neurosurgery Residency Core Curriculum as determined by the ADHOC Committee on Core Curriculum of the Society of Neurological Surgeons and the Congress of Neurological Surgeons Committee on Education has defined objective guidelines for progress as it relates to neurovascular surgery. At the junior level, residents are expected to acquire knowledge related to normal vascular anatomy, both intracranial and extracranial, and syndromes of ischemia such as strokes. Furthermore, they should gain an understanding of the physiology of autoregulation in the cerebral vasculature. Clinically, the junior resident should be able to diagnose hemorrhages, vasculopathies, infarctions, and relevant therapeutic windows with the aid of the physical exam and appropriate diagnostic studies. In the management of neurovascular patients at this level, the resident should understand the pathophysiology of entities such as cerebral vasospasm, its prevention, and ischemic thresholds. Also at the junior level, the trainee is expected to develop a basic skill set, including those commonly found in the neurosurgical critical care setting such as arterial lines and Swan Ganz catheters, ventriculostomy catheters, and lumbar drains. In addition, the junior trainee acquires the skills to perform basic operations, including exposure of the cervical carotid artery, craniotomies for the evacuation of intracranial clots, and the pterional craniotomy for simple aneurysms. At this point, the trainee also begins to teach these fundamental skills.

Into the middle level of training, skills for independent management decisions are acquired, and the trainee begins to focus on outcome generation and to check his or her own actions appropriately. Observation of local practices is considered within the context of the current literature and information from organized conferences, leading to the initial development of critical thinking. With an increasing supervisory role, the mid-level trainee develops individual personality traits for effective leadership. In addition, increased clinical responsibilities require an increasing sense of urgency and prioritization skills for multiple, concurrent problems. At this point, the operative skill set is also expanded to include the use of frameless stereotactic neuronavigational systems. The mid-level trainee begins to assist in all cases, allowing for first-hand observation of the basic surgical techniques required for cerebrovascular surgery such as the Sylvian fissure split, carotid endarterectomy, aneurysm dissection and clipping, and arteriovenous malformation (AVM) dissection.

As the neurovascular trainee enters the senior years of training, accumulation of skills, knowledge, and experience naturally leads to further sophistication in critical evaluation of the literature and a more mature understanding of the nuances of local practices within the context of the field generally. This results in increased creativity and formulation of individual hypotheses relating to both academic and clinical practices. The senior-level trainee assumes an increased role as teacher, especially as the senior person in the absence of an attending. This often requires the delineation of independent treatment plans guided by the appropriate interpretation of diagnostic studies. In the OR, the senior-level trainee begins to conceptualize more-sophisticated surgical techniques such as various avenues of exposure and proximal and distal control. In addition, the trainee acquires the skills to execute a pterional craniotomy, split the Sylvian fissure, perform non-complex neurovascular operations, and assist in complex ones. Specifically, proficiency is developed in the use of the fenestrated sucker, bipolar forceps, micro-needle holder and suture, as well as aneurysm clip appliers. Finally, the senior-level trainee is introduced to increased administrative responsibilities and additional clinical duties.

Skills Laboratory

The value of a skills laboratory was demonstrated in the late 1970s and early 1980s when trainees were trying to gain the techniques necessary for the extracranial to intracranial (ECIC) bypass. The concept was further validated with the focus on cranial base surgical exposures. Such a practice environment allowed for the repetition of movements in the context of relevant anatomy, modestly recapitulating the OR environment. Our general and orthopedic surgical colleagues have institutionalized this concept with their more formalized endoscopic technologies courses. These learning laboratories have even allowed for the measurement of indices of performance and competence. At the least, a cerebrovascular trainee should be able to take advantage of the practice effect of repeatedly splitting the cadaveric Sylvian fissure, anastomosing the left rat carotid artery to the right one, and drilling out the far lateral approach.

Acquiring Expertise in Microvascular Neurosurgery: The Cognitive Psychology Viewpoint

So far, the discussion has been limited to the period of initial development of the neurovascular surgeon. From this point, a progression occurs sequentially through increasing levels of expertise.[6] The focus of the residency-training program is to bring the *novice* to the level of *competence*. Within the context of surgical skills, competence is acquiring the ability to perform procedures safely within a reasonable time. Society demands this level of expertise. As further training and practice is acquired, *proficiency* is achieved, where performance is expert in terms of task quality, efficiency, and outcome. In our current educational system, enrollment in a fellowship program is a key factor in accelerating the process. Aptitude, environment, and opportunity may coalesce in the development of the *expert*, who by virtue of his or her level of knowledge and skill is recognized as an authority. The ultimate level of *master* is reserved for those who produce masterpieces

The learning of neurovascular surgery can be understood from the perspective of the cognitive psychologist.[6] Indeed, in FITT's (Frequency, Intensity, Type, and Time) Stages of Cognitive Skill, the initial *conceptualization stage* is marked by the acquisition of skills and understanding of tasks (**Fig. 27–1**). This is the role of the residency and fellowship. Next, control processes are developed and strategies refined in the *associative stage.* Many refer to this stage as "experience gaining." The implication is that this stage, to the extent that it is lengthy, results in increasing expertise. Clearly, that is wrong or the oldest surgeons would invariably have the best results. Finally, the *proficiency stage* is reached when automatic processing is achieved.

Automatic processing of a psychomotor skill occurs when the physical procedure is performed efficiently, ostensibly without the mental component. Shifting a

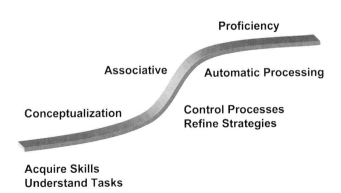

FIGURE 27–1 The figure depicts FITT's (Frequency, Intensity, Type, and Time) stages of cognitive skill.

standard transmission in an automobile is an example. Automatic processing of highly evolved skills that then produce repeatedly the desired result is what has been termed in sports "being in the zone."[8,9] The expert or master cerebrovascular surgeon should at least occasionally experience that level.

Central to successful neurovascular surgery is a specific set of coordinated mental and physical abilities, or psychomotor skills, including reaction time, control precision, aiming, multi-limb coordination, eye–hand speed, rapid sequencing, and visual–spatial perception. Some have written that separate from the manual skills of a surgeon is the concept of judgment. As a separate component, judgment can somehow allow someone with mediocre technical skills to obtain better outcomes. A more functional approach to surgical expertise recognizes that judgment is incorporated in each movement, task, or skill.

The acquisition of these skills and judgment during the quest for proficiency occurs through the process of *self-regulation*.[10] This is defined as a self-imposed set of rules allowing for adaptation and optimization of performance through supervision and control of learning and through transfer and modification of previously acquired knowledge. The "previously acquired knowledge" component is conventionally referred to as "experience." To the extent that "experienced" practitioners can fail to get consistently good outcomes, self-regulation is the missing ingredient.

A key element in self-regulation is the *metacognitive experience*.[10,11] In the case of the expert surgeon, alternatives typically exist at key points in a habitual sequence. An error is detected when this process is disrupted and no habitual response exists. Thus, successful completion of the operation is impossible. The elite athlete or expert surgeon acknowledges an understanding of the movement and its consequences, personal limitations, the environment, motor feedback, and cognitive strategies to create an innovative solution. At times, metacognitive experience will cause the surgeon to stop an operation when outmatched by the task. At the novice level, this results in a minimally effective procedure affectionately known as a "peek and shriek."

■ Microvascular Neurosurgery: Forces Affecting the Future

The paradigm for the treatment of neurovascular diseases is changing, with endovascular methods making rapid inroads as an alternative to traditional microsurgery.[12] This is resulting in a significant decrease in the number of cases traditionally treated by microsurgical means, including aneurysms, bypass procedures,

and carotid endarterectomy. In addition, sociopolitical forces are affecting the very nature of residency training in neurosurgery. Both will surely affect both the development and ultimate role of microvascular neurosurgeons.

■ Evolving Paradigms in the Management of Neurovascular Disease

Endovascular surgery is playing an increasing role in the therapy of intracranial aneurysms and arteriovenous malformations, carotid stenosis, and other cerebrovascular disorders. The impact of this modality on strategies for patient management is indisputable. A variety of factors, including market forces and technological advances, are driving this transformation.

For example, we recently reviewed the surgical records at our institution from 1995 (the year after detachable aneurysm coils gained approval by the United States Food and Drug Administration) to 2003.[13] The numbers of cerebral aneurysms treated by craniotomy and microsurgery (parent vessel occlusion or selective clip ligation) versus endovascular surgery (parent vessel occlusion or selective aneurysm coil embolization) were compared for each year. The analysis was stratified according to aneurysm location (anterior vs. posterior circulation). The total number of cerebral aneurysms treated ranged from 104 to 145 each year. The percentage of all aneurysms treated by endovascular means increased steadily, and more are currently being treated with this modality than with open surgery (**Fig. 27–2**).

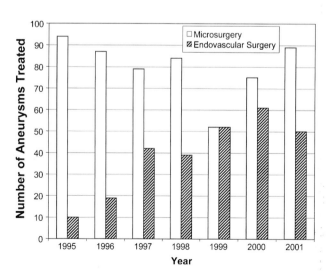

FIGURE 27–2 Aneurysms treated by conventional microsurgical versus endovascular means at the University of Southern California, 1995–2000.

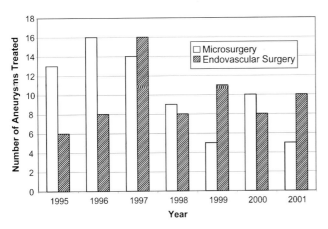

FIGURE 27–3 Posterior circulation aneurysms treated by conventional microsurgical versus endovascular means at the University of Southern California, 1995–2000.

In the stratified analysis, this trend was true of both anterior circulation and posterior circulation aneurysms (**Fig. 27–3**). An informal survey conducted at a recent national meeting confirms that these developments are not unique to our institution. At many centers in Europe, for instance, fewer than 20% of aneurysms are presently being treated with open microsurgical methods.

We have identified two major forces influencing this evolving paradigm. The first concerns refinements of endovascular techniques such as balloon remodeling or stent-assisted coil embolization, facilitated by recent device enhancements such as the advent of intracranial stents. The second major influence underlying this trend is increased awareness of treatment options, including preferences among referring physicians, patients, and their family members. Several studies suggest that outcomes might be more favorable after endovascular therapy than after craniotomy.[13A]

Implications of Endovascular Techniques for Training Neurovascular Surgeons

Endovascular surgery is utilized increasingly in the management of cerebral aneurysms, while the percentage of cases treated with microsurgery is declining. Evolution of endovascular instrumentation and methodologies, as well as increased awareness of treatment options among patients and physicians, accounts for this transformation. Extrapolation of these trends suggests the possibility that, in the near future, the majority of aneurysms will be treated by endovascular means. The impact of this modality on the treatment of AVMs, carotid stenosis, and other cerebrovascular disorders is also indisputable.

The consequence of these evolving paradigms is that neurosurgical residents in training will be exposed to fewer cases of cerebrovascular disease treated by conventional (open surgical) methods. The significance of this fact for resident education and the implications for requisite fellowship training remain uncertain.

■ Residency Training in the New Millenium: Impact of Work Hour Limitations

In 1984, the unfortunate death of Libby Zion in a New York emergency room triggered scrutiny into the impact of resident fatigue on patient care.[14] Allegations that the excessive workloads and long hours demanded of house staff led to a preventable death started a grand jury investigation, culminating in a mandatory reduction in resident work hours for the state of New York.[15] These regulations became institutionalized in 1987. The controversy surrounding the relationship between resident fatigue and preventable medical errors intensified in 1999 when a report issued by the Institute of Medicine shocked the nation by alleging that up to 98,000 Americans die each year because of preventable medical errors. At the same time, political pressures from within the medical profession were at work to improve the quality of life of house staff. The Committee of Interns and Residents, the largest union representative for physicians in training, was working to limit the workloads and hours for its constituency.

In July 2002, the Accreditation Council for Graduate Medical Education (ACGME) passed a set of regulations limiting the number and distribution of work hours for all residency training programs, regardless of specialty. These rules went into effect in July 2003 and stipulated that house staff would not be permitted to work more than 80 hours each week and that each shift be less than 30 consecutive hours.

Many issues have been raised over the impact that a mandatory reduction in work hours will have on residency education. In particular, surgical specialties, which have had a long tradition of lengthy training programs and arduous work schedules, have resisted these changes. While some critics cite the long hours in surgical training as simply an unnecessary relic of tradition or a "rite of passage," others point to the responsibility and training gained from following individual patients over the course of their acute hospitalization.

Based upon the experiences in New York State, preliminary studies have investigated the impact of these regulations on residency training. In a study of General Surgery house staff at two New York City hospitals the mean number of hours worked was reduced from 101 to 86 hours.[16] The survey also found that 85% of residents experienced improvements in their quality of life but 76% also felt that continuity of care for patients had been negatively impacted. Written board examination scores improved in this longitudinal cohort, and the number of cases performed over the span of residency appeared to increase modestly.

Within the field of neurological surgery, there have been a variety of responses. Because of the nature of neurosurgical care, with frequent emergencies and long surgical procedures, restrictions on work hours have generally been viewed as detrimental to the educational experience. Specifically, the development of both cognitive and technical skills in neurovascular surgery may be negatively affected by the profound changes occurring in training programs. This may be particularly important in the field of cerebrovascular disease because of the unpredictable and time-sensitive nature of catastrophic clinical events.

The first issue relating specifically to neurovascular surgery is the unpredictability of cerebrovascular events. Because most centers are treating ruptured aneurysms urgently to prevent rebleeding, the operative intervention frequently occurs in a nonelective manner. Prior to the duty hours' limitations this did not pose a problem from an educational standpoint. Put simply, the training opportunity from the senior resident's viewpoint was typically that the benefits from being involved in these surgeries far outweighed the costs of having to stay in the hospital after a night on call. However, in the new training paradigm the decision of which resident, if any, will participate in a given surgical case may be determined by the mandate to send postcall house staff home. Because the learning opportunity in complex cerebrovascular cases is clearly highest for senior-level residents, this may lead to lost training opportunities if junior-level house staff or no residents are involved in these cases.

The second area where duty hours' restrictions may impact on the educational experience is in the pre- and posthospital care of cerebrovascular patients. Again, because many of these surgeries are not elective, patients are often admitted after their transfer from an outside hospital or a visit to the emergency room. Thus, the initial evaluation frequently is conducted at odd hours. This preoperative interface between resident physician and patient is critical, not only from the viewpoint of resident training but also because it gives the resident who will participate in the operative treatment the opportunity to establish a rapport with the patient.

More importantly, the care of patients following subarachnoid hemorrhage is complex. Effective cognitive and technical skills for treating posthemorrhage complications can only be acquired through first-hand experience. A "shift work" mentality lends itself to poor patient care in the face of acute clinical events, as alterations in neurological function can be initially quite subtle. For the physician unaware of a patient's baseline neurological status, perceived alterations in consciousness can go undetected or be needlessly worked-up.

While the mandated reduction in work hours for house staff is substantially altering the nature of surgical training in America, European neurosurgical programs are working under significantly greater restraints. Under Directive 2000/34/EC, the maximum weekly working time will be capped at 48 hours.[17] These changes will occur over a 5- to 8-year transition period that began in 2004, but some countries already employ stricter regulations, such as Denmark with its 35-hour cap.

The ultimate impact of these new regulations on the training of neurovascular surgeons remains unknown. Cerebrovascular patients require expert care 24 hours a day, 7 days a week. In the academic environment, residents currently deliver much of this care. Physicians-in-training are expected to develop a sense of responsibility for their patients, and professionalism dictates that this does not start and stop at designated shift changes. However, no one individual can be available to his or her patients at all times. Ultimately, a delicate balance must be struck between the competing factors of physician fatigue and quality of life versus training experience and continuity of care.

■ Fellowships: Credentialing and Accreditation

Fellowships fulfill two separate objectives. Residents seek "fellowships" because of deficiencies in their own training programs. The fellowship then serves as a normative process bringing the residents experience with a certain discipline up to the level of competence or to the level of comparable to other trainees at similar stages in training. For the purpose of this discussion, we restrict our definition of fellowship to the acquisition of advanced skills. The implication is that the advanced training will lead ultimately to the development of proficiency with the required surgical skills and a more advanced grounding in the scientific underpinnings of the discipline. The goals are to facilitate subspecialization and/or the attainment of an academic position. The fellowship environment is no different from an idealized residency training experience. Imperatives include an active research effort, either clinical or basic, and a volume of cases that allows for the simultaneous training of residents while the fellow gains advanced leadership, technical, and strategic skills.

The Residency Review Committee for Neurosurgery attempts to adjudicate the impact of a fellowship on the existing training program by requiring the program director to report on the number of cases available. By establishing certain minimum criteria based on available statistics from all 94 residency training programs, resident experience with, in this case, vascular disorders will remain adequate.

The question is frequently asked whether a fellowship is needed if a resident is trained in a high-volume environment. Certainly, the public relations aspect of evidence of advanced training should not be discounted. As a practical matter, residency and fellowship have different goals. Residency training brings the trainee to the level of competence. If one accepts the hierarchical scale of novice, competent, proficient, expert, and master, fellowship theoretically can bring the trainee to the level of proficiency. To the extent a fellow can be expected to reach that level depends on aptitude and the limitations of the individual's own learning curve. The ability to become expert in something as demanding as vascular neurosurgery transcends any reasonably structured training program, because the expert has had to perform a substantial number of complex cases to bring their psychomotor skill set up to the metacognitive level.

Thus, the fellowship is only the start to reaching a higher level of practice. A strong mentor in a busy practice situation with advanced teaching skill may very well be able to recapitulate the fellowship environment and develop partners that produce highly acceptable outcomes. This is how many of us trained in an era before organized fellowships gained proficiency. There is no reason the model would not work today.

■ The Future

Key questions for the future include whether the complete neurovascular surgeon has both endovascular and open vascular skills, and can skill sets be maintained if they are not utilized frequently. Although there are examples of the expert practitioner with advanced skills in open and interventional vascular techniques (Nick Hopkins, Professor of Neurosurgery S.U.N.Y. Buffalo comes to mind), the fact that these skills do not overlap in a psychomotor sense and the fact that they are performed in separate environments, causes most practitioners to gravitate toward a single focus. As endovascular technologies advance, more pathologies can be treated leading to more time spent in the radiology suite. Furthermore, as expertise grows more cases become available leading to the natural tendency to divide duties among those primarily assigned to the OR and others assigned to the radiology department. As more neurosurgeons learn endovascular techniques, it is conceivable that members of large teams could alternate duties to maintain a high level of both skills. Until there is a viable alternative to open surgery for *all* cases of disease processes currently treated by microvascular techniques, it is imperative that the skills required for safe and successful surgical treatment continue to be taught, developed, maintained, and advanced.

■ References

1. Dandy WE. Intracranial aneurysm of the internal carotid artery. Ann Surg 1938;107:654–659
2. Apuzzo ML, Liu CY. *Quid Novi?* In the realm of ideas—the neurosurgical dialectic. Clin Neurosurg 2002;49:157–185
3. Apuzzo ML, Liu CY. Reinventing neurosurgery—surgery of the human cerebrum: a collective modernity. Clin Neurosurg 2002;49:27–89
4. Apuzzo ML, Liu CY. 2001: Things to come. Neurosurgery 2001;49:765–778
5. Liu CY, Apuzzo ML. The genesis of neurosurgery and the evolution of the operative environment: Part I—prehistory to 2003. Neurosurgery 2003;52:3–19
6. Giannotta SL. Cerebrovascular surgical skills: learning them, teaching them. Donaghey Lecture: Annual Meeting of the Association of Neurological Surgeons; April, 2003; San Diego, CA
7. Humara M. Personnel selection in athletic programs. Athletic Insight [serial online]. 2000; Volume 2, Issue 2. Available at: http://www.athleticinsight.com/Vol2Iss2/Personnel.htm. Accessed July 18, 2000
8. Marr AJ. Commentary: in the zone—a biobehavioral theory of the flow experience. Athletic Insight [serial online]. 2001; Volume 3, Issue 1. Available at: http://www.athleticinsight.com/Vol3Iss1/Commentary.htm. Accessed May 10, 2002
9. Tolson J. Into the zone. US News World Rep 2000;Jul 3:38–45
10. Behncke L. Self-Regulation: A brief review. Athletic Insight [serial online]. 2002; Volume 4, Issue 1. Available at: http://www.athleticinsight.com/Vol4Iss1/SelfRegulation.htm. Accessed Jan 8, 2003
11. Lee K, Chen L. The development of metacognitive knowledge of basic motor skill: walking. J Genet Psychol 1996;157:361–375
12. Hopkins LN, Lanzino G, Guterman LR. Treating complex nervous system vascular disorders through a "needle stick": origins, evolution, and future of neuroendovascular therapy. Neurosurgery 2001;48:463–475
13. Amar AP, Giannotta SL, Larsen DW, Teitelbaum GP. Evolving paradigms in the management of cerebrovascular disease. Paper presented at: Annual Meeting of the Joint Section of Cerebrovascular Surgery; 2003; Phoenix, AZ
13A. Molyneux AJ, Kerr RS, Yu LM, Claske M, et al. International subarachnoid Aneurysm Trial (ISAT) Collaborative Group. ISAT of neurosurgical clipping versus endovascular coiling in 2143 patients with ruptured intracranial aneurysms: a randomized comparison of effects on survival, dependancy, seizures, rebleeding, subgroups, and aneurysm occlusion. Lancet 2005; 366(9488):783–785.
14. Asch D, Parker R. Sounding board: the Libby Zion case. N Engl J Med 1988;318:771–775
15. Recommendations of the New York State Department of Health's Ad Hoc Advisory Committee on Emergency Services. In: Greater New York Hospital Association. New York, NY; 1987
16. Barden C, Specht M, McCarter M, Daly J, Fahey T. Effects of limited work hours on surgical training. J Am Coll Surg 2002;195:531–538
17. Lazarides MK, Polychronids A, Simopoulos E. Effects of limited work hours on surgical training: a European aspect. J Ann Coll Surg 2003;196(4):661–662

28

Developing the Endovascular and Neurovascular Specialists of the Future

CAMERON G. MCDOUGALL

Objectives: After completing this chapter, the reader should be able to identify the personal characteristics, residency training environment, and fellowship standards needed to gain competency in endovascular techniques required to treat neurovascular diseases.

Accreditation: The AANS* is accredited by the Accreditation Council for Continuing Medical Education (ACCME) to sponsor continuing medical education for physicians.

Credit: The AANS designates this educational activity for a maximum of 15 credits in Category 1 credit toward the AMA Physician's Recognition Award. Each physician should claim only those hours of credit that he/she spent in the educational activity.

The Home Study Examination is online on the AANS Web site at: http://www.aans.org/education/books/controversy.asp

* The acronym AANS refers to both the American Association of Neurological Surgeons and the American Association of Neurosurgeons.

Training matters. As with other medical and surgical subspecialties, producing adequate numbers of individuals competently trained in endovascular surgical neuroradiology (ESN) requires creating an appropriate training infrastructure. The American Council for Graduate Medical Education (ACGME) defines ESN as "a subspecialty that uses catheter technology, radiologic imaging, and clinical expertise to diagnose and treat diseases of the central nervous system." This subspecialty exists as a distinct entity because the ACGME recognizes that "the unique clinical and invasive nature of this subspecialty requires special training and skills."[1] Inherent in this definition is the understanding that ESN is more than a set of technical skills. If ESN is to endure as a distinct entity, training programs must create not only competent clinicians for today's needs but also thoughtful physicians capable of leading and developing the subspecialty in the future.

Questions regarding what constitutes a competently trained individual and how a trainee acquires such

competency are considered in this chapter. The topics covered include a brief look at the development of ESN as a distinct discipline, a discussion of data that might influence the establishment of training standards, the standards as they currently exist, and finally, some thoughts regarding training objectives for the future.

It is clear that endovascular techniques are maturing into an integral component in the overall management of neurovascular disease. These techniques likely will continue to improve and be increasingly used in the near future. Previous chapters in this monograph have discussed the wide and expanding role of ESN. The impact of the changes brought about by endovascular techniques should not be underestimated. Currently about half of all cerebral aneurysms in North America and Europe receive endovascular treatment. Carotid stenting has recently been approved in the United States. Over time, it will replace carotid endarterectomy for most patients. Undoubtedly, stenting techniques will rapidly be adapted to the vertebral and intracranial arteries. Likewise, endovascular stroke therapies are increasingly promising for the treatment of acute ischemic stroke. Despite the short history of ESN, much has been accomplished, and there is every reason to expect even more rapid development in the future.

■ Birth of a Subspecialty

Endovascular surgical neuroradiology developed as a subspecialty because of the dedicated efforts of talented and imaginative individuals. Many of the early efforts were born out of desperation, hoping to treat terrible afflictions that throughout history have defied effective treatment. Some of these conditions are now treated routinely; others remain a challenge. Over time, a distinct body of knowledge has been acquired, and this body of knowledge comprises the subspecialty of ESN. This knowledge, this skill set, has been developed at a high price. The learning curve climbed as the techniques developed leaving behind a legacy not only of heroic successes, but also of tragic failures. We are indebted to those who suffered because of our failures but who, in the process, taught us how we might succeed in the future. The penultimate goal of a training program is to use wisely the priceless lessons learned during this development for the betterment of the human condition; to create a training program is to honor the debt we owe to those we have failed in the past, and on their behalf, to deliver a gift of healing knowledge to future practitioners who will pick up where we leave off.

As a skill set emerges into a distinct field of expertise, standards of practice are eventually recognized and incorporated into training programs. To appreciate how the current training requirements were established, one must understand how the field developed. Traditionally, neurologists and neurosurgeons have managed cerebrovascular diseases. Although there has been more consensus than not, each specialty has had its own approach and limitations. The division of expertise between the specialties has not always been clear, and controversies have arisen regarding the different approaches adapted by the two specialties.

Endovascular techniques were first introduced in a report by Luessenhop and Spence in 1960.[2] Similar pioneering work was initiated in the former Soviet Union and in Europe by individuals such as Serbinenko[3] and Debrun and coworkers,[4,5] who began to report their work in English language publications in the late 1960s and early 1970s. Simultaneously, in America, groups such as Hieshima and coworkers,[6] Kerber and coworkers,[7,8] and Berenstein and Kricheff[9,10] were beginning to publish their own work on developing endovascular techniques for the neurovascular system. This novel situation of neuroradiologists treating neurovascular conditions previously managed by neurologists and neurosurgeons was the beginning of ESN. Fundamentally, the three specialties were linked in this endeavor because each possessed only a portion of the skills and knowledge necessary for clinical success.

■ Developing Training Standards

The definition of what constitutes training is always changing. In the United States, training requirements for a medical specialty or subspecialty typically are defined by the ACGME. These requirements are discussed later in this chapter. In practice, many specialty areas often find themselves at odds with one another with respect to the management of conditions that overlap specialty fields. In this setting, involved organizations often promulgate "guidelines" or "standards" that are believed to define accepted medical practices with respect to a given condition.

Inevitably, establishing training standards is controversial. There is no assurance that standards established by one specialty organization will be agreed to or respected by a second organization. Ultimately, a balance must be struck between ensuring clinical competency and the practical constraints of time, expense, and resources. Training must occur in an environment where adequate supervision is available to ensure that the well-being of patients is not compromised. Trainees must have adequate components of cognitive knowledge and technical expertise.

Technical proficiency in ESN begins with mastery of cerebral and spinal angiography. All catheter-based neurovascular interventions begin and end with diagnostic angiography. Many of the risks of angiography overlap with those of the international procedures. In addition to the technical elements of performing angiography, interpretation of the diagnostic studies demands in-depth knowledge of neurovascular anatomy and pathology. With respect to the purely technical components of diagnostic neuroangiography, appropriate training and experience enhance the safety of this procedure. Permanent neurological deficits related to diagnostic cerebral angiography have ranged from 0.3 to 5.7%.[8,11–24]

In a prospective study examining 1000 patients undergoing cerebral angiography, 1% of the patients suffered a neurological deficit, and the deficit persisted in half of them. This study was performed in a high-volume teaching hospital where the cerebral angiography was performed by dedicated neuroradiologists. In this study, 9 of 10 patients suffering neurological complications had a history of prior stroke or transient ischemic attack. This finding suggests that patients with clinically significant atherosclerosis have a significantly increased risk for neurological complications.[15] Cases with neurological complications were also associated with increased procedural time and increased doses of contrast.

Addressing the learning curve for cerebral angiography, Dion et al noted that the fluoroscopy time needed for cerebral angiography decreased linearly until 100 diagnostic cases had been performed.[11] This finding is particularly relevant because operator risk factors for ischemic complications include increased procedural and fluoroscopy time, increased number of catheters used, and performance of arch aortography.[18,21] These factors are typically related to the operator's experience. An analysis of 5000 angiograms showed that the neurological complication rate of fellowship-trained specialists is 0.5%; this is slightly less than that of nonfellowship-trained angiographers and much less than the 2.8% complication rate seen with trainees under supervision.[18–20]

Evaluation of the complication rates associated with trainees suggests that an individual may need to perform 200 angiograms to gain sufficient clinical competence.[11] Learning curves are equally long for cerebrovascular interventions, for example, for carotid angioplasty and stenting[23] and coil embolization of intracranial aneurysms.[25]

As a relatively new field of endeavor, the parent specialties of ESN have yet to establish specific training standards that require defined numbers of procedures. However, it is likely that these standards will develop as training needs become more refined. The American College of Radiology has published guidelines regarding standards for the performance of diagnostic cervicocerebral angiography in adults.[26]

A collaborative panel of the American Society of Interventional and Therapeutic Neuroradiology, the American Society of Neuroradiology, and the Society of Interventional Radiology published explicit and detailed guidelines for the performance of cervical carotid angioplasty and stent placement.[27] As a prerequisite to carotid stenting, the recommendations require the operator to have sufficient angiographic experience to perform cervicocerebral angiography safely and to obtain appropriate stent training. The operator can meet the diagnostic portion of the training if he or she has performed at least 200 diagnostic cervicocerebral angiograms or alternatively 100 angiograms plus a documented experience in peripheral vascular interventions as required by the American Heart Association. After the requirements for cervicocerebral angiography have been met, carotid stent training can be accomplished with the following experience: noncarotid stenting (25 cases) plus a comprehensive carotid stenting course (16 hours) in addition to four supervised cases with acceptable outcomes. Alternatively, the trainee may perform 10 supervised carotid stent cases as the primary operator with acceptable success.

Parallels can be taken from other fields of expertise. Influential societies overseeing catheter-based coronary interventions, such as the American College of Cardiology (ACC), have acknowledged the learning curve involved in interventional procedures. The ACC requires individuals to complete diagnostic coronary angiography training before training for coronary interventions.[28] One year of dedicated training is mandated. During this time, the trainee must perform a minimum of 300 coronary angiograms, after which he or she may start training for interventional procedures. An additional 8 months and 250 procedures are required to complete the technical component of an interventional cardiology training program.[28]

In a similar fashion, recent collaboration among neuroscience specialties has led to the recognition of the need for "adequate cognitive training" for those who would perform catheter-based cervicocerebral diagnostic and interventional procedures. This cognitive training includes four critical components: (1) formal training that imparts an adequate depth of cognitive knowledge of the brain and its associated pathophysiological vascular processes; (2) adequate procedural skill achieved by repetitive supervised training by a qualified instructor; (3) diagnostic acumen achieved by studying, performing, and correctly interpreting a large number of diagnostic procedures with proper tutelage; and (4) adequate diagnostic procedural skills and knowledge.

Although these principles—understanding the end organ, knowing how to recognize its pathological state, and possessing the technical abilities necessary to perform the required diagnostic and therapeutic procedures—may seem almost intuitive, specific criteria must be defined and met to achieve these laudable objectives. At the time of this writing, these specific criteria remain the subject of debate.

■ The American Council for Graduate Medical Education Training Requirements

In recognition of the complexity and level of specialization required to perform neurovascular interventions safely, the ACGME has recognized ESN as a distinct subspecialty. This recognition was propelled through years of effort on the part of many individuals, most notably R.T. Higashida, L.N. Hopkins, A. Berenstein, V.V. Halbach, and C. Kerber.[1,29] Although debate continues regarding training standards for particular components of ESN, the ACGME has defined training program requirements for this subspecialty. The training requirements as stated in this document are the result of a consensus among specialties and they may require modification over time.

Details of the ACGME training requirements are available online.[1] The program permits entry to appropriately trained individuals from a background of neurology, neurosurgery, or neuroradiology. All candidates are required to have at least 12 months of training, preferably consecutively, in neuroradiology. The details of the objectives for this "preparatory training" before starting an ESN fellowship are itemized by the ACGME on the downloadable document. During this period of preparation, candidates must gain skills and knowledge in catheter techniques. Both neurosurgical and neurology candidates must acquire a minimum of 3 months training in basic radiology skills. Neurology candidates also must complete a minimum of 3 months of neurosurgical experience and have completed an ACGME-accredited 1-year vascular neurology program. Neuroradiologists must spend 3 months of clinical experience in an ACGME-accredited neurological surgery program. Some of these preparatory requirements may be obtained during electives throughout the respective residency programs.

With respect to the 1-year requirement for ESN after the preparatory year, the specific details again can readily be reviewed online or downloaded.[1] The program requires training and experience in the following areas: signs and symptoms of disorders amenable to diagnosis and treatment by endovascular surgical neuroradiology techniques, neurological examinations to evaluate patients with neurological disorders, the pathophysiology and natural history of these disorders, the indications and contraindications to endovascular surgical neuroradiology procedures, the clinical and technical aspects of endovascular surgical neuroradiology procedures, medical and surgical alternatives, preoperative and postoperative management of endovascular patients, neurointensive care management, the fundamentals of imaging physics and radiation biology, and the interpretation of radiographic studies pertinent to the practice.

Training that includes instruction in the material relevant to ESN under the following categories is also required: basic anatomical and physiological knowledge; technical aspects of endovascular surgical neuroradiology; pharmacology; the coagulation cascade; brain and spinal cord arteriovenous malformations; fistulas of the brain, spine, and spinal cord; head and neck vascular malformations; ischemic stroke; cerebral aneurysms; tumors of the head, neck, spine, and central nervous system; revascularization for occlusive vascular diseases; embolization for epistaxis or other causes of hemorrhage; invasive functional testing; and balloon test occlusion.

The sponsoring institution must have a patient population sufficient to provide a variety and experience commensurate with the training objectives. The minimum number of therapeutic endovascular surgical neuroradiology procedures required by the ACGME to provide this experience is 100 cases per year.

■ Considerations for the Future

In the end, the inescapable conclusion is that ESN is a clinical subspecialty. It involves the management of patients with neurovascular and related diseases. Practitioners cannot effectively work as technicians and leave the clinical decision-making to allied clinicians. Rather they must accept an equal role with other neurovascular team members, and as such, they must be fully responsible for their treatment decisions. This can only happen if trainees are equipped with sufficient clinical skills to allow them to make sound decisions. Conversely, if training programs focus excessively but narrowly on the procedures or the technology alone, the larger picture will be missed. Although the subspecialty is driven by technology, it is essential to avoid being seduced by technology: Technology is not the end goal, it is only a means to the end. The goal is continual improvement in patient care. Residency and fellowship programs must fashion specialists who are knowledgeable about the conditions that they treat, comfortable with the latest techniques in treating these conditions, and confident enough to develop ever more innovative therapies for the betterment of our patients.

■ Acknowledgment

The author is greatly indebted to J. J. Connors III for his assistance in preparing this manuscript.

■ References

1. Program ACGME. Requirements for Residency Education in Endovascular Surgical Neuroradiology. Chicago, IL: American Council for Graduate Medical Education; 2003. Available at: www.acgme.org/acWebsite/downloads/RRC_progReq/422pr403.pdf. Accessed December 15, 2005
2. Luessenhop AJ, Spence WT. Artificial embolization of cerebral arteries. Report of use in a case of arteriovenous malformation. JAMA 1960;172:1153–1155
3. Serbinenko FA. Balloon catheterization and occlusion of major cerebral vessels. J Neurosurg 1974;41(2):125–145
4. Debrun G, Lacour P, Caron JP, et al. Inflatable and released balloon technique experimentation in dog—application in man. Neuroradiology 1975;9(5):267–271
5. Debrun G, Lacour P, Caron JP, et al. Detachable balloon and calibrated-leak balloon techniques in the treatment of cerebral vascular lesions. J Neurosurg 1978;49(5):635–649
6. Hieshima GB, Mehringer CM, Grinnell VS, et al. Emergency occlusive techniques. Surg Neurol 1978;9(5):293–302
7. Kerber C. Balloon catheter with a calibrated leak. A new system for superselective angiography and occlusive catheter therapy. Radiology 1976;120(3):547–550
8. Kerber CW, Cromwell LD, Drayer BP, Bank WO. Cerebral ischemia. I. Current angiographic techniques, complications, and safety. AJR Am J Roentgenol 1978;130(6):1097–1103

9. Berenstein A, Krischeff II. Catheter and material selection for transarterial embolization: technical considerations. I. Catheters. Radiology 1979;132(3):619–630

10. Berenstein A, Krischeff II. Therapeutic vascular occlusion. J Dermatol Surg Oncol 1978;4(11):874–880

11. Dion JE, Gates PC, Fox AJ, Barnett HJ, Blom RJ. Clinical events following neuroangiography: a prospective study. Stroke 1987; 18(6):997–1004

12. Earnest F, Forbes G, Sandok BA, et al. Complications of cerebral angiography: prospective assessment of risk. AJR Am J Roentgenol 1984;142(2):247–253

13. Endarterectomy for asymptomatic carotid artery stenosis. Executive Committee for the Asymptomatic Carotid Atherosclerosis Study. JAMA 1995;273(18):1421–1428

14. Grzyska U, Freitag J, Zeumer H. Selective cerebral intraarterial DSA. Complication rate and control of risk factors. Neuroradiology 1990;32(4):296–299

15. Heiserman JE, Dean BL, Hodak JA, et al. Neurologic complications of cerebral angiography. AJNR Am J Neuroradiol 1994;15(8):1401–1407

16. Horowitz MB, Duton K, Purdy PD. Assessment of complication types and rates related to diagnostic angiography and interventional neuroradiologic procedures. Interventional Neuroradiology 1998;4:27–37

17. Johnston DC, Chapman KM, Goldstein LB. Low rate of complications of cerebral angiography in routine clinical practice. Neurology 2001;57(11):2012–2014

18. Mani RL, Eisenberg RL. Complications of catheter cerebral arteriography: analysis of 5,000 procedures. II. Relation of complication rates to clinical and arteriographic diagnoses. AJR Am J Roentgenol 1978;131(5):867–869

19. Mani RL, Eisenberg RL. Complications of catheter cerebral arteriography: Analysis of 5,000 procedures. III. Assessment of arteries injected, contrast medium used, duration of procedure, and age of patient. AJR Am J Roentgenol 1978;131(5):871–874

20. Mani RL, Eisenberg RL, McDonald EJ Jr, Pollock JA, Mani JR. Complications of catheter cerebral arteriography: Analysis of 5,000 procedures. I. Criteria and incidence. AJR Am J Roentgenol 1978;131(5):861–865

21. McIvor J, Steiner TJ, Perkin GD, Greenhalgh RM, Rose FC. Neurological morbidity of arch and carotid arteriography in cerebrovascular disease. The influence of contrast medium and radiologist. Br J Radiol 1987;60(710):117–122

22. Moran CJ, Milburn JM, Cross DT III, et al. Randomized controlled trial of sheaths in diagnostic neuroangiography. Radiology 2001;218(1):183–187

23. Vitek JJ. Femoro-cerebral angiography: analysis of 2,000 consecutive examinations, special emphasis on carotid arteries catheterization in older patients. Am J Roentgenol Radium Ther Nucl Med 1973;118(3):633–647

24. Willinsky RA, Taylor SM, TerBrugge K, et al. Neurologic complications of cerebral angiography: prospective analysis of 2,899 procedures and review of the literature. Radiology 2003;227(2): 522–528

25. Singh V, Gress DR, Higashida RT, et al. The learning curve for coil embolization of unruptured intracranial aneurysms. AJNR Am J Neuroradiol 2002;23(5):768–771

26. American College of Radiology. American College of Radiology: Standard for the performance of diagnostic cervicocerebral angiography in adults. In: American College of Radiology, ed. American College of Radiology Standards 2000–2001. Reston, VA: American College of Radiology; 2000:415–426

27. Barr JD, Connors JJ III, Sacks D, et al. Quality improvement guidelines for the performance of cervical carotid angioplasty and stent placement. AJNR Am J Neuroradiol 2003;24(10):2020–2034

28. Creager MA, Cooke JP, Olin JW, et al. Revised Recommendations for Training in Adult Cardiovascular Medicine Core Cardiology Training II (COCATS 2; Revision of the 1995 COCATS Training Statement). Bethesda, MD: American College of Cardiology; 2003. Available at: http://www.acc.org/clinical/training/COCATS2 .pdf.6-4-2003 Accessed December 15, 2005

29. Higashida RT, Hopkins LN, Berenstein A, Halbach VV, Kerber C. Program requirements for residency/fellowship education in neuroendovascular surgery/interventional neuroradiology: a special report on graduate medical education. AJNR Am J Neuroradiol 2000;21(6):1153–1159

Index

Page numbers followed by an italic *f* or *t* indicate the entry on that page is in a figure or table.